ECG WORKOUT

EXERCISES
IN ARRYTHMIA
INTERPRETATION

SEVENTH EDITION

ECG WORKOUT

EXERCISES IN ARRHYTHMIA INTERPRETATION

Jane Huff, RN, CCRN

Education Coordinator, Critical Care Unit
Arrhythmia Instructor
Advanced Cardiac Life Support (ACLS) Instructor
Preceptor-Mentor, Critical Care Unit
Unity Health White County Medical Center
Searcy, Arkansas

SEVENTH EDITION

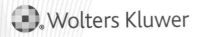
. Wolters Kluwer

Philadelphia • Baltimore • New York • London
Buenos Aires • Hong Kong • Sydney • Tokyo

Executive Editor: Shannon W. Magee
Product Development Editor: Maria M. McAvey
Developmental Editor: Julie Vitale
Production Project Manager: David Orzechowski
Design Coordinator: Stephen Druding
Manufacturing Coordinator: Kathleen Brown
Senior Marketing Manager: Mark Wiragh
Prepress Vendor: SPi Global

7th edition

Library of Congress Cataloging-in-Publication Data
　Names: Huff, Jane, RN, author.
　Title: ECG workout : exercises in arrhythmia interpretation / Jane Huff.
　Description: 7th edition. | Philadelphia : Wolters Kluwer, [2017]
　Identifiers: LCCN 2016008681 | ISBN 9781469899817 (paperback)
　Subjects: | MESH: Arrhythmias, Cardiac—diagnosis | Electrocardiography |
　Problems and Exercises
　Classification: LCC RC685.A65 | NLM WG 18.2 | DDC 616.1/207547—dc23 LC record available at http://lccn.loc.gov/2016008681

This book is dedicated to my heavenly Father for His guidance and love.

Preface

ECG Workout: Exercises in Arrhythmia Interpretation, Seventh Edition, was written to assist physicians, nurses, medical and nursing students, paramedics, emergency medical technicians, telemetry technicians, and other allied health personnel in acquiring the knowledge and skills essential for identifying basic arrhythmias. It may also be used as a reference for ECG review for those already knowledgeable in ECG interpretation.

The text is written in a simple manner and illustrated with figures, tables, boxes, and ECG tracings. Each chapter is designed to build on the knowledge base from the previous chapters so that the beginning student can quickly understand and grasp the basic concepts of electrocardiography. An effort has been made not only to provide *good quality ECG tracings* but also to provide a sufficient number and variety of ECG practice strips so the learner feels confident in arrhythmia interpretation. There are *over 600 practice strips—more than any book on the market*.

Chapter 1 provides a discussion of basic anatomy and physiology of the heart. The electrical basis of electrocardiology is discussed in Chapter 2. The components of the ECG tracing (waveforms, intervals, segments, and complexes) are described in Chapter 3. This chapter also includes practice tracings on waveform identification. Cardiac monitors, lead systems, lead placement, ECG artifacts, and troubleshooting monitor problems are discussed in Chapter 4.

A step-by-step guide to rhythm strip analysis is provided in Chapter 5, in addition to practice tracings on rhythm strip analysis. The individual rhythm chapters (Chapters 6 through 9) include a description of each arrhythmia, arrhythmia examples, causes, and management protocols.

Current advanced cardiac life support (ACLS) guidelines are incorporated into each arrhythmia chapter as applicable to the rhythm discussion. Each arrhythmia chapter also includes approximately 100 practice strips. Chapter 10 presents a general discussion of cardiac pacemakers (types, indications, function, pacemaker terminology, malfunctions, and pacemaker analysis), along with practice tracings. Chapter 11 is a posttest consisting of a mix of rhythm strips that can be used as a self-evaluation tool or for testing purposes.

The text has been thoughtfully revised and expanded to include new figures, updated boxes and tables, additional glossary terms, and even more practice rhythm strips. New to this edition, *pull-out arrhythmia summary cards with rhythm strip examples* on each arrhythmia group can be found in the back of the book to use as a guide to interpret the practice strips at the end of each chapter. *Skillbuilder rhythm strips* appear immediately following the practice rhythm strips in Chapters 7, 8, and 9. Each Skillbuilder section provides a mix of strips that test not only your understanding of information learned in that arrhythmia chapter but also the concepts and skills learned in the chapter(s) immediately preceding it. For example, the Skillbuilder strips in Chapter 7 (Atrial Arrhythmias) include atrial rhythm strips as well as strips on sinus arrhythmias (covered in Chapter 6). The skillbuilder strips in Chapter 8 (Junctional Arrhythmias and AV Blocks) include junctional and AV block strips as well as strips on sinus and atrial arrhythmias. The skillbuilder strips in Chapter 9 (Ventricular Arrhythmias and Bundle-Branch Block) include a mix of all the arrhythmias covered in Chapters 6 through 9. Such practice with mixed strips will enhance your ability to differentiate between rhythm groups as you progress through the book—a definite advantage when you get to the posttest. *Pull-out flashcards* are included in the back of the book to further challenge your ability to identify different types of arrhythmias.

The ECG tracings included in this book are actual strips from patients. Above each rhythm strip are 3-second indicators for rapid-rate calculation. For precise rate calculation, an *ECG conversion table for heart rate* is printed on the inside back cover. For convenience, a removable plastic version is also attached to the inside back cover. The heart rates for regular rhythms listed in the answer keys were determined by the precise rate calculation method and will not always coincide with the rapid-rate calculation method. Rate calculation methods are discussed in Chapter 5.

The author and publisher have made every attempt to check the content, especially drug dosages and management protocols, for accuracy. Medicine is continually changing, and the reader has the responsibility to keep informed of local care protocols and changes in emergency care procedures.

Contents

ECG WORKOUT

EXERCISES IN ARRYTHMIA INTERPRETATION

SEVENTH EDITION

one

Anatomy and Physiology of the Heart

Description and Location of the Heart

The heart is a hollow, four-chambered muscular organ that lies in the middle of the thoracic cavity between the lungs, behind the sternum, in front of the spinal column, and just above the diaphragm (Figure 1.1). The top of the heart (the base) is at approximately the level of the second intercostal space. The bottom of the heart (the apex) is formed by the tip of the left ventricle and is positioned just above the diaphragm to the left of the sternum at the fifth intercostal space, midclavicular line. There, the apex can be palpated during ventricular contraction. This physical examination landmark is referred to as the *point of maximal impulse* (PMI) and is an indicator of the heart's position within the thorax.

The heart is tilted forward and to the left so that the right side of the heart lies toward the front. About two-thirds of the heart lies to the left of the body's midline and one-third extends to the right. The average adult heart is approximately 12 cm long, 8 cm wide, and 6 cm thick—a little larger than a normal-sized fist. Heart size and weight are influenced by age, weight, body build, frequency of exercise, and heart disease.

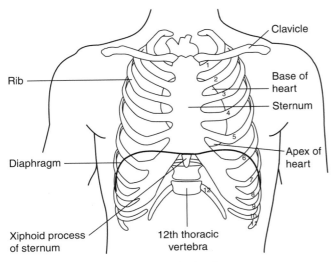

Figure 1.1 Location of the heart in the thorax.

Function of the Heart

The heart is the hardest working organ in the body. The heart functions primarily as a pump to circulate blood and supply the body with oxygen and nutrients. Each day, the average heart beats over 100,000 times. During an average lifetime, the human heart will beat more than 3 billion times.

The heart is capable of adjusting its pump performance to meet the needs of the body. As needs increase, as with exercise, the heart responds by accelerating the heart rate to propel more blood to the body. As needs decrease, as with sleep, the heart responds by decreasing the heart rate, resulting in less blood flow to the body.

The heart consists of:
- four chambers
  - two atria that receive incoming blood
  - two ventricles that pump blood out of the heart
- four valves that control the flow of blood through the heart
- an electrical conduction system that conducts electric impulses to the heart, resulting in muscle contraction

Heart Surfaces

There are four main heart surfaces to consider when discussing the heart: *anterior, posterior, inferior*, and *lateral* (Figure 1.2).
- anterior—the front
- posterior—the back
- inferior—the bottom
- lateral—the side

The surfaces of the heart are used to reference its position in relation to other structures within the thorax, and to describe the location of damage, as in myocardial infarction.

Structure of the Heart Wall

The heart wall is arranged in three layers (Figure 1.3):
- the *pericardium*—the outermost layer
- the *myocardium*—the middle muscular layer
- the *endocardium*—the inner layer

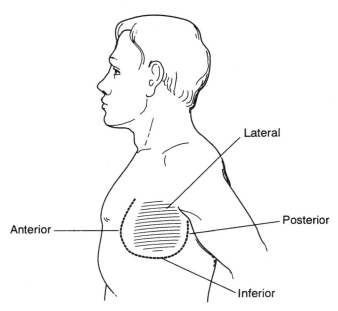

Figure 1.2   Heart surfaces.

The **_pericardium_** encloses and protects the heart and consists of:

1. *Fibrous pericardium*—an outer tough, fibrous sac, which comes in direct contact with the covering of the lung (the pleura) and is attached to the center of the diaphragm inferiorly, to the sternum anteriorly, and to the esophagus, trachea, and main bronchi posteriorly. This position anchors the heart to the chest and prevents it from shifting about in the thorax.
2. *Serous pericardium*—an inner, fluid-secreting membrane, which forms two layers:
   a. the parietal layer—lines the inner surface of the fibrous sac

   b. the visceral layer (also called epicardium)—lines the outer surface of the heart muscle (the myocardium)

Between the two layers of the serous pericardium is the pericardial space or cavity. This space provides room for the heart to contract and relax. The pericardial space is filled with approximately 10 to 30 mL of thin, clear fluid (the pericardial fluid) secreted by the serous layers. The pericardial fluid provides lubrication, preventing friction as the heart beats. In certain conditions, the accumulation of fluid, blood, or exudates can accumulate in the pericardial space and interfere with ventricular filling and the heart's ability to contract. If indicated, a pericardiocentesis (aspiration of the fluid) may be done.

The **_myocardium_** is the thick, middle, muscular layer that makes up the bulk of the heart wall. This layer is composed primarily of cardiac muscle cells and is responsible for the heart's ability to contract.

The **_endocardium_** is a thin layer of tissue that lines the inner surface of the heart muscle and the heart chambers. Extensions and folds of this tissue form the valves of the heart.

Circulatory System

The circulatory system is a network of blood vessels through which the nutrient fluids (blood) of the body circulate. This system consists of two separate circuits, the pulmonary circuit and the systemic circuit.

The **_pulmonary circuit_** is a small circuit and includes blood vessels within the lung and those carrying blood between the heart and lungs. The **_systemic circuit_** is a large circuit and includes the coronary circulation, blood vessels within the body, and those carrying blood to and from the body. The two circuits are designed so that blood flow is pumped from one circuit to the other.

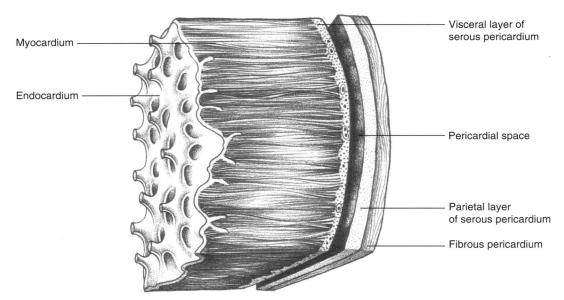

Figure 1.3   Heart wall.

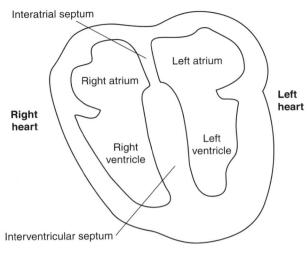

Figure 1.4   Chambers of the heart.

Heart Chambers

The interior of the heart consists of four hollow chambers (Figure 1.4). The two upper chambers, the ***right atrium*** and the ***left atrium***, are divided by a wall called the interatrial septum. The two lower chambers, the ***right ventricle*** and the ***left ventricle***, are divided by a thicker wall called the interventricular septum. The two septa divide the heart into two pumping systems—a right heart and a left heart.

The right heart pumps venous (deoxygenated) blood through the pulmonary arteries into the lungs (Figure 1.5). Oxygen and carbon dioxide exchange takes place in the alveoli of the lungs, and arterial (oxygenated) blood returns through the pulmonary veins to the left heart. The left heart then pumps arterial blood through the aorta and on to all parts of the body.

Blood flow within the body is designed so that arteries transport arterial blood and veins transport venous blood. An exception to this rule is within the pulmonary circulation where pulmonary arteries transport venous blood from the right heart to the lungs and pulmonary veins transport arterial blood from the lungs to the left heart.

The thickness of the walls in each chamber is related to the workload performed by that chamber. Both atria are low-pressure chambers serving as blood-collecting reservoirs for the ventricles. They add a small amount of force to the moving blood. Therefore, their walls are relatively thin. The walls of the ventricles are thicker and more muscular than the atria. The right ventricle pumps blood a fairly short distance to the lungs against a relatively low resistance to flow and therefore has a thicker wall than the atria, but not as thick as the left ventricle The left ventricle has the thickest wall because it must eject blood through the aorta against a much greater resistance to flow (the arterial pressure in the systemic circulation).

Heart Valves

There are four valves in the heart: the ***tricuspid valve***, separating the right atrium from the right ventricle; the ***pulmonic valve***, separating the right ventricle from the pulmonary arteries; the ***mitral valve***, separating the left atrium from the left ventricle; and the ***aortic valve***, separating the left ventricle from the aorta (see Figure 1.5). The primary function of the valves is to allow blood flow in one direction through the heart's chambers and prevent a backflow of blood (regurgitation). Changes in chamber pressure govern the opening and closing of the heart valves.

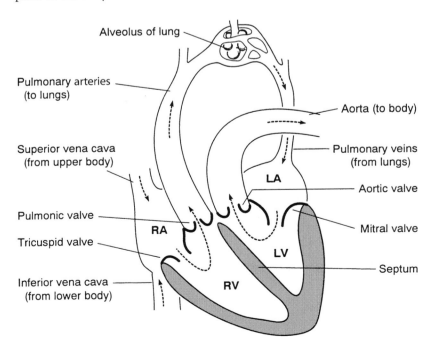

Figure 1.5   Chambers, valves, and blood flow. *RA*, right atrium; *RV*, right ventricle; *LA*, left atrium; *LV*, left ventricle.

The tricuspid and mitral valves separate the atria from the ventricles and are referred to as the **atrioventricular (AV) valves**. These valves serve as inflow valves for the ventricles. The tricuspid valve consists of three valve cusps or leaflets and is larger in diameter than the mitral valve. The tricuspid valve directs blood flow from the right atrium to the right ventricle. The mitral valve (or bicuspid valve) has only two cusps. The mitral valve directs blood flow from the left atrium to the left ventricle. Both valves are encircled by tough, fibrous rings (valve rings). The leaflets of the AV valves are attached to thin strands of fibrous cords called *chordae tendineae* (heart strings) (Figure 1.6). The chordae tendineae are then attached to papillary muscles, which arise from the walls and floor of the ventricles. During ventricular filling (diastole) when the AV valves are open, the valve leaflets, the chordae tendineae, and the papillary muscles form a funnel, promoting blood flow into the ventricles. As pressure increases during ventricular contraction (systole), the valve cusps close. Backflow of blood into the atria is prevented by contraction of the papillary muscles and the tension in the chordae tendineae. Dysfunction of the chordae tendineae or a papillary muscle can cause incomplete closure of an AV valve. This may result in a regurgitation of blood from the ventricle into the atrium, leading to cardiac compromise. The first heart sound (S1) is produced by closure of the tricuspid and mitral valves. S1 is best heard at the apex of the heart located on the left side of the chest, fifth intercostal space, midclavicular line.

The aortic and pulmonic valves are composed of three cup-shaped cusps of approximate equal size in the shape of a half-moon and are referred to as the **semilunar (SL) valves**. These valves serve as outflow valves for the ventricles. Like the AV valves, the rims of the SL valves are supported by valve rings. The pulmonic valve directs blood flow from the right ventricle to the pulmonary arteries. The aortic valve directs blood flow from the left ventricle to the aorta. As pressure decreases during ventricular relaxation (diastole), the valve cusps close. Backflow of blood into the ventricles is prevented because of the fibrous strength of the cusps, their close approximation, and their shape. The second heart sound (S2) is produced by closure of the aortic and pulmonic valves. S2 is best heard over the second intercostal space on the left or right side of the sternum.

Blood Flow through the Heart and Lungs

Blood flow through the heart and lungs can be traced from the right side of the heart to the left side of the heart (see Figure 1.5). The right atrium receives venous blood from the superior vena cava, the inferior vena cava, and the coronary sinus. The superior vena cava returns blood from the upper body. The inferior vena cava returns blood from the lower body. The coronary sinus returns blood from the capillary beds of the myocardium.

As the right atrium fills with blood, the pressure in the chamber increases. When pressure in the right atrium exceeds that of the right ventricle, the tricuspid valve opens, allowing blood to flow into the right ventricle. As the right ventricle fills with blood, the pressure in that chamber increases, forcing the tricuspid valve shut and the pulmonic valve open, ejecting blood into the pulmonary arteries and onto the lungs. In the lungs, the blood collects oxygen and excretes carbon dioxide.

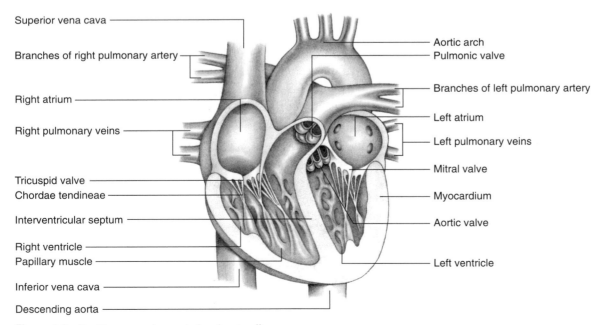

Figure 1.6 Papillary muscles and chordae tendineae.

The left atrium receives arterial blood from the pulmonary circulation via the pulmonary veins. As the left atrium fills with blood, the pressure in the chamber increases. When pressure in the left atrium exceeds that of the left ventricle, the mitral valve opens, allowing blood to flow into the left ventricle. As the left ventricle fills with blood, the pressure in that chamber increases, forcing the mitral valve shut and the aortic valve open, ejecting blood into the aorta and throughout the body where the body releases oxygen to the cells and collects carbon dioxide.

Although blood flow can be traced from the right side of the heart to the left side of the heart, it is important to realize that the heart works as two pumps (the right heart and the left heart) working simultaneously. As the right atrium receives venous blood from the systemic circulation, the left atrium receives arterial blood from the pulmonary circulation. As the atria fill with blood, the pressure in the chambers increases. When pressure in the atria exceeds that of the ventricles, the AV valves open, allowing blood to flow into the ventricles. Toward the end of ventricular filling, the atria contract, pumping the remaining atrial blood into the ventricles. Atrial contraction accounts for an additional 20% to 30% to ventricular filling volume

and is called the ***atrial kick***. In normal heart rhythms, the atria contract before the ventricles, completely filling the ventricles before ventricular contraction. In some abnormal heart rhythms, the atria do not regularly contract and empty normally. The loss of this atrial kick may result in incomplete filling of the ventricles and a reduction in cardiac output (the amount of blood pumped out of the heart). As the ventricles fill with blood, the pressure in the ventricles begins to increase. Once ventricular pressure exceeds the pressure in the circulation, the AV valves close and the SL valves open. The ventricles contract simultaneously, ejecting blood through the pulmonic valve into the pulmonary circulation and through the aortic valve into the systemic circulation.

Coronary Circulation

The blood supply to the heart is supplied by the ***right coronary artery***, ***the left coronary artery***, ***and their branches*** (Figure 1.7). There is some individual variation in the pattern of coronary artery branching, but in general, the right coronary artery supplies the right side of the heart and the left coronary artery supplies the left side of the heart.

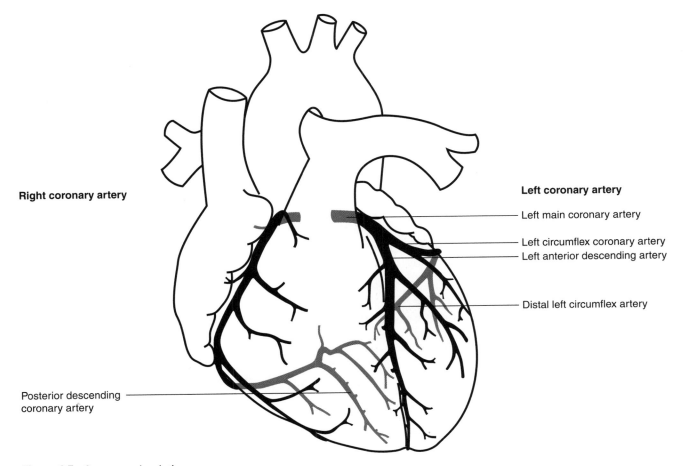

Right coronary artery

Left coronary artery

Left main coronary artery

Left circumflex coronary artery
Left anterior descending artery

Distal left circumflex artery

Posterior descending coronary artery

Figure 1.7   Coronary circulation.

The right coronary artery arises from the right aortic cusp, extends down the right side of the heart, travels inferiorly, and ends posteriorly. It supplies the right atrium and the right ventricle. In 90% of individuals, the right coronary artery also supplies the inferior wall of the left ventricle, the posterior one-third of the interventricular septum, the AV node, and the bundle of His. In 55% of hearts, it supplies the SA node.

The left coronary artery arises from the left aortic cusp and consists of the left main coronary artery (a short stem), which divides into the left anterior descending (LAD) coronary artery and the left circumflex coronary artery. The LAD coronary artery travels downward over the left side of the heart and circles the apex to end behind it. The left circumflex coronary artery travels along the lateral aspect of the left ventricle and ends posteriorly. The LAD supplies the anterior wall of the left ventricle, a portion of the lateral wall of the left ventricle, the anterior two-thirds of the interventricular septum, and the right and left bundle branches. The left circumflex coronary artery supplies the left atrium and the lateral and posterior walls of the left ventricle. In 10% of individuals, the left circumflex coronary artery also supplies the inferior wall of the left ventricle, the posterior one-third of the interventricular septum, the AV node, and the bundle of His. In 45% of hearts, it supplies the SA node. Table 1.1 summarizes the coronary artery distribution to the myocardium and conduction system (discussed in Chapter 2).

If an obstruction occurs in one of the main coronary arteries, secondary blood vessels (collateral vessels) may enlarge and anastomose to each other to form a vascular network around the occluded vessel. This vascular network is called the **collateral circulation** (Figure 1.8). The collateral circulation develops best (greater number of coronary collaterals with larger caliber vessels) in the presence of a slow evolution of coronary obstruction. Collateral circulation potentially offers an important alternative source of blood supply when the original vessel fails to provide sufficient blood.

Coronary artery dominance is the term used to describe coronary vasculature and refers to the distribution of the terminal portion of the arteries. The artery that supplies the posterior descending artery determines the coronary dominance.

- If the posterior descending artery is supplied by the right coronary artery, then the coronary circulation is classified as "right dominant."
- If the posterior descending artery is supplied by the left circumflex artery, then the coronary circulation is classified as "left dominant."
- If the posterior descending artery is supplied by both the right coronary artery and the left circumflex artery, then the coronary circulation is classified as "codominant."

Approximately 70% of the populations are right dominant, 20% are codominant, and 10% are left dominant.

Cardiac Innervation

The heart is under the control of the autonomic nervous system located in the medulla oblongata, a part of the brain stem. The autonomic nervous system regulates functions of the body that are involuntary, or not under conscious control, such as blood pressure and heart rate. It includes the **sympathetic nervous system** and the **parasympathetic**

table 1.1 Coronary Arteries

Coronary artery and its branches	Portion of myocardium supplied	Portion of conduction system supplied
Right coronary artery		
	Right atrium	Sinoatrial (SA) node (55%)*
	Right ventricle	Atrioventricular (AV) node and bundle of His (90%)*
	Inferior wall of left ventricle (90%)*	
	Posterior one-third of interventricular septum (90%)*	
Left coronary artery		
Left anterior descending (LAD)	Anterior wall of left ventricle	Right and left bundle branches
	Portion of lateral wall of left ventricle	
	Anterior two-thirds of interventricular septum	
Circumflex	Left atrium	SA node (45%)*
	Lateral wall of left ventricle	AV node and bundle of His (10%)*
	Posterior wall of left ventricle	
	Inferior wall of left ventricle (10%)*	
	Posterior one-third of interventricular septum (10%)*	

* = of population.

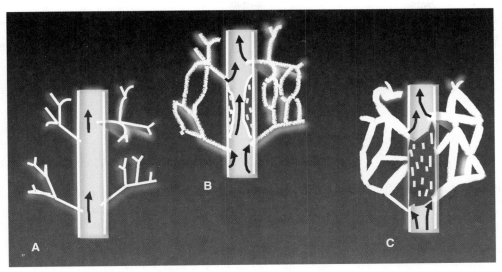

Figure 1.8 Collateral circulation forming around a vessel occlusion. **A.** Normal vessel. **B.** Partially occluded vessel. **C.** Completely occluded vessel. (Illustration by Brandy Huff Tarini.)

nervous system, each producing opposite effects when stimulated. Stimulation of the sympathetic nervous system results in the release of norepinephrine, a neurotransmitter, which accelerates the heart rate, speeds conduction through the AV node, and increases the force of ventricular contraction. This system prepares the body to function under stress (the "fight or flight" response). Stimulation of the parasympathetic nervous system results in the release of acetylcholine, a neurotransmitter, which slows the heart rate, decreases conduction through the AV node, and causes a small decrease in the force of ventricular contraction. This system regulates the calmer functions of the body (the "rest and digest" response). Normally, a balance is maintained between the accelerator effects of the sympathetic system and the inhibitory effects of the parasympathetic system.

two

Electrophysiology

Cardiac Cells

The heart is composed of thousands of cardiac cells. The cardiac cells are long and narrow and divide at their ends into branches. These branches connect with branches of adjacent cells, forming a branching and anastomosing network of cells. At the junctions where the branches join together is a specialized cellular membrane of low electrical resistance, which permits rapid conduction of electrical impulses from one cell to another throughout the cell network. Stimulation of one cardiac cell initiates stimulation of adjacent cells and ultimately leads to cardiac muscle contraction.

There are two basic kinds of cardiac cells in the heart: the myocardial *muscle cells* (or working cells) and the myocardial *pacemaker cells*. The muscle cells are contained in the muscular layer of the walls of the atria and ventricles. The muscle cells are permeated by contractile filaments, which, when electrically stimulated, produce myocardial muscle contraction followed by muscle relaxation. The pacemaker cells are found in the electrical conduction system of the heart and are responsible for the spontaneous generation of electrical impulses.

Cardiac cells have four primary cell characteristics:

- **Automaticity**—the ability of the pacemaker cells to generate their own electrical impulses spontaneously; this characteristic is specific to the pacemaker cells.
- **Excitability**—the ability of the cardiac cells to respond to an electrical impulse; this characteristic is shared by all cardiac cells.
- **Conductivity**—the ability of cardiac cells to conduct an electrical impulse; this characteristic is shared by all cardiac cells.
- **Contractility**—the ability of cardiac cells to cause cardiac muscle contraction; this characteristic is specific to the muscle cells.

Depolarization and Repolarization

Cardiac cells are surrounded and filled with an electrolyte solution. An electrolyte is a substance whose molecules dissociate into charged particles (ions) when placed in water, producing positively and negatively charged ions. The two major ions that affect cardiac function are sodium and potassium. Potassium (K^+) is the primary ion inside the cell and sodium (Na^+) is the primary ion outside the cell. Sodium plays a major role in depolarization of the myocardium. Potassium plays a vital part in both myocardial depolarization and repolarization.

A membrane separates the inside of the cardiac cell (intracellular) from the outside (extracellular). There is a constant movement of ions across the cardiac cell membrane. Differences in concentrations of these ions determine the cell's electric charge. The distribution of ions on either side of the membrane is determined by several factors:

- Membrane channels (pores)—The cell membrane has openings through which ions pass back and forth between the extracellular and intracellular spaces. Some channels are always open; others can be opened or closed; still others can be selective, allowing one kind of ion to pass through and excluding all others. Membrane channels open and close in response to a stimulus.
- Concentration gradient—Particles in solution move, or diffuse, from areas of higher concentration to areas of lower concentration. In the case of uncharged particles, movement proceeds until the particles are uniformly distributed within the solution.
- Electrical gradient—Charged particles also diffuse, but the diffusion of charged particles is influenced not only by the concentration gradient but also by an electrical gradient. Like charges repel; opposite charges attract. Therefore, positively charged particles tend to flow toward negatively charged particles and negatively charged particles toward positively charged particles.
- Sodium-potassium pump—The sodium-potassium pump is a mechanism that actively transports ions across the cell membrane against its electrochemical gradient. This pump helps to reestablish the resting concentrations of sodium and potassium after cardiac depolarization.

Electrical impulses are the result of the flow of ions (primarily sodium and potassium) back and forth across the cardiac cell membrane (Figure 2.1). Normally, there is an ionic difference between the two sides. In the resting cardiac cell, there are more negative ions inside the cell than outside the cell. When the ions are so aligned, the resting cell is called polarized. During this time, no electrical activity is occurring and a straight line (isoelectric line) is recorded on the ECG (see Figure 2.5).

Once a cell is stimulated, the membrane permeability changes. Potassium begins to leave the cell, increasing cell permeability to sodium. Sodium rushes into the cell, causing the inside of the cell to become more positive than negative (cell is depolarized). Muscle contraction follows

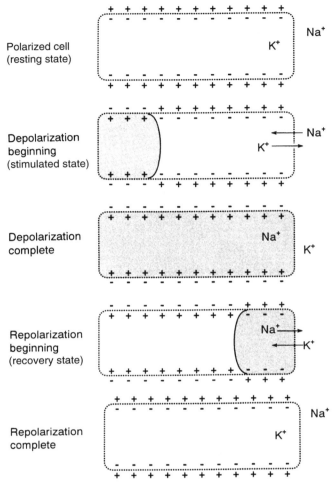

Figure 2.1 Depolarization and repolarization of a cardiac cell.

Polarized cell
(resting state)

Depolarization
beginning
(stimulated state)

Depolarization
complete

Repolarization
beginning
(recovery state)

Repolarization
complete

depolarization. Depolarization and muscle contraction are not the same. Depolarization is an electrical event that results in muscle contraction, a mechanical event.

After depolarization, the cardiac cell begins to recover. The sodium-potassium pump is activated to actively transport sodium out of the cell and move potassium back into the cell. The inside of the cell becomes more negative than positive (cell is repolarized) and returns to its resting state. The cardiac cell is now ready to be stimulated again.

Depolarization of one cardiac cell acts as a stimulus on adjacent cells and causes them to depolarize. Propagation of the electrical impulses from cell to cell produces an electric current that can be detected by skin electrodes and recorded as waves or deflections onto graph paper, called the ECG.

Electrical Conduction System of the Heart

The heart is supplied with an electrical conduction system that generates and conducts electrical impulses along specialized pathways to the atria and ventricles, causing them

to contract (Figure 2.2). The system consists of the **sino-atrial node (SA node)**, the **interatrial tract (Bachmann bundle)**, the **internodal tracts**, the **atrioventricular node (AV node)**, the **bundle of His**, the **right bundle branch**, the **left bundle branch**, and the **Purkinje fibers.**

The SA node is located in the wall of the upper right atrium near the inlet of the superior vena cava. Specialized electrical cells, called pacemaker cells, in the SA node discharge impulses at an intrinsic rate of 60 to 100 times a minute. An intrinsic rate is the rate at which a pacemaker of the heart normally generates impulses. Pacemaker cells are located at other sites along the conduction system, but the SA node is normally in control and is called the pacemaker of the heart because it possesses the highest level of automaticity (its intrinsic firing rate is greater than that of the other pacemaker sites). Pacemaker cells in the AV junction generate electrical impulses at 40 to 60 times per minute. Pacemaker cells in the ventricles generate electrical impulses at a much slower rate (30 to 40 times per minute or less). In general, the further away the impulse originates from the SA node, the slower the intrinsic rate.

Other areas of the heart can take over pacemaker control of the heart by discharging impulses more rapidly than does the SA node. Or if the SA node generates impulses too slowly or stops functioning entirely, or if the conduction of impulses are blocked for any reason, then these pacemaker sites may assume pacemaker control at their intrinsic firing rate.

As the electrical impulse leaves the SA node, it is conducted to the left atria by way of the interatrial tract and through the right atria via the internodal tracts, causing electrical stimulation (depolarization) and contraction of the atria. The impulse is then conducted to the AV node located in the lower right atrium near the interatrial septum. The AV node relays the electrical impulses from the atria to the ventricles. It provides the only normal conduction pathway between the atria and the ventricles. The AV node has three main functions:

- To slow conduction of the electrical impulse through the AV node to allow time for the atria to contract and empty its contents into the ventricles (atrial kick) before the ventricles contract. This delay in the AV node is represented on the ECG tracing as the flat line of the PR interval.
- To serve as a backup pacemaker, if the SA node fails, at a rate of 40 to 60 beats per minute.
- To block some of the impulses from being conducted to the ventricles when the atria rate is rapid, thus protecting the ventricles from dangerously fast rates.

After the delay in the AV node, the impulse moves through the bundle of His. The bundle of His divides into two important conducting pathways called the right bundle branch and the left bundle branch. The right bundle branch conducts the electrical impulse to the right ventricle. The left bundle branch divides into two divisions: the anterior fascicle, which carries the electrical impulse to the anterior

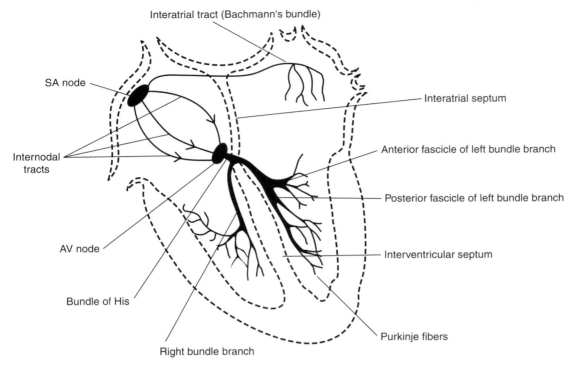

Figure 2.2 Electrical conduction system of the heart.

wall of the left ventricle, and the posterior fascicle, which carries the electrical impulse to the posterior wall of the left ventricle. Both bundle branches terminate in a network of conduction fibers called Purkinje fibers. These fibers make up an elaborate web that carry the electrical impulses directly to the ventricular muscle cells. The ventricles are capable of serving as a backup pacemaker at a rate of 30 to 40 beats per minute (sometimes less). Transmission of the electrical impulses through the conduction system is slowest in the AV node and fastest in the His-Purkinje system (bundle of His, bundle branches, and Purkinje fibers).

Waveforms

The heart's electrical activity is represented on the monitor or ECG tracing by three basic waveforms: the *P wave*, the *QRS complex*, and the *T wave* (Figure 2.3). A U wave is sometimes present. Between the waveforms are the following segments and intervals: the PR interval, the PR segment, the ST segment, and the QT interval. Although the letters themselves have no special significance, each component represents a particular event in the depolarization-repolarization cycle.

The P wave represents atrial depolarization, the spread of the electrical impulse throughout the right and left atria. A waveform representing atrial repolarization is not seen on the ECG because atrial repolarization occurs during ventricular depolarization and is hidden in the QRS complex.

The PR interval represents the time from the onset of atrial depolarization to the onset of ventricular depolarization. The PR segment, a part of the PR interval, is the short isoelectric line between the end of the P wave and the beginning of the QRS complex. It is used as a baseline to evaluate elevation or depression of the ST segment.

The QRS complex represents ventricular depolarization, the spread of the electrical impulse throughout the right and left ventricle. The ST segment represents early ventricular repolarization. The T wave represents ventricular repolarization. The U wave, which isn't always present, represents late ventricular repolarization. The QT interval

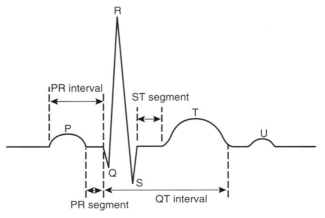

Figure 2.3 Relationship of the electrical conduction system to the ECG.

represents total ventricular activity (the time from the onset of ventricular depolarization to the end of ventricular repolarization).

The Cardiac Cycle

A cardiac cycle consists of one heartbeat or **one PQRST sequence**. It represents a sequence of atrial contraction and relaxation followed by ventricular contraction and relaxation. The basic cycle repeats itself again and again (Figure 2.4). Regularity of the cardiac rhythm can be assessed by measuring from one heartbeat to the next (from one R wave to the next R wave, also called the R-R interval). Between cardiac cycles is the isoelectric line (baseline), the flat line in the ECG during which electrical activity is absent (Figure 2.5). Any waveform above the isoelectric line is considered a positive (upright) deflection and any waveform below this line a negative (downward) deflection. A deflection having both a positive and negative component is called a biphasic deflection. This basic concept can be applied to the P wave, the QRS complex, and the T-wave deflections.

Waveforms and Current Flow

A monitor lead, or ECG lead, provides a view of the heart's electrical activity between two points or poles (a positive pole and a negative pole). The direction in which the electric current flows determines how the waveforms appear on the ECG tracing (Figure 2.6). An electric current flowing toward the positive pole will produce a **positive deflection**; an electric current traveling toward the negative pole produces a **negative deflection**. Current flowing away from the poles will produce a **biphasic deflection** (both positive and negative). Biphasic deflections may be equally positive and negative, more negative than positive, or more positive than negative (depending on the angle of current flow to the positive or negative pole).

The size of the wave deflection depends on the magnitude of the electrical current flowing toward the individual pole. The magnitude of the electrical current is determined by how much voltage is generated by depolarization of a particular portion of the heart. The QRS complex is normally larger than the P wave because depolarization of the

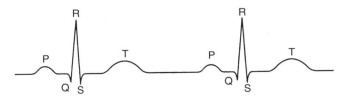

Figure 2.4 The cardiac cycle.

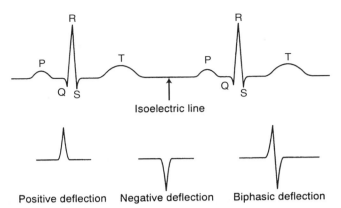

Figure 2.5 Relationship between waveforms and the isoelectric line.

larger muscle mass of the ventricle generates more voltage than does depolarization of the smaller muscle mass of the atria.

Refractory Periods of the Cardiac Cycle

Refractoriness is a term used to describe the extent to which a cell is able to respond to a stimulus. In the heart, refractoriness is divided into two phases (Figure 2.7):

- **Absolute refractory period**—During the absolute refractory period, the cardiac cell is unable to respond to an electrical stimulus. This period extends from the onset of the QRS complex to the peak of the T wave. During this time, the cardiac cells have depolarized and are in the process of repolarizing. Because the cardiac cells have not repolarized to their threshold

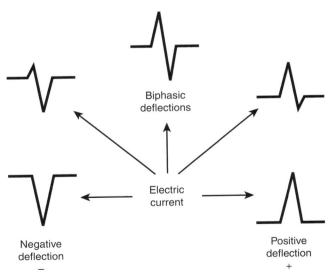

Figure 2.6 Relationship between current flow and waveform deflections.

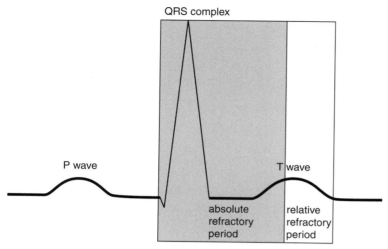

Figure 2.7 Refractory periods.

potential (the level at which a cell must be repolarized before it can be depolarized again), they cannot respond to further stimulation no matter how strong the stimulus.

- **Relative refractory period**—During the relative refractory period, the cardiac cells have repolarized sufficiently to respond to a strong stimulus. This period corresponds to the downslope of the T wave (from the peak of the T wave to the end of the T wave). The relative refractory period is also called the vulnerable period of repolarization. A strong stimulus occurring during the vulnerable period may usurp the primary pacemaker of the heart (usually the SA node) and take over pacemaker control. An example might be a premature ventricular contraction (PVC) that falls during the vulnerable period and takes over control of the heart in the form of ventricular tachycardia.

ECG Graph Paper

The PQRST sequence is recorded on special graph paper made up of horizontal and vertical lines (Figure 2.8). The horizontal lines measure the duration (width) of the waveform in seconds of time. Each small square measured horizontally represents 0.04 second in time. The width of the QRS complex in Figure 2.9 extends across for 2 small squares and represents 0.08 second (0.04 second × 2 squares). The vertical lines measure the amplitude or voltage (the height or depth of a wave or complex) in millimeters (mm). Each small square represents 1 mm in height or depth. The height of the QRS complex in Figure 2.9 extends upward from baseline 16 small squares and represents 16 mm voltage (1 mm × 16 squares).

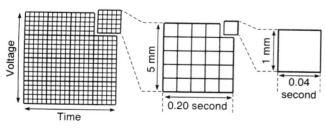

Figure 2.8 Electrocardiographic paper.

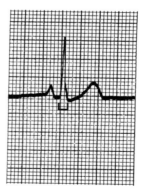

Figure 2.9 QRS width, 0.08 second; QRS height, 16 mm.

three

Waveforms, Intervals, Segments, and Complexes

Much of the information that the ECG tracing provides is obtained from the examination of the three principal waveforms (the P wave, the QRS complex, and the T wave) and their associated segments and intervals. Assessment of these data provides the facts necessary for an accurate cardiac rhythm interpretation.

P Wave

The first deflection of the cardiac cycle, the P wave, is caused by depolarization of the right and left atria (Figure 3.1). The first half of the P wave represents depolarization of the right atrium; the second half reflects depolarization of the left atrium. The waveform begins as the deflection leaves baseline and ends when the deflection returns to baseline. *A normal sinus P wave originates in the sinus node and travels through normal atria, resulting in normal depolarization*.

Characteristics of a normal P wave include the following:

- Smooth and round
- Positive in lead II
- 0.5 to 2.5 mm in height
- 0.10 second or less in duration (width)
- One sinus P wave to each QRS complex

There are *two types of abnormal P waves*:

- **The impulse originates in the sinus node and travels through enlarged atria, resulting in abnormal depolarization of the atria.** Abnormal atrial depolarization results in abnormal-looking P waves. Impulses traveling through an enlarged right atrium (right atrial hypertrophy) result in P waves that are typically tall and peaked but may be biphasic in some leads. The abnormal P wave in right atrial enlargement is sometimes referred to as P pulmonale because the atrial enlargement that it signifies is common with chronic pulmonary diseases such as chronic

obstructive pulmonary disease (COPD) and asthma. Impulses traveling through an enlarged left atrium (left atrial hypertrophy) result in P waves that are typically wide and notched (M shaped) but may be biphasic in some leads. The term P mitrale is used to describe the abnormal P waves seen in left atrial enlargement because they are typically associated with severe mitral stenosis.

- **The impulse originates in an ectopic site.** The term ectopic means away from its original location. Therefore, an ectopic P wave arises from a site other than the SA node and will produce abnormal P waves. Ectopic sites include the atria and the AV junction. P waves from the atria are usually positive and may appear small and pointed, biphasic, as a small squiggle, wavy, or sawtooth in appearance. Occasionally atrial P waves are negative (inverted) if the ectopic site is close to the AV junction. P waves from the AV junction are always negative and may precede or follow the QRS complex or be hidden within the QRS complex and not visible. Examples of P waves are shown in Figure 3.2.

PR Interval

The PR interval (sometimes abbreviated PRI) represents the time from the onset of atrial depolarization to the onset of ventricular depolarization. The PR interval (Figure 3.3) includes a P wave and the short isoelectric line (PR segment) that follows it. The PR interval is measured from the beginning of the P wave as it leaves baseline to the beginning of the QRS complex. The duration of the normal PR interval is 0.12 to 0.20 seconds.

Abnormal PR intervals may be short or prolonged:

- **Short PR interval**—A short PR interval is less than 0.12 second and may be seen if the electrical impulse originates in an ectopic site in the AV junction. A shortened PR interval may also occur if the electrical impulse progresses from the atria to the ventricles through one of several abnormal conduction pathways (called accessory pathways) that bypass a part or all of the AV node. Wolff-Parkinson-White syndrome (WPW) is an example of such an accessory pathway.
- **Prolonged PR interval**—A prolonged PR interval is greater than 0.20 second and indicates that the impulse was delayed longer than normal in the AV node. Prolonged PR intervals are seen in first-degree AV block. Examples of PR intervals are shown in Figure 3.4.

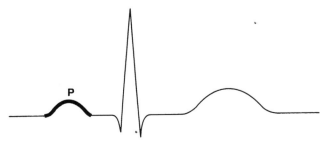

Figure 3.1 The P wave.

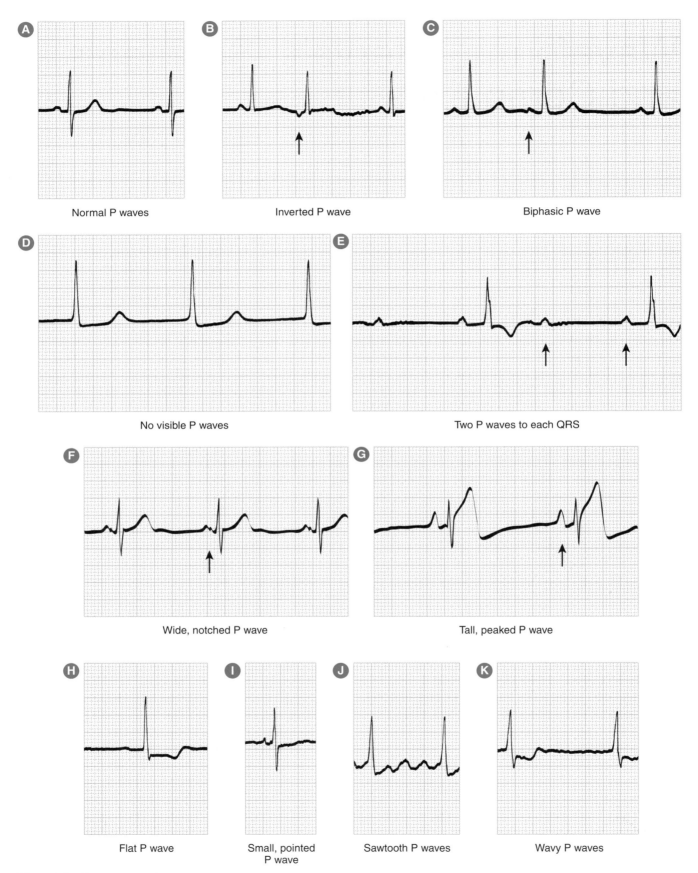

Figure 3.2   P wave examples.

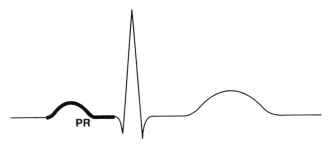

Figure 3.3 The PR interval.

Figure 3.5 The QRS complex.

QRS Complex

The QRS complex (Figure 3.5) represents depolarization of the right and left ventricles. Ventricular depolarization triggers contraction of the ventricles.

The QRS complex is composed of three wave deflections: the **Q wave**, the **R wave**, and the **S wave**. The R wave is a positive waveform; the Q wave is a negative waveform that precedes the R wave; and the S wave is a negative waveform that follows the R wave. The normal QRS complex is predominantly positive in lead II (a positive lead) with a duration of 0.10 second or less.

The QRS is measured from the beginning of the QRS complex (as the first wave of the complex leaves baseline) to the end of the QRS complex (when the last wave of the complex begins to level out into the ST segment). The point where the QRS complex meets the ST segment is called the J point (junction point). Finding the beginning of the QRS complex usually isn't difficult. Finding the end of the QRS complex, however, is at times a challenge because of elevation or depression of the ST segment. Remember, the QRS complex ends as soon as the straight line of the ST segment begins, even though the straight line may be above or below baseline.

Although the term QRS complex is used, not every QRS complex contains a Q wave, R wave, or S wave. Many variations exist in the configuration of the QRS complex (Figure 3.6). Whatever the variation, the complex is still called the QRS complex. For example, you might see a QRS complex with a Q and an R wave, but no S wave (Figure 3.6, example B), an R and S wave without a Q wave (Figure 3.6, example C), or an R wave without a Q wave or an S wave (Figure 3.6, example D). If the entire complex is negative (Figure 3.6, example F), it is termed a QS complex (not a negative R wave because R waves are always positive). It's also possible to have more than one R wave (Figure 3.6, example I) and more than one S wave (Figure 3.6, example J). The second R wave is called R prime and is written R′. The second S wave is called S prime and is written S′. To be labeled separately, a wave must cross the baseline. A wave that changes direction but doesn't cross the baseline is called a notch (Figure 3.6, example E shows a notched R, and Figure 3.6, example K shows a notched S).

Capital letters are used to designate waves of large amplitude (5 mm or more), and lower case letters are used to designate waves of small amplitude (less the 5 mm). This allows

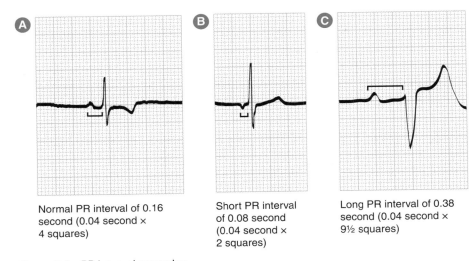

Normal PR interval of 0.16 second (0.04 second × 4 squares)

Short PR interval of 0.08 second (0.04 second × 2 squares)

Long PR interval of 0.38 second (0.04 second × 9½ squares)

Figure 3.4 PR interval examples.

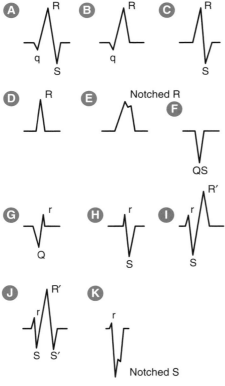

Figure 3.6   QRS variations.

you to visualize a complex mentioned in a textbook when illustrations aren't available. For example, if a complex is described in a text as having an rS waveform, the reader can easily picture a complex with a small r wave and a big S wave.

An abnormal QRS complex is wide with a duration of 0.12 seconds or more. An abnormally wide QRS complex may result from the following:

- An electrical impulse that has originated in an ectopic site in the ventricles—This is the most common cause of a wide QRS complex.
- A block in the conduction of impulses through the right or left bundle branch (bundle branch block)—This is the second most common cause of a wide QRS complex.
- An electrical impulse that has arrived early (as with premature beats) at the bundle branches before repolarization is complete, allowing the electrical impulse to initiate depolarization of the ventricles earlier than usual. The cells have not repolarized to threshold level, causing conduction of the impulse to be slow, resulting in a wide QRS complex.
- An electrical impulse that has been conducted from the atria to the ventricles through an abnormal accessory conduction pathway that bypasses the AV node allowing the electrical impulse to initiate depolarization of the ventricles earlier than usual. The cells have not depolarized to threshold level, causing conduction of the impulse to be slow, resulting in a wide QRS complex.

Examples of QRS complexes are shown in Figure 3.7.

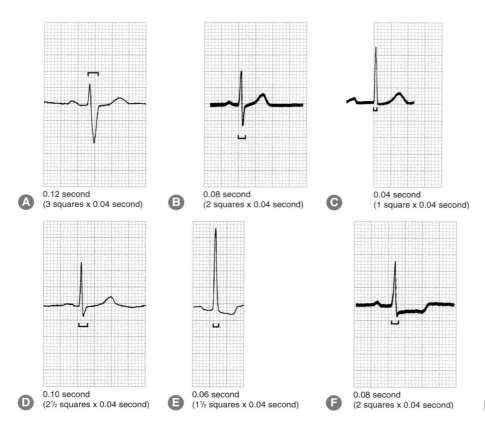

A 0.12 second
(3 squares x 0.04 second)

B 0.08 second
(2 squares x 0.04 second)

C 0.04 second
(1 square x 0.04 second)

D 0.10 second
(2½ squares x 0.04 second)

E 0.06 second
(1½ squares x 0.04 second)

F 0.08 second
(2 squares x 0.04 second)

Figure 3.7   QRS examples.

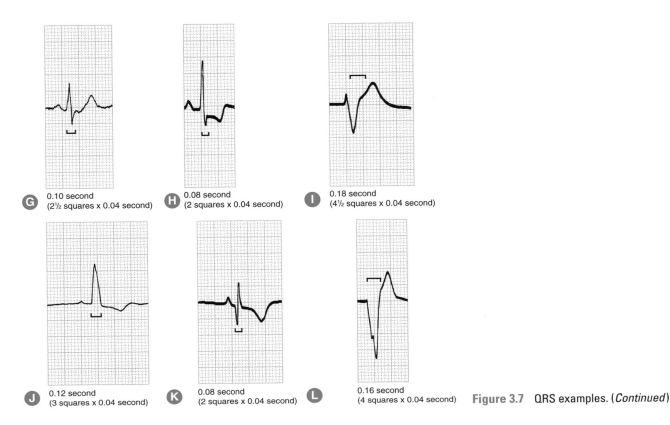

(G) 0.10 second
(2½ squares × 0.04 second)

(H) 0.08 second
(2 squares × 0.04 second)

(I) 0.18 second
(4½ squares × 0.04 second)

(J) 0.12 second
(3 squares × 0.04 second)

(K) 0.08 second
(2 squares × 0.04 second)

(L) 0.16 second
(4 squares × 0.04 second)

Figure 3.7 QRS examples. (*Continued*)

ST Segment

The ST segment represents early ventricular repolarization. The ST segment is the flat line between the QRS complex and the T wave (Figure 3.8). Normally, the ST segment is positioned at baseline (the isoelectric line). The ST segment may be displaced above baseline (elevated ST segment) or below baseline (depressed ST segment). The PR segment is normally used as a baseline reference to evaluate the degree of displacement of the ST segment from the isoelectric line. To determine the degree of displacement, start measuring at a point 0.04 second (1 small square) past the J point. ST segment elevation or depression is considered abnormal if the displacement is greater than 1 mm from baseline.

Elevated ST segments may be horizontal (straight across), convex (rounded upward), or concave (rounded inward).

Common causes include ST elevation myocardial infarction (STEMI), coronary artery spasm (Prinzmetal angina), acute pericarditis, ventricular aneurysm, early repolarization pattern (a form of myocardial repolarization seen in normal healthy individuals that produces ST segment elevation closely mimicking that of acute myocardial infarction (MI) or pericarditis), hyperkalemia, and hypothermia.

Depressed ST segments may be horizontal, downsloping, or sagging. Common causes include myocardial ischemia, non-ST elevation MI (non-STEMI), reciprocal ECG changes associated with STEMI, hypokalemia, and digitalis effect. Digitalis causes a sagging ST segment depression with a characteristic "scooped-out" appearance. Examples of ST segments are shown in Figure 3.9.

T Wave

The T wave represents ventricular repolarization. The normal T wave begins as the deflection gradually slopes upward from the ST segment and ends when the waveform returns to baseline (Figure 3.10). Normal T waves are rounded and slightly asymmetrical (with the first part of the T wave gradually sloping to the peak and returning more abruptly to baseline), positive in lead II (a positive lead), with an amplitude less than 5 mm. The T wave always follows the QRS complex (repolarization always follows depolarization).

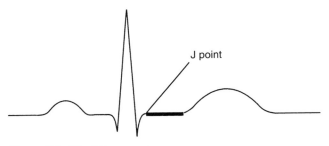

J point

Figure 3.8 The ST segment.

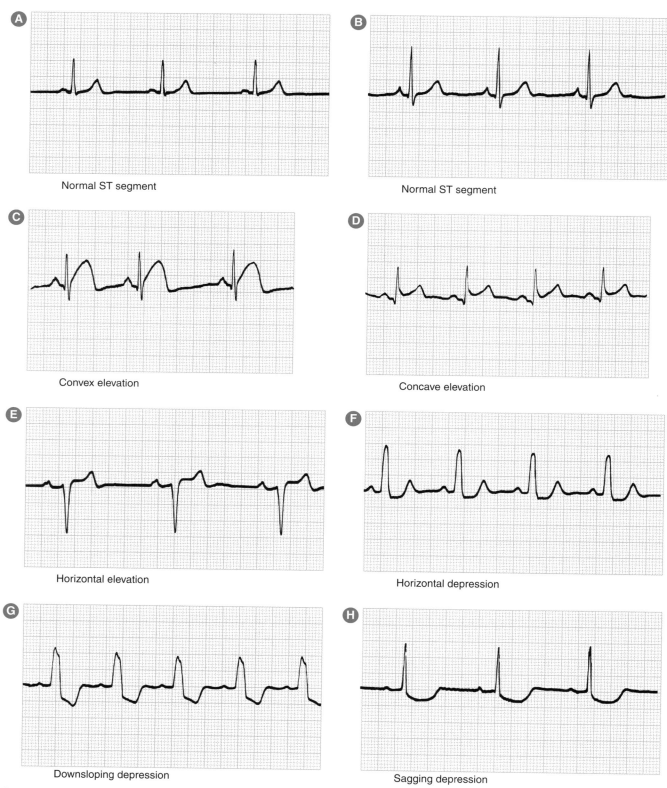

Figure 3.9   ST segment examples.

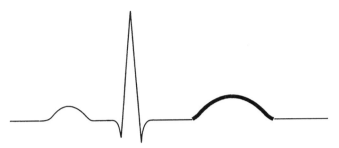

Figure 3.10 The T wave.

Abnormal T waves may be abnormally tall, flat, inverted, or biphasic. Common causes include myocardial ischemia, acute MI, pericarditis, hyperkalemia, ventricular enlargement, bundle branch block, and subarachnoid hemorrhage. Significant cerebral disease, such as subarachnoid hemorrhage, may be associated with deeply inverted T waves

(called cerebral T waves). Examples of T waves are shown in Figure 3.11.

QT Interval

The QT interval represents the time between the onset of ventricular depolarization and the end of ventricular repolarization. The QT interval is measured from the beginning of the QRS complex to the end of the T wave (Figure 3.12). Duration of the QT interval can be determined by multiplying the number of small squares in the QT interval by 0.04 second (Figure 3.13). The length of the QT interval varies according to age, sex, and particularly heart rate. The QT interval is more prolonged with slow heart rates. The determination of the QT interval should be made in a lead where the T wave is most prominent and should not include the U wave. Accurate

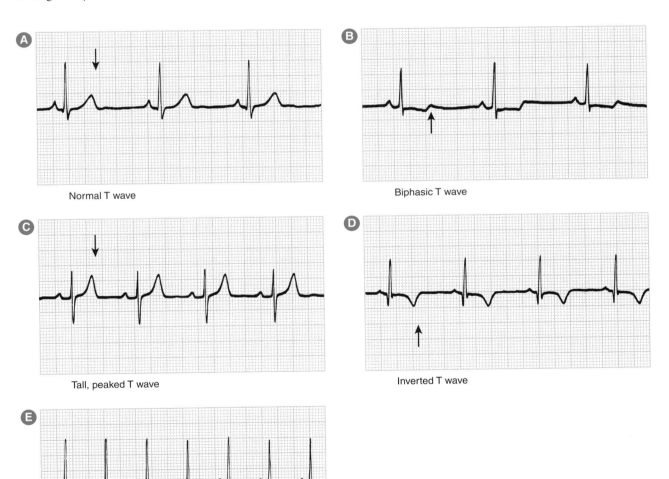

Figure 3.11 T wave examples.

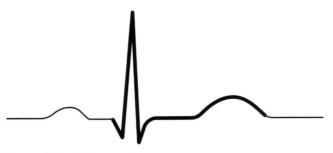

Figure 3.12 QT interval.

measurement of the QT interval can be done only when the rhythm is regular for at least two cardiac cycles before the measurement.

Generally speaking, the **normal QT interval should be less than half the R-R interval** (the distance between two consecutive R waves) when the rhythm is regular. To determine if the QT interval is normal or prolonged (see Figure 3.13):

- Count the number of small boxes in the R-R interval and divide by two.
- Count the number of small boxes in the QT interval.
- Compare the difference—If the QT interval measures less than half the R-R interval, it is normal; if the QT interval measures the same as half the R-R interval, it is considered borderline; if the QT interval measures longer than half the R-R interval, it is prolonged.

A prolonged QT interval indicates a delay in ventricular repolarization. Delayed ventricular repolarization results in a lengthened relative refractory period (vulnerable period), which puts the ventricles at risk for life-threatening arrhythmias such as torsades de pointes ventricular tachycardia (discussed in Chapter 9).

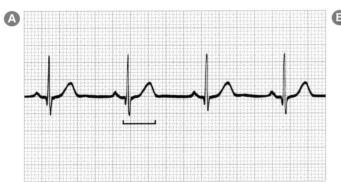

1. Number of small square between R waves = 22. Half of 22 = 11.
2. Number of small squares in QT interval = 9
3. Compare the difference: QT interval is less than half the R-R interval (9 small squares are less than 11 small squares). QT interval is normal for this heart rate. (Duration of QT interval: 9 squares × 0.04 second = 0.36 second)

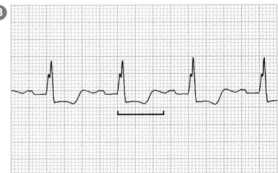

1. Number of small squares between R–waves = 20. Half of 20 = 10.
2. Number of small squares in QT interval = 13
3. Compare the difference: QT interval is more than half the R-R interval (13 small squares are more than 10 small squares). QT interval is prolonged for this heart rate. (Duration of QT interval: 13 squares × 0.04 second = 0.52 second)

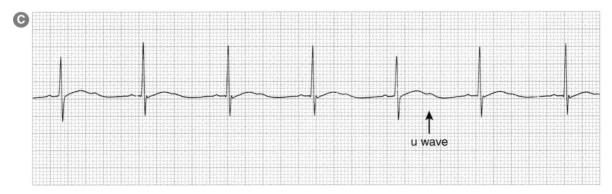

This strip has a small u wave immediately after the T wave. The end of the T wave cannot be determined for sure, so measurement of the QT interval would be inaccurate.

Figure 3.13 QT interval examples.

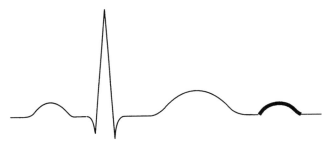

Figure 3.14 The U wave.

U Wave

The U wave is a small deflection sometimes following the T wave (Figure 3.14). Neither its presence nor its absence is considered abnormal. The U wave represents late repolarization of the ventricles, probably a small segment of the ventricles.

The waveform begins as the deflection leaves baseline and ends when the deflection returns to baseline. Normal U waves are small, rounded, and symmetrical, positive in lead II (a positive lead), with a height of 1.5 mm or less, and smaller than the preceding T wave. The U wave can best be seen when the heart rate is slow.

In general, a U wave 2 mm or more in height is considered abnormal. A common cause of a large U wave is a low serum potassium level (hypokalemia). A large U wave may occasionally be mistaken for a P wave, but usually, a comparison of the morphology of both waveforms will help differentiate the U wave from the P wave. If two P waves are present (seen in some heart blocks), the P waves will look the same (in size, shape, and direction), and the P-P interval (the distance between two consecutive P waves) will be regular.

Examples of U waves are shown in Figure 3.15.

Common causes include low serum levels of potassium, magnesium, calcium, and thiamine; consumption of alcohol in high concentrations; hypothermia; hypothyroidism; bradycardia; myocardial ischemia; and hereditary long QT syndrome. A prolonged QT interval may also be drug induced. Medications that can lengthen the QT interval include certain antibiotics, antidepressants, antihistamines, diuretics, heart medications, cholesterol-lowering drugs, and diabetes medications, as well as some antifungal and antipsychotic drugs. It can also occur without a known cause (idiopathic).

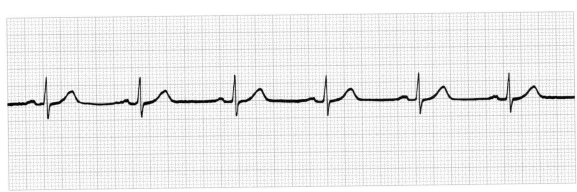

ECG without U wave

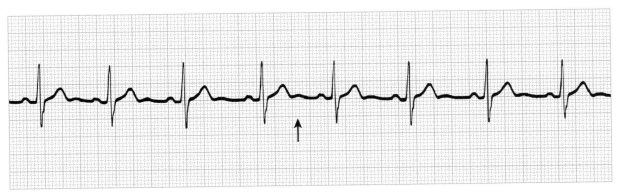

ECG with U wave

Figure 3.15 U wave examples.

WAVEFORM PRACTICE: LABELING WAVES

For each of the following rhythm strips (strips 3-1 through 3-14), label the P, Q, R, S, T, and U waves in one cardiac cycle. Some of the strips may not have all of these waveforms. Check your answers with the answer key in the back of the book.

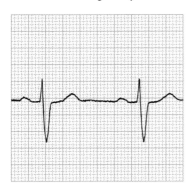

Strip 3.1

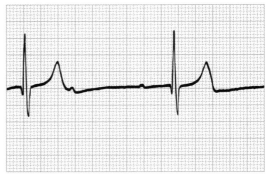

Strip 3.5

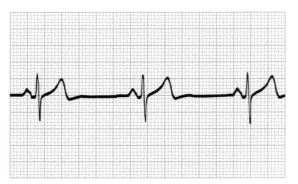

Strip 3.2

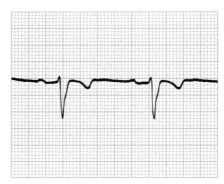

Strip 3.6

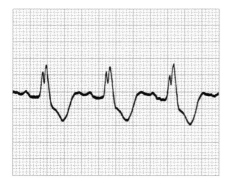

Strip 3.3

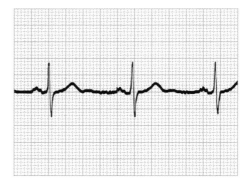

Strip 3.7

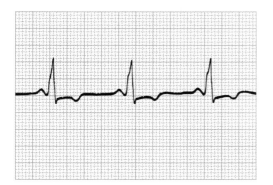

Strip 3.4

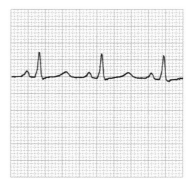

Strip 3.8

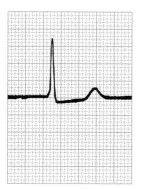

Strip 3.9

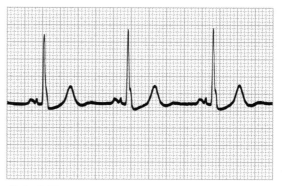

Strip 3.12

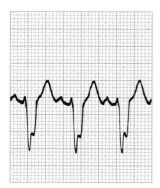

Strip 3.10

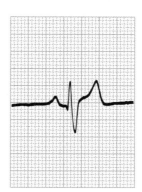

Strip 3.13

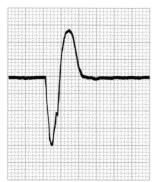

Strip 3.11

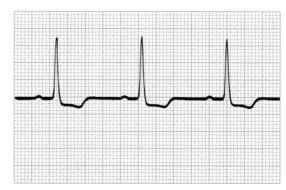

Strip 3.14

four

Cardiac Monitors

Purpose of ECG Monitoring

The electrocardiogram (ECG) is a recording of the electrical activity of the heart. The ECG records two basic electrical processes:

- **Depolarization**—the spread of the electrical stimulus through the heart muscle, producing the P wave from the atria and the QRS complex from the ventricles

- **Repolarization**—the recovery of the stimulated muscle to the resting state, producing the ST segment, the T wave, and the U wave

The depolarization-repolarization process produces electrical currents that are transmitted to the surface of the body. This electrical activity is detected by electrodes attached to the skin. After the electric current is detected, it is amplified, displayed on a monitor screen (oscilloscope), and recorded on ECG graph paper as waves and complexes. The waveforms can then be analyzed in a systematic manner and the "cardiac rhythm" identified.

Bedside monitoring allows continuous observation of the heart's electrical activity and is used to identify arrhythmias (disturbances in rate, rhythm, or conduction), evaluate pacemaker function, and evaluate the response to medications (for example, antiarrhythmics). Continuous cardiac monitoring is useful in monitoring patients in critical care units, cardiac step-down units, surgery suites, outpatient surgery departments, emergency departments, and postanesthesia recovery units.

Types of ECG Monitoring

There are two types of ECG monitoring: *hardwire* and *telemetry*. With hardwire monitoring (bedside monitoring), electrode pads (conductive gel discs) are placed on the patient's chest and connected to a lead wire cable that is attached to a stationary bedside monitor. With telemetry monitoring (portable monitoring), electrode pads are placed on the patient's chest and connected to leads that are attached to a portable monitor transmitter.

- **Hardwire monitoring**—Hardwire monitoring uses either a five-lead wire system or a three-lead wire system. With the five-lead wire system (Figure 4.1), five electrode pads and five lead wires are used. One electrode is placed below the right clavicle (2nd interspace, right midclavicular line), one below the left clavicle (2nd interspace, left midclavicular line), one on the right lower rib cage (8th

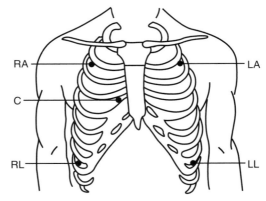

Figure 4.1 Hardwire monitoring, five-lead system. This illustration shows you where to place the electrodes and attach lead wires using a five-lead wire system. The lead wires are color-coded as follows:
- White—right arm (RA)
- Black—left arm (LA)
- Green—right leg (RL)
- Red—left leg (LL)
- Brown—chest (C)

Leads placed in the arm and leg positions as shown allow you to view leads, I, II, III, AVR, AVL, and AVF. To view chest leads V_1-V_6, the chest lead must be placed in the specific chest lead position desired. In this example, the brown chest lead is in V_1 position.

interspace, right midclavicular line), one on the left lower rib cage (8th interspace, left midclavicular line), and one in a chest lead position (V_1-V_6).

The six chest lead positions (Figure 4.2) include:
- V_1—4th interspace, right sternal border
- V_2—4th interspace, left sternal border
- V_3—midway between V_2 and V_4
- V_4—5th interspace, left midclavicular line
- V_5—5th interspace, left anterior axillary line
- V_6—5th interspace, left midaxillary line

The right arm (RA) lead is attached to the electrode pad below the right clavicle, the left arm (LA) lead to the electrode pad below the left clavicle, the right leg (RL) lead to the electrode pad on the right lower rib cage, the left leg (LL) lead to the electrode pad on the left lower rib cage, and the chest lead to the electrode pad of the specific chest position desired (V_1-V_6).

With the five-lead wire system for hardwire monitoring, you can continuously monitor two leads using a lead selector on the monitor. Leads placed in the arm and leg

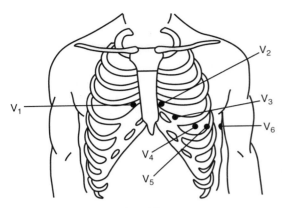

Figure 4.2 Chest lead positions.

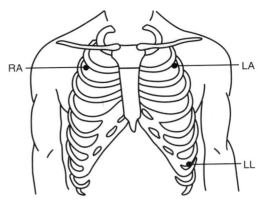

Figure 4.3 Hardwire monitoring, three-lead wire system. This illustration shows you where to place the electrodes and attach lead wires using a three-lead wire system. The lead wires are color-coded as follows:
- White—right arm (RA)
- Black—left arm (LA)
- Red—left leg (LL)

Leads placed in this position will allow you to monitor leads I, II, or III using the lead selector on the monitor.

positions (limb leads) allow you to view leads I, II, III, AVR, AVL, and AVF. To view chest leads V_1-V_6, the chest lead must be placed in the specific chest lead position desired. Generally, a limb lead (usually I, II, or III) and a chest lead (usually V_1 or V_6) are chosen to be monitored.

With the three-lead wire system (Figure 4.3), three electrode pads and three lead wires are used. One electrode pad is placed below the right clavicle (2nd interspace, right midclavicular line), one below the left clavicle (2nd interspace, left midclavicular line), and one on the left lower rib cage (8th interspace, left midclavicular line). The RA lead is attached to the electrode pad below the right clavicle, the LA lead is attached to the electrode pad below the left clavicle, and the LL lead is attached to the electrode pad on the lower left rib cage. You can continuously monitor one lead (either limb leads I, II, or III) by turning the lead selector on the monitor. Although you can't monitor chest leads (V_1-V_6) with a three-lead wire system, you can monitor modified chest leads that provide similar information. To monitor the modified chest leads, reposition the LL lead to the approximate position for the chest lead you want to monitor and turn the lead selector on the monitor to

lead III. Examples of modified chest lead V_1 (MCL_1) and V_6 (MCL_6) are shown in Figure 4.4.

Telemetry monitoring—Wireless monitoring, or telemetry, gives your patient more freedom than hardwire monitoring. Instead of being connected to a bedside monitor, the patient is connected to a portable monitor transmitter, which can be placed in a pajama pocket or in a telemetry pouch. Telemetry monitoring systems are available in a five-lead wire system and a three-lead wire system.

The five-lead wire system for telemetry (Figure 4.5) is connected in the same manner as the five-lead wire system for hardwire monitoring with the four limb lead positions (RA, LA, RL, and LL) in the conventional positions and the chest leads placed in the desired V_1-V_6 location. With this system, you can monitor any one of the 12 leads using a

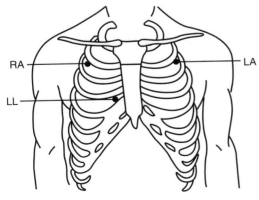

Modified Chest Lead V₁ (MCL₁)

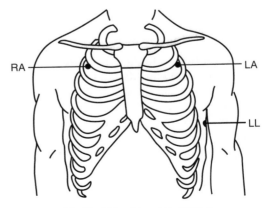

Modified Chest Lead V₆ (MCL₆)

Figure 4.4 Hardwire monitoring, three-lead wire system: Leads MCL_1 and MCL_6. Modified chest leads can be monitored with the three-lead wire system by repositioning the left leg (LL) lead to the chest position desired and turning the lead selector on the monitor to lead III.

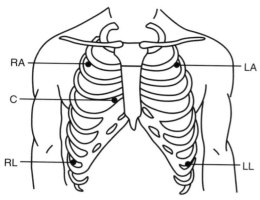

Figure 4.5   Telemetry monitoring, five-lead wire system. This illustration shows you where to place the electrodes and attach lead wires using a five-lead wire system. The lead wires are color-coded as follows:

- White—right arm (RA)
- Black—left arm (LA)
- Green—right leg (RL)
- Red—left leg (LL)
- Brown—chest (C)

With the five-lead wire system for telemetry monitoring, you can monitor any of the 12 leads using a lead selector on the monitor. Leads placed in the conventional limb positions allow you to view leads I, II, III, AVR, AVL, and AVF. To view chest leads V_1 to V_6, the chest lead must be placed in the specific chest lead desired.

lead selector on the monitor. Leads placed in the limb positions as shown in Figure 4.5 allow you to view leads I, II, III, AVR, AVL, or AVF. To view chest leads V_1-V_6, the chest lead must be placed in the specific chest lead position desired.

The three-lead wire system for telemetry (Figure 4.6) uses three electrodes and three lead wires. The lead wires are connected to positive, negative, and ground connections on the telemetry transmitter and attached to electrode pads placed in specific lead positions (leads I, II, III, MCL_1, and MCL_6). Only one lead position can be monitored at a time, and a lead selector on the monitor isn't available.

Applying Electrode Pads

Proper attachment of the electrode pads to the skin is the most important step in obtaining a good quality ECG tracing. Unless there is good contact between the skin and the electrode pad, distortions of the ECG tracing (artifacts) may appear. An artifact is any abnormal wave, spike, or movement on the ECG tracing that isn't generated by the electrical activity of the heart. The procedure for attaching the electrodes is as follows:

- **Choose monitor lead position**. It's helpful to assess the 12-lead ECG to ascertain which lead provides the best QRS complex voltage and P wave identification.
- **Prepare the skin**. Clip the hair from the skin using a clipper: hair interferes with good contact between the electrode pad and the skin. Using a dry washcloth, wipe site free of

loose hair. If the patient is perspiring and the electrodes won't stay adhered to the skin, prep skin surface with liquid adhesive, allow to dry, and reapply electrode pad.

- **Attach the electrode pads**. Remove pads from packaging and check them for moist conductive gel: dried gel can cause loss of the ECG signal. Place an electrode pad on each prepared site, pressing firmly around periphery of the pad and avoiding bony areas, such as the clavicles or prominent rib markings.
- **Connect the lead wires to the electrode pads**.

Troubleshooting Monitor Problems

Many problems may be encountered during cardiac monitoring. The most common problems are related to patient movement, interference from equipment in or near the patient's room, weak ECG signals, poor choice of monitor lead or electrode placement, and poor contact between the skin and electrode pad. Monitor problems can cause artifacts on the ECG tracing, making identification of the cardiac rhythm difficult or triggering false monitor alarms (false high rate alarms and false low rate alarms). Some problems are potentially serious and require intervention, whereas others are temporary, non–life-threatening occurrences that will correct themselves. The nurse and monitor technician need to be proficient in recognizing monitoring problems, identifying probable causes, and seeking solutions to correct the problem The most common monitoring problems are:

False high rate alarms—High-voltage artifact potentials are commonly interpreted by the monitor as QRS complexes and activate the high rate alarm. Most high-voltage artifacts are related to muscle movement from the patient turning in bed or moving the extremities (Figure 4.7). Seizure activity can also produce high-voltage artifact potentials (Figure 4.8). Implanted electrical devices such as the gastric pacemaker (for patients with gastroparesis), which intermittently delivers high-frequency electrical impulses to the stomach wall to stimulate gastric motility, may also activate the high rate alarm on the monitor (Figure 4.9). Tall T waves caused by increased potassium or elevation of the ST segment and T wave caused by acute myocardial infarction may activate the high rate alarm. The monitor counts both the R wave and the T wave, doubling the heart rate. An example of elevation of the ST-T portion of the cardiac cycle is shown in Figure 4.10.

False low rate alarms—Any disturbance in the transmission of the electrical signal from the skin electrode to the monitoring system can activate a false low rate alarm. This problem is usually caused by ineffective contact between the skin and the electrode-lead wire system, resulting from dried conductive gel, a loose electrode, or a disconnected lead wire (Figures 4.11 and 4.12). Low-voltage QRS complexes can also activate the low rate alarm. If the ventricular waveforms aren't tall enough, the monitor detects no electrical activity and will cause the low rate alarm to activate. This problem can be continuous (Figure 4.13) or intermittent (Figure 4.14).

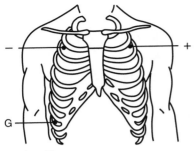

Lead I

Negative lead – 2nd interspace
right midclavicular line

Positive lead – 2nd interspace
left midclavicular line

Ground lead – 8th interspace
right midclavicular line

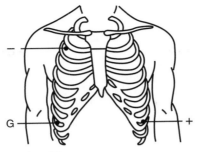

Lead II

Negative lead – 2nd interspace
right midclavicular line

Positive lead – 8th interspace
left midclavicular line

Ground lead – 8th interspace
right midclavicular line

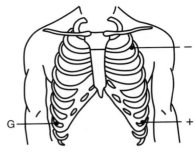

Lead III

Negative lead – 2nd interspace
left midclavicular line

Positive lead – 8th interspace
left midclavicular line

Ground lead – 8th interspace
right midclavicular line

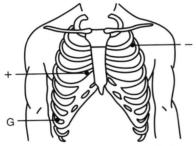

Modified Chest Lead V$_1$ (MCL$_1$)

Negative lead – 2nd interspace
left midclavicular line

Positive lead – 4th interspace
right sternal border

Ground lead – 8th interspace
right midclavicular line

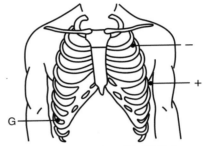

Modified Chest Lead V$_6$ (MCL$_6$)

Negative lead – 2nd interspace
left midclavicular line

Positive lead – 5th interspace
left midaxillary line

Ground lead – 8th interspace
right midclavicular line

Figure 4.6 Telemetry monitoring: three-lead wire system. The three-lead wire system uses three electrode pads and three lead wires. The lead wires are connected to positive, negative, or ground connections on the telemetry transmitter and attached to specific lead positions (lead I, lead II, lead III, lead MCL$_1$, or lead MCL$_6$). Only one lead position can be monitored at a time. A lead selector isn't available.

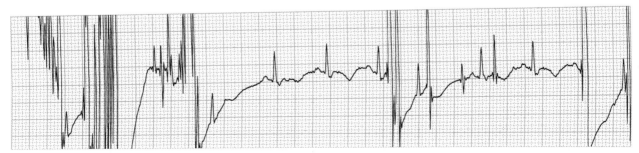

Figure 4.7 High rate alarm. *Cause:* Patient turning in bed or extremity movement. *Solution:* Problem is usually intermittent and no correction is necessary. Movement artifact can be reduced by avoiding placement of electrode pads in areas where extremity movement is greatest (bony areas such as the clavicles).

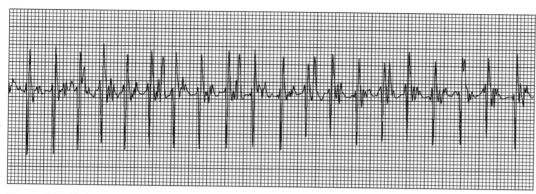

Figure 4.8   High rate alarm. *Cause:* Seizure activity can activate the high rate alarm on the monitor.

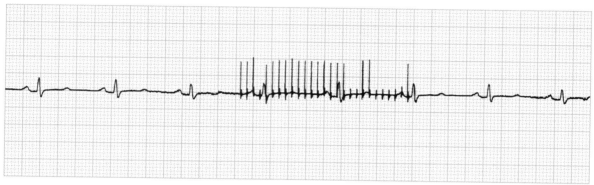

Figure 4.9   High rate alarm. *Cause:* High-frequency electrical impulses from a gastric pacemaker may activate the high rate alarm on the monitor.

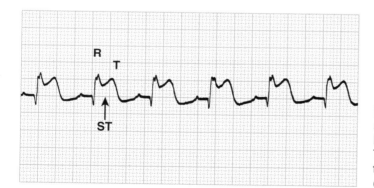

Figure 4.10   High rate alarm. *Cause:* An elevated ST segment and T wave related to an acute MI may activate the high rate alarm. The monitor counts both the R wave and the T wave and doubles the rates. *Solution:* Change monitor lead to one that does not have elevation in the ST-T portion of the cardiac cycle.

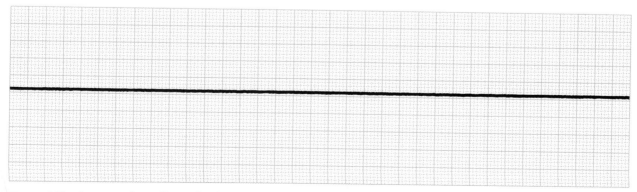

Figure 4.11   Low rate alarm. *Cause:* Continuous straight line related to dried conductive gel, disconnected lead wire, or disconnected electrode pad. *Solution:* Check electrode system; re-prep and reattach electrodes and leads as necessary. *Note:* A straight line may also indicate the absence of electrical activity in the heart; the patient must be evaluated immediately for the presence of a pulse.

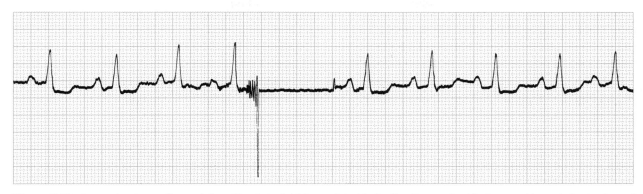

Figure 4.12   Low rate alarm. *Cause:* Intermittent straight line related to ineffective contact between skin and electrode pad. *Solution:* Make sure hair is clipped and electrode pad is placed on clean, dry, skin; if diaphoresis is a problem, prep skin surface with liquid adhesive, allow to dry, and reapply electrode pad.

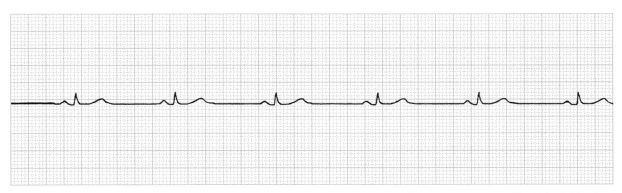

Figure 4.13   Low rate alarm. *Cause:* Continuous low-voltage QRS complexes. *Solution:* Turn up amplitude (gain) knob on monitor or change lead positions.

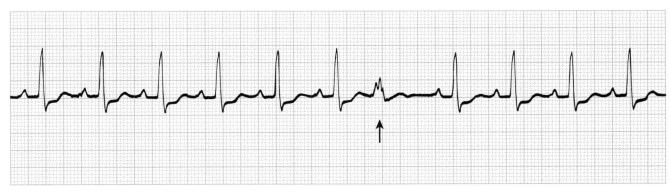

Figure 4.14   Low rate alarm. *Cause:* Intermittent low-voltage QRS complexes as seen in strip above. *Solution:* If the problem is frequent and activates the low rate alarm, change lead position.

Muscle tremors—Muscle tremors can occur in tense, nervous patients, those shivering from being cold, or those having a chill from increased temperature. The ECG baseline has an uneven, coarsely jagged appearance, obscuring the waveforms on the ECG tracing. The problem may be continuous (Figure 4.15) or intermittent (Figure 4.16).

Telemetry-related interference—Telemetry-related artifacts occur when the ECG signals are poorly received over a telemetry monitoring system. Weak ECG signals are caused by weak batteries or by the transmitter being used in the outer fringes of the reception area for the telemetry receiver, resulting in sharp spikes or straight lines on the ECG tracing (Figure 4.17).

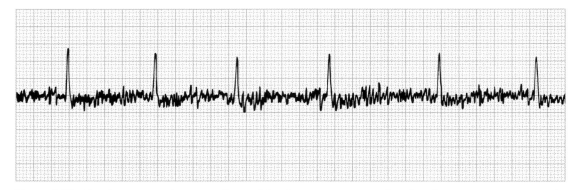

Figure 4.15   Continuous muscle tremor. *Cause:* Muscle tremors are usually related to tense or nervous patients of those shivering from cold or a chill. *Solution:* Treat cause.

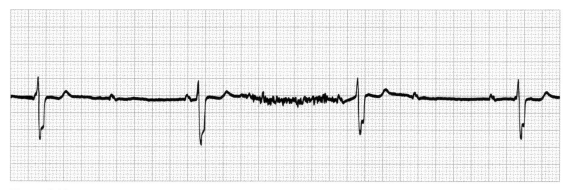

Figure 4.16   Intermittent muscle tremor. *Cause:* Muscle tremors that occur intermittently. *Solution:* Correction is usually unnecessary. *Note*: In this strip, the patient has two P waves preceding each QRS complex (second-degree atrioventricular block, Mobitz II). If the muscle tremors were continuous (as in Figure 4.15), you would be unable to identify this serious arrhythmia.

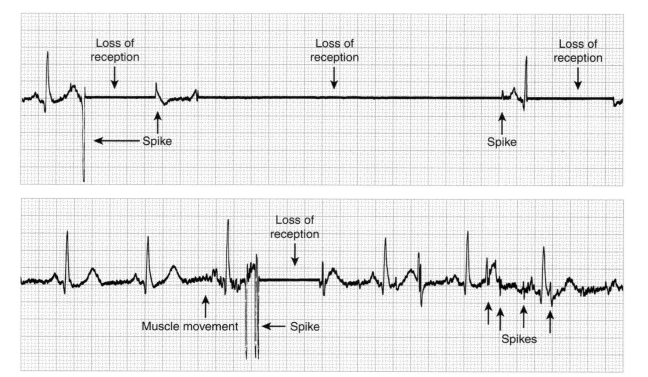

Figure 4.17   Telemetry-related interference. *Cause:* ECG: signals are poorly received over the telemetry system causing sharp spikes and sometimes loss of signal reception. The problem is usually related to weak batteries or the transmitter being used in the outer fringes of the reception area for the telemetry receiver. *Solution:* Change batteries; keep patient within reception range.

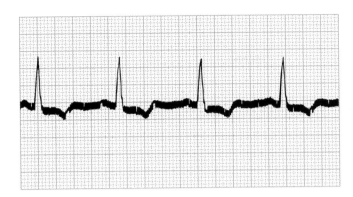

Figure 4.18 Electrical interference (AC interference). *Cause:* Patients using electrical equipment (electric razor, hair dryer), multiple electrical equipment in use in the room, improperly grounded equipment, loose electrical connections, or exposed wiring. *Solution:* If patient is using electrical equipment, problem is transient and will correct itself. If patient is not using electrical equipment, unplug all equipment not in continuous use, remove from service and report any equipment with breaks or wires showing, and ask the electrical engineer to check the wiring.

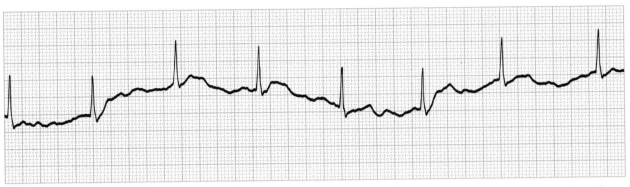

Figure 4.19 Wandering baseline. *Cause:* Exaggerated respiratory movements usually seen in patients in respiratory distress (patients with chronic obstructive pulmonary disease). *Solution:* Avoid placing electrode pads in areas where movements of the accessory muscles are most exaggerated (which can be anywhere on the anterior chest wall). Place the pads on the upper back if necessary.

Electrical interference (AC interference)—Electrical interference (Figure 4.18) most often occurs when a patient is using an electrical device such as an electric razor or hair dryer. AC interference may also occur when multiple pieces of equipment are plugged into the same electrical receptacle, when improperly grounded equipment is in use, or when loose electrical connections or exposed wiring is present. This type of interference consists of a continuous series of fine, even, rapid spikes that can obscure the waveforms on the ECG tracing.

Wandering baseline—A wandering baseline (Figure 4.19) is a monitor pattern that wanders up and down on the monitor screen or ECG tracing and is caused by exaggerated respiratory movements commonly seen in patients with severe pulmonary disease such as COPD. This type of artifact makes it difficult to identify the cardiac rhythm as well as changes in the ST segment and T wave.

five

Analyzing a Rhythm Strip

There are five basic steps to be followed in analyzing a rhythm strip. Each step should be followed in sequence. Eventually, this will become a habit and will enable you to identify a strip quickly and accurately.

Step 1: Determine Regularity (Rhythm) of R Waves

Starting at the left side of the rhythm strip, place an index card above the first two R waves (Figure 5.1). Using a sharp pencil, mark on the index card above the two R waves. Measure from R wave to R wave across the rhythm strip, marking on the index card any variation in R wave regularity. If the rhythm varies by 0.12 second (3 small squares) or more between the shortest and longest R wave variation marked on the index card, the rhythm is irregular. If the rhythm doesn't vary or varies by less than 0.12 second, the rhythm is considered regular.

Calipers may also be used, instead of an index card, to determine regularity of the rhythm strip. R-wave regularity is assessed in the same manner as with the index card, by placing the two caliper points on top of two consecutive R waves and proceeding left to right across the rhythm strip, noting any variation in the R-R regularity.

The author prefers the index card method, because each R-wave variation (however slight) can be marked and measured to determine if a 0.12-second or greater variance exists between the shorter and longer R-wave variations. With calipers, a variation in the R-wave regularity may be noted, but without marking and measuring between the shortest and longest R-wave variation, there is no way to determine how irregular the rhythm is. Examples of rhythm measurements are shown in Figures 5.2 to 5.4.

Step 2: Calculate the Heart Rate

This measurement will always refer to the ventricular rate unless the atrial and ventricular rates differ, in which case both will be given. The ventricular rate is usually determined by looking at a 6-second rhythm strip. The top of the electrocardiogram paper is marked at 3-second intervals; two intervals equal 6 seconds (Figure 5.5). Several methods can be used to calculate heart rate. These methods differ according to the regularity or irregularity of the rhythm.

Regular Rhythms

Two methods can be used to calculate heart rate in regular rhythms.

- **Rapid rate calculation**—Count the number of R waves in a 6-second strip (Figure 5.6) and multiply by 10 (6 seconds × 10 = 60 seconds, or the heart rate per minute). The R waves must be counted within the 6-second markers (some strips in this book are longer than 6 seconds). This method provides an approximate heart rate in beats per minute, is fast and simple, and can be used with both regular and irregular rhythms. If you only have a 3-second strip, count the number of R waves in a 3-second strip and multiply by 20 (3 seconds × 20 = 60 seconds or the heart rate per minute).
- **Precise rate calculation**—Count the number of small squares between two consecutive R waves (Figure 5.7) and refer to the conversion table printed on the inside back cover of the book. A removable conversion table is also provided. Although this method is accurate, it can be used only for regular rhythms. If a conversion table isn't available, divide the number of small squares between the two consecutive R waves into 1,500 (the number of small squares in a 1-minute rhythm strip). The heart rates for regular rhythms in the answer keys were determined by the precise rate calculation method.

Irregular Rhythms

Only rapid rate calculation is used to calculate heart rate in irregular rhythms. Count the number of R waves in a 6-second strip and multiple by 10 (Figure 5.8), or count the number of R waves in a 3-second strip and multiply by 20.

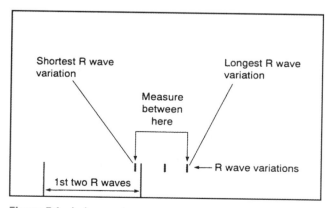

Figure 5.1 Index card.

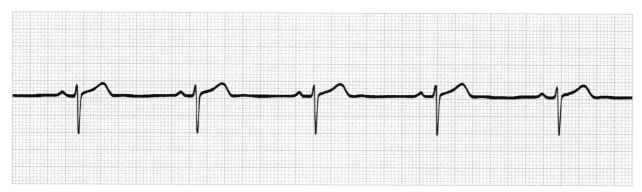

Figure 5.2   Regular rhythm; R-R intervals do not vary.

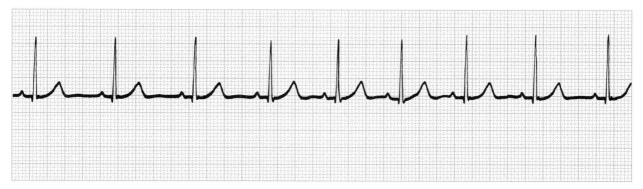

Figure 5.3   Irregular rhythm; R-R intervals vary by 5 squares (0.20 second).

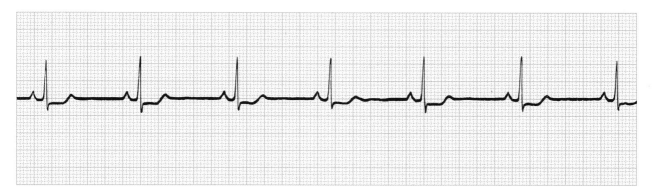

Figure 5.4   Regular rhythm; R-R intervals by 1½ squares (0.06 second).

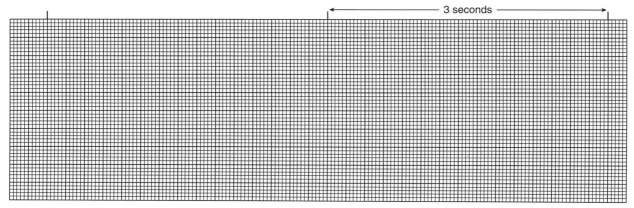

Figure 5.5   ECG graph paper.

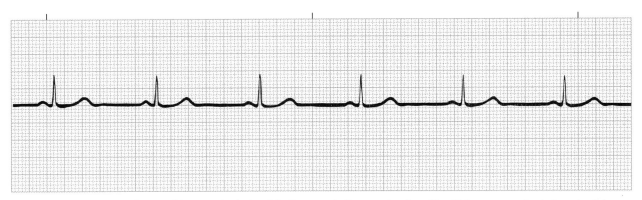

Figure 5.6 Regular rhythm: rapid rate calculation (six R waves in 6 second strip × 10 = 60 beats per minute heart rate).

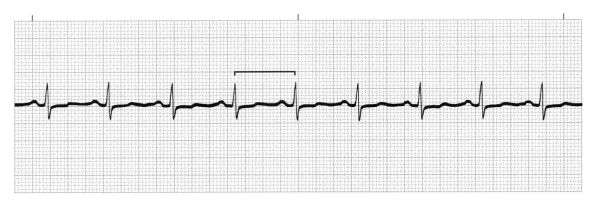

Figure 5.7 Regular rhythm: precise rate calculation (17 small squares between two consecutive R waves = 88 beats per minute heart rate).

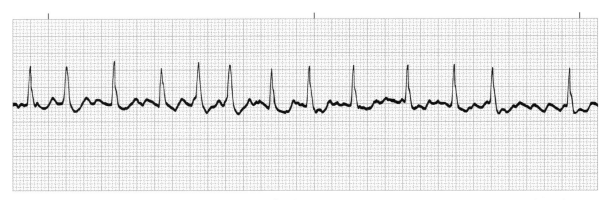

Figure 5.8 Irregular rhythm: rapid rate calculation (12 R waves in 6 second strip × 10 = 120 beats per minute heart rate).

Other Hints

When rhythm strips have a premature beat (Figure 5.9), the premature beat isn't included in the calculation of the heart rate. The premature beat is a beat from a different pacemaker site in the heart and must be assessed separately. In this example, the basic rhythm is regular and the heart rate is 68 beats per minute (22 small squares between R waves = 68).

When rhythm strips have more than one rhythm on a 6-second strip (Figure 5.10), rates must be calculated for each rhythm. This will aid in the identification of each rhythm. In the example, the first rhythm is irregular and the heart rate is 120 beats per minute (6 R waves in

3 seconds × 20 = 120). The second rhythm is regular and the heart rate is 250 beats per minute (6 small squares between two consecutive R waves = 250). A rhythm consists of three or more consecutive beats, has the same appearance, and may be regular or irregular.

When a rhythm covers less than 3 seconds on a rhythm strip (Figure 5.11), rate calculation is difficult, but not impossible. In the example, the first rhythm takes up half of a 3-second interval. There are only two R waves. Therefore, you can't determine if the rhythm is regular or irregular. In this situation, multiply the two R waves by 40 (1½ second × 40 = 60 seconds or the heart rate per minute) to obtain an

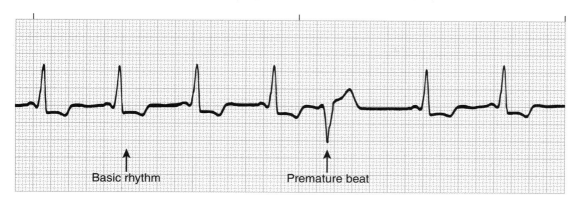

Figure 5.9   Basic rhythm with premature beat.

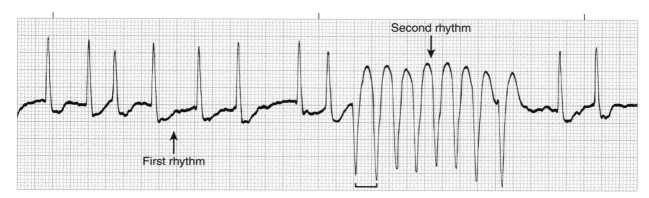

Figure 5.10   Rhythm strip with two different rhythms.

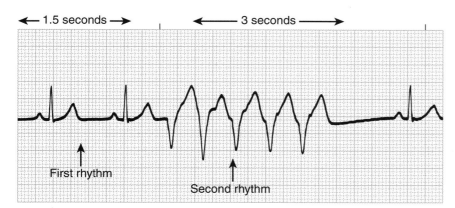

Figure 5.11   Calculating rate when a rhythm covers less than 3 seconds.

approximate heart rate of 80 beats per minute. The second rhythm is regular, with a heart rate of 167 beats per minute (9 small squares between R waves = 167).

As you have seen, rhythm strips may have one rhythm (Figures 5.6 to 5.8) with one answer. Rhythm strips may also have a rhythm with a beat from another pacemaker site (Figure 5.9) or have two different rhythms (Figures 5.10 and 5.11) with more than one answer. Each beat from a different pacemaker site and each rhythm must be analyzed separately. When interpreting a rhythm strip, describe the basic underlying rhythm first, then

add additional information such as normal sinus rhythm with one premature ventricular contraction (PVC) (Figure 5.9).

Step 3: Identify and Examine P Waves

Analyze the P waves. One P wave should precede each QRS complex and should be identical (or near identical) in size, shape, and position. In Figure 5.12, there is one P wave to each QRS complex, and all P waves are the same in size,

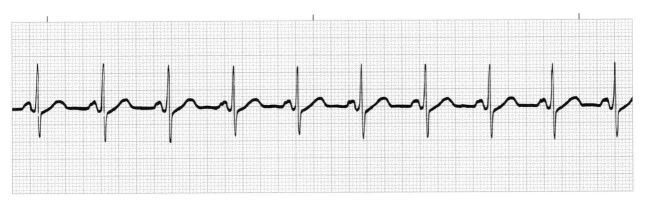

Figure 5.12 P waves have the same appearance across strip.

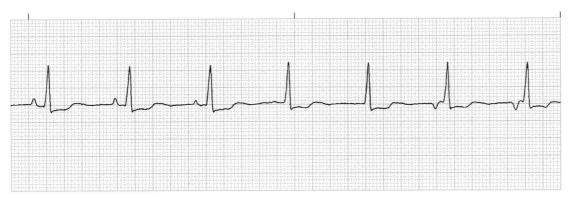

Figure 5.13 P waves differ in appearance across strip.

shape, and position. In Figure 5.13, there is one P wave to each QRS complex, but the P waves vary in size, shape, and position across the rhythm strip.

Step 4: Measure the PR Interval

Measure from the beginning of the P wave as it leaves baseline to the beginning of the QRS complex. Count the number of small squares contained in this interval and multiply by 0.04 second. In Figure 5.14, the PR interval is 0.16 second (4 small squares × 0.04 second = 0.16 second).

Step 5: Measure the QRS Complex

Measure from the beginning of the QRS complex as it leaves baseline until the end of the QRS complex when the ST segment begins. Count the number of small squares in this measurement and multiply by 0.04 second. In Figure 5.15, the QRS complex takes up 3 small squares and represents 0.12 second (3 small squares × 0.04 second = 0.12 second). In Figure 5.16, the QRS complex takes up 2½ small squares and represents 0.10 second (2½ small squares × 0.04 second = 0.10 second).

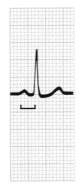

Figure 5.14 PR interval 0.16 second.

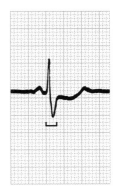

Figure 5.15 QRS complex 0.12 second.

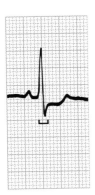

Figure 5.16   QRS complex 0.10 second.

box 5.1   Rhythm Strip Analysis

1. Determine regularity (rhythm).
2. Calculate rate.
3. Examine P waves.
4. Measure PR interval.
5. Measure QRS complex.

If rhythm strips are analyzed using a systematic step-by-step approach (Box 5.1), accurate interpretation will be achieved most of the time.

MEASUREMENT PRACTICE: MEASURING PR INTERVALS AND QRS COMPLEXES

Instructions: The intervals and complexes have been marked to help you learn where to begin and where to end. Count the number of small squares marked and multiply by 0.04 second. Check your measurement answers with the answer key in the appendix.

PR Intervals

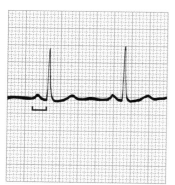

Strip 5.1

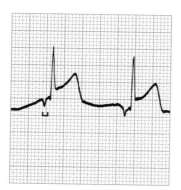

Strip 5.2

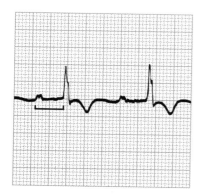

Strip 5.3

QRS Complexes

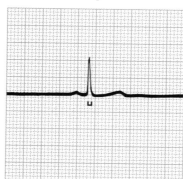

Strip 5.4

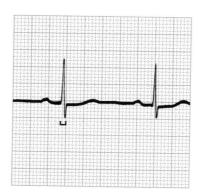

Strip 5.5

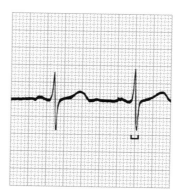

Strip 5.6

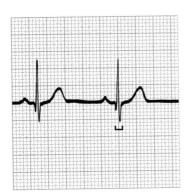

Strip 5.7

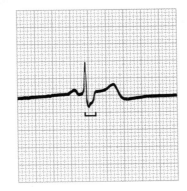

Strip 5.8

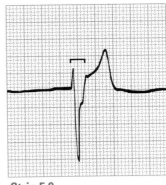

Strip 5.9

RHYTHM STRIP PRACTICE: ANALYZING RHYTHM STRIPS

Instructions: Analyze the following rhythm strips using the five-step process discussed in this chapter. Check your answers with the answer key in the appendix.

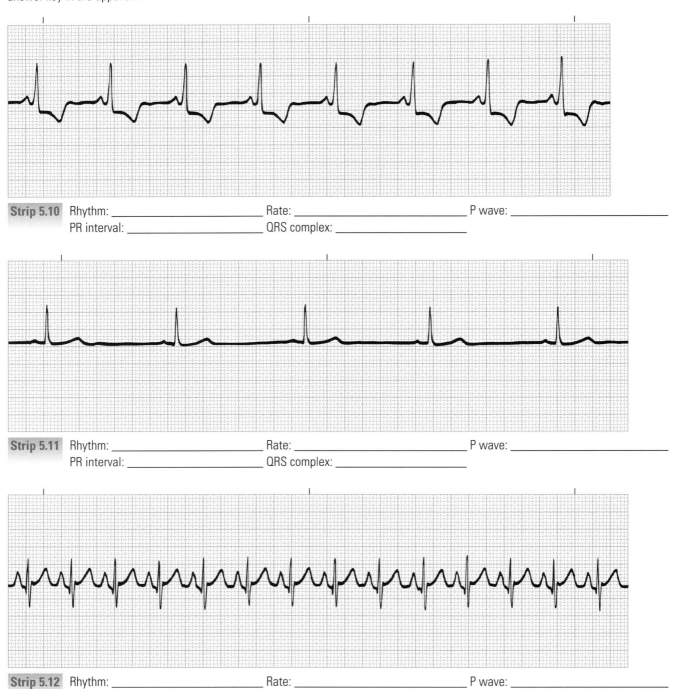

Strip 5.10 Rhythm: _____ Rate: _____ P wave: _____

PR interval: _____ QRS complex: _____

Strip 5.11 Rhythm: _____ Rate: _____ P wave: _____

PR interval: _____ QRS complex: _____

Strip 5.12 Rhythm: _____ Rate: _____ P wave: _____

PR interval: _____ QRS complex: _____

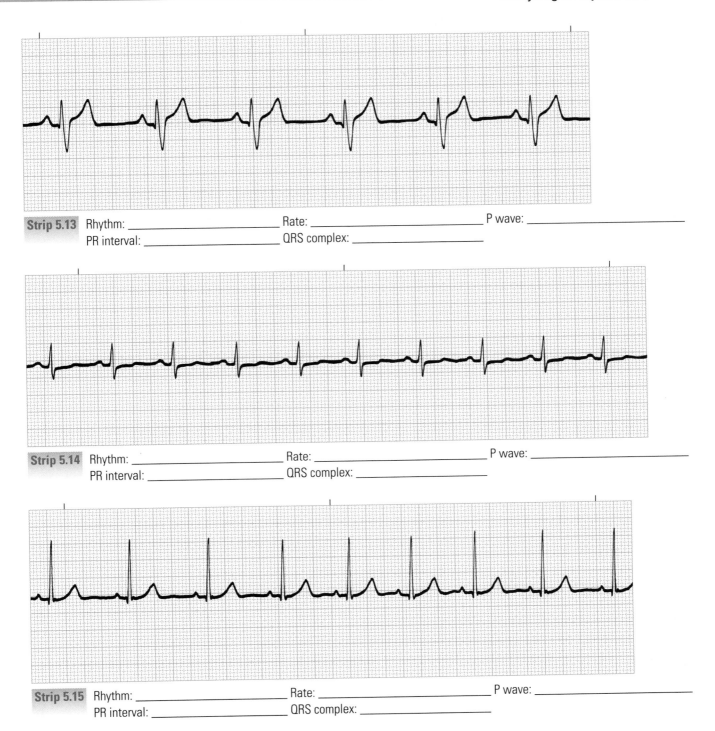

Strip 5.13 Rhythm: _____ Rate: _____ P wave: _____
PR interval: _____ QRS complex: _____

Strip 5.14 Rhythm: _____ Rate: _____ P wave: _____
PR interval: _____ QRS complex: _____

Strip 5.15 Rhythm: _____ Rate: _____ P wave: _____
PR interval: _____ QRS complex: _____

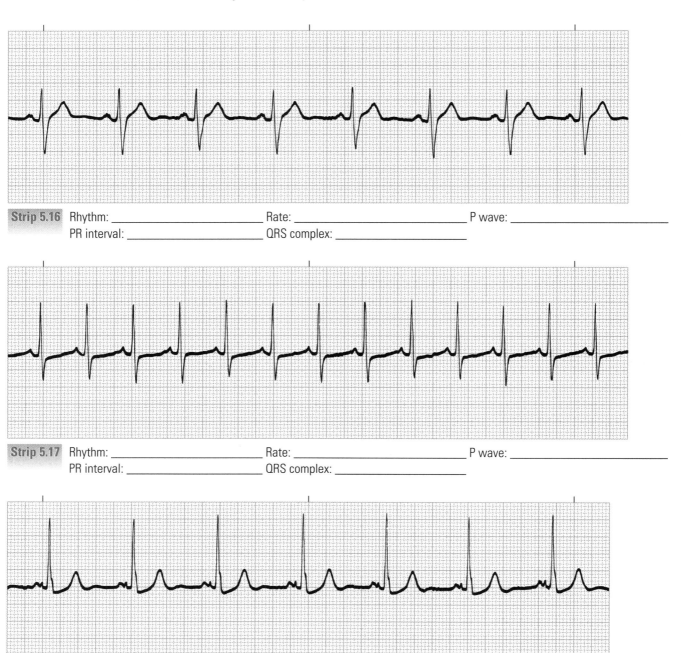

Strip 5.16   Rhythm: _____   Rate: _____   P wave: _____
PR interval: _____   QRS complex: _____

Strip 5.17   Rhythm: _____   Rate: _____   P wave: _____
PR interval: _____   QRS complex: _____

Strip 5.18   Rhythm: _____   Rate: _____   P wave: _____
PR interval: _____   QRS complex: _____

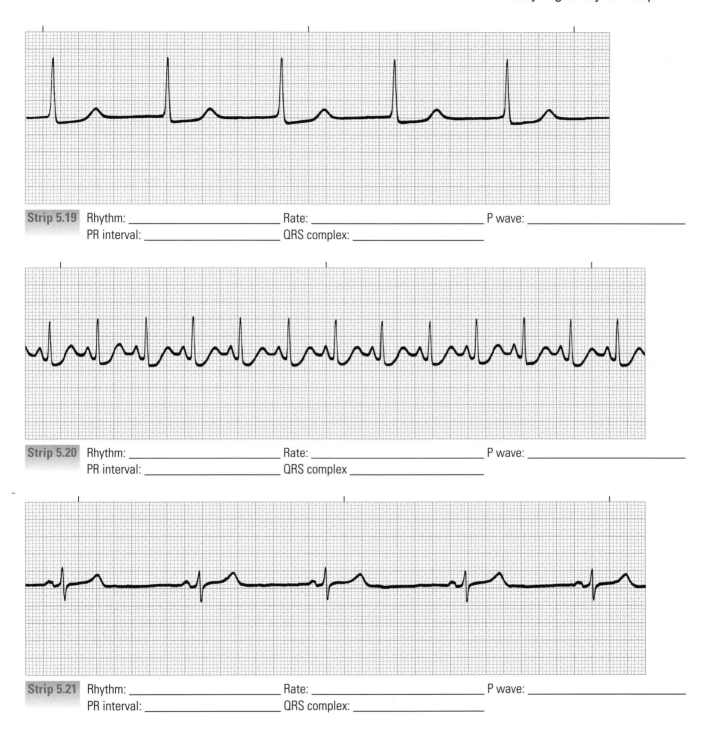

Strip 5.19 Rhythm: _____ Rate: _____ P wave: _____
PR interval: _____ QRS complex: _____

Strip 5.20 Rhythm: _____ Rate: _____ P wave: _____
PR interval: _____ QRS complex _____

Strip 5.21 Rhythm: _____ Rate: _____ P wave: _____
PR interval: _____ QRS complex: _____

six

Sinus Arrhythmias

Overview

Broadly defined, a cardiac arrhythmia (also called dysrhythmia) is any deviation from the normal pattern of the heartbeat (normal sinus rhythm). There are many different types of arrhythmias. Most arrhythmias are harmless, but some can be serious or even life threatening. Sinus arrhythmias (Figure 6.1) result from disturbances in impulse discharge or impulse conduction from the sinus node. The sinus node retains its role as pacemaker of the heart but discharges impulses too fast (sinus tachycardia) or too slow (sinus bradycardia); discharges impulses irregularly (sinus arrhythmia); or fails to discharge an impulse (sinus arrest), or the impulse discharged is blocked as it exits the sinus node (sinus exit block).

Normal Sinus Rhythm

Normal sinus rhythm (Figure 6.2 and Box 6.1) reflects the heart's normal electrical activity. The SA node normally initiates impulses at a rate of 60 to 100 beats per minute. Since this rate is faster than other pacemaker sites in the conduction system, the SA node retains control as the primary pacemaker of the heart. Sinus rhythm originates in the SA node, and the impulse follows the normal conduction pathway through the atria, the AV node, the bundle branches, and the ventricles, resulting in normal atrial and ventricular depolarization.

Normal sinus rhythm is regular with a heart rate between 60 and 100 beats per minute. The P waves are normal in size, shape, and direction and positive in lead II (a positive lead), with one P wave preceding each QRS complex. The duration of the PR interval and the QRS complex is within normal limits. Normal sinus rhythm is the normal rhythm of the heart. No treatment is indicated.

box 6.1	Normal Sinus Rhythm: Identifying ECG Features
Rhythm:	Regular
Rate:	60 to 100 beats/minute
P waves:	Normal in size, shape, and direction; positive in lead II; one P wave precedes each QRS complex
PR interval:	Normal (0.12 to 0.20 second)
QRS complex:	Normal (0.10 second or less)

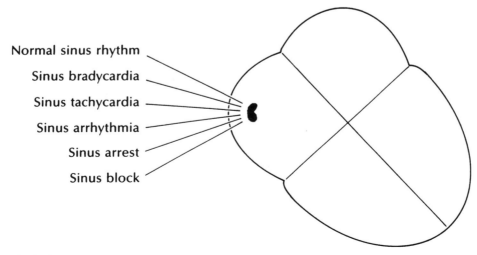

Figure 6.1 Sinus arrhythmias.

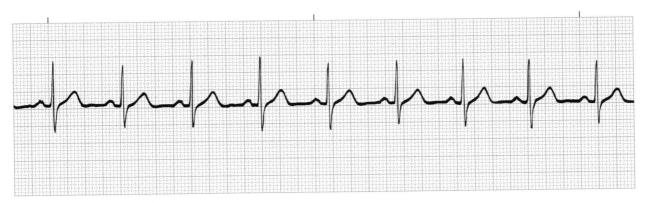

Figure 6.2	**Normal sinus rhythm.**
Rhythm:	Regular
Rate:	79 beats/minute
P waves:	Sinus
PR interval:	0.16 to 0.18 second
QRS complex:	0.06 to 0.08 second.

Sinus Tachycardia

Sinus tachycardia (Figure 6.3 and Box 6.2) is a rhythm that originates in the sinus node and discharges impulses regularly at a rate between 100 and 160 beats per minute. The P waves are normal in size, shape, and direction and positive in lead II (a positive lead), with one P wave preceding each QRS complex. The duration of the PR interval and the QRS complex is within normal limits. The distinguishing feature of this rhythm is the sinus origin and the rate between 100 and 160 beats per minute.

Sinus tachycardia is a normal response of the heart to the body's demand for increased blood flow, as in exercise and exertion. The sinus node increases its rate in response to the needs of the body. When these needs no longer exist, the heart rate slows down.

box 6.2 Sinus Tachycardia: Identifying ECG Features

Rhythm:	Regular
Rate:	100 to 160 beats/minute
P waves:	Normal in size, shape, and direction; positive in lead II; one P wave precedes each QRS complex
PR interval:	Normal (0.12 to 0.20 second)
QRS complex:	Normal (0.10 second or less)

Sinus tachycardia may occur with any of the following:
- Exercise, exertion
- Intake of stimulants such as caffeine, nicotine, cocaine, or amphetamine
- Drug withdrawal

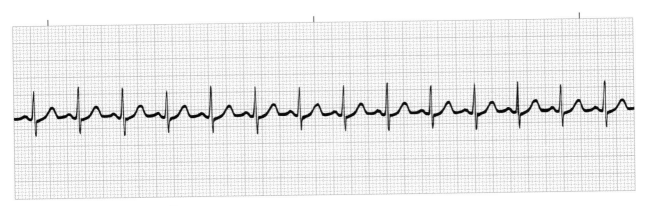

Figure 6.3	**Sinus tachycardia.**
Rhythm:	Regular
Rate:	125 beats/minute
P waves:	Sinus
PR interval:	0.12 to 0.14 second
QRS complex:	0.04 to 0.06.

- Increase in catecholamine release resulting from anxiety, excitement, pain, or stress
- Increased metabolic conditions (hyperthermia, hyperthyroidism)
- Anemia
- Hypoxia, hypovolemia, hypotension or shock, heart failure
- Myocardial ischemia or acute MI
- Pulmonary embolism
- Drugs that increase sympathetic tone (epinephrine, dopamine, isoproterenol, nitroprusside) or drugs that decrease parasympathetic tone (atropine)

Sinus tachycardia is usually a benign arrhythmia that resolves on its own. Sinus tachycardia begins and ends gradually in contrast to other tachycardias that begin and end suddenly. Treatment is directed at correcting the underlying cause. Simple therapies such as treatment of pain, anxiety, fever, hypoxia, or volume replacement may be all that is needed to resolve the arrhythmia. Persistent sinus tachycardia may require more aggressive treatment. An increased heart rate increases the workload of the heart and its oxygen requirements and may cause a decreased stroke volume leading to a decrease in cardiac output. In addition, heart rates higher than normal decrease the amount of time the heart spends in diastole, leading to a decrease in coronary artery perfusion (coronary arteries are perfused during diastole). Sinus tachycardia that persists can be one of the first signs of early heart failure.

Sinus Bradycardia

Sinus bradycardia (Figure 6.4 and Box 6.3) is a rhythm that originates in the SA node and discharges impulses regularly at a rate between 40 and 60 beats/minute. The P waves are normal in size, shape, and direction and positive in lead II (a positive lead), with one P wave preceding each QRS complex. The duration of the PR interval and the QRS complex is within normal limits. The distinguishing feature of this

box 6.3	Sinus Bradycardia: Identifying ECG Features
Rhythm:	Regular
Rate:	40 to 60 beats/minute
P waves:	Normal in size, shape, and direction; positive in lead II; one P wave precedes each QRS complex
PR interval:	Normal (0.12 to 0.20 second)
QRS complex:	Normal (0.10 second or less)

rhythm is the sinus origin and a heart rate between 40 and 60 beats/minute.

Sinus bradycardia is the normal response of the heart to relaxation or sleeping when the parasympathetic effect on cardiac automaticity dominates over the sympathetic effect. It is common among trained athletes who may have a resting or sleeping pulse rate as low as 35 beats/minute. Mild bradycardia may actually be beneficial in some patients (e.g., in acute MI) because of the decrease in the workload on the heart.

Sinus bradycardia may occur with any of the following:
- During sleep and in healthy, well-conditioned individuals such as athletes
- In acute inferior wall MI involving the right coronary artery, which usually supplies the SA node
- As a reperfusion rhythm after coronary angioplasty or after treatment with thrombolytics
- Sleep apnea
- Hypoxia
- Decreased metabolic conditions (hypothermia, hypothyroidism)
- High serum potassium (hyperkalemia)
- Pain
- Hypoglycemia

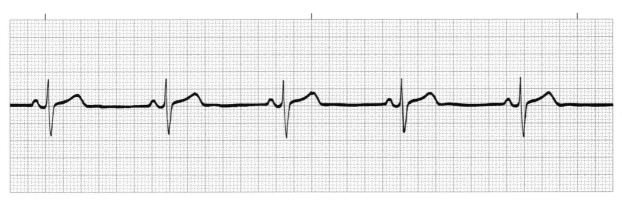

Figure 6.4   **Sinus bradycardia.**

Rhythm:	Regular
Rate:	45 beats/minute
P waves:	Sinus
PR interval:	0.16 to 0.18 second
QRS complex:	0.08 to 0.10 second.

- Pericarditis, pericardial tamponade
- Vagal stimulation from pain, gagging, vomiting, bearing down (Valsalva maneuver), carotid sinus pressure, or carotid sinus hypersensitivity syndrome
- Vasovagal reaction from pain, gagging, vomiting, fright, or sudden stressful situations. A vasovagal reaction is an extreme body response that causes a marked decrease in heart rate (caused by vagal stimulation) and a marked decrease in blood pressure (caused by vasodilation). The combination of extreme bradycardia (sometimes less than 30 beats/minute) and hypotension may result in fainting (vasovagal syncope). The situation is usually reversed when the individual is placed in a recumbent position, thereby increasing venous return to the heart. If fainting occurs with the individual in a recumbent position, it can usually be reversed with leg elevation.
- Sudden movement from recumbent to an upright position (common in the elderly)
- Increased intracranial pressure (a sudden appearance of sinus bradycardia in a patient with cerebral edema or subdural hematoma is an important clinical observation)
- Drugs such as digitalis, beta-blockers, or calcium channel blockers

Sinus bradycardia does not require treatment unless the patient becomes symptomatic. Symptoms requiring treatment include hypotension (systolic BP less than 90 mm Hg), syncope, reduced consciousness or cognitive function, decreased urine output, and development of heart failure. If sinus bradycardia persists, the treatment of choice is atropine, a drug that increases the heart rate by decreasing parasympathetic tone. The usual dose is 0.5 mg IV push every 5 minutes until the bradycardia is resolved or a maximum dose of 3 mg is given. Atropine should not be given too slowly or in doses less than 0.5 mg as this can further decrease the heart rate instead of increasing it. If the rhythm still does not resolve after the atropine is administered, a transcutaneous (external) or transvenous pacemaker may be needed. Hypotension can be corrected with either a dopamine drip or an epinephrine drip. All medications that cause a decrease in heart rate should be reviewed and discontinued if indicated. For chronic symptomatic bradycardia, permanent pacing may be indicated.

Sinus Arrhythmia

Sinus arrhythmia (Figure 6.5 and Box 6.4) is a rhythm that originates in the sinus node and discharges impulses irregularly. The heart rate may be normal (60 to 100 beats/minute) or slow (less than 60 beats/minute). If the heart rate is less than 60/minute, the rhythm is often interpreted as sinus arrhythmia with a bradycardic rate (Figure 6.6). The P waves are normal in size, shape, and direction and positive in lead II (a positive lead), with one P wave preceding each QRS complex. The duration of the PR interval and QRS complex is within normal limits. The distinguishing feature of this rhythm is the sinus origin and the rhythm irregularity.

box 6.4	Sinus Arrhythmia: Identifying ECG Features
Rhythm:	Irregular
Rate:	Normal (60 to 100 beats/minute) or slow (less than 60 beats/minute)
P waves:	Normal in size, shape, and direction; positive in lead II; one P wave precedes each QRS complex
PR interval:	Normal (0.12 to 0.20 second)
QRS complex:	Normal (0.10 second or less)

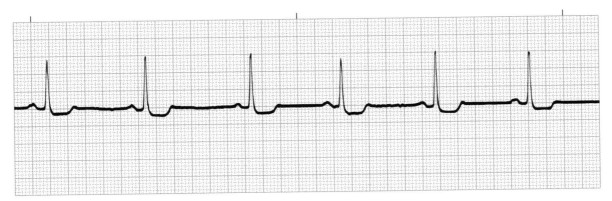

Figure 6.5   Sinus arrhythmia.

Rhythm:	Irregular
Rate:	60 beats/minute
P waves:	Sinus
PR interval:	0.16 to 0.20 second
QRS complex:	0.04 to 0.08 second
Comment:	ST segment depression is present.

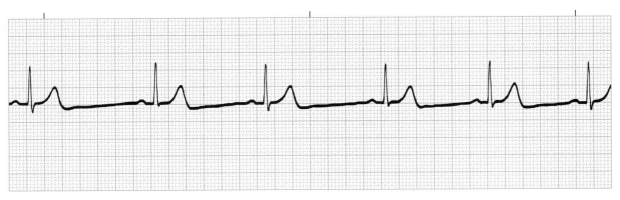

Figure 6.6   Sinus arrhythmia with a bradycardic rate.

Rhythm:	Irregular
Rate:	40 beats/minute
P waves:	Sinus
PR interval:	0.16 to 0.20 second
QRS complex:	0.04 to 0.08 second

Sinus arrhythmia is a normal physiological phenomenon most common in children and young adults. It is caused by the changes in vagal tone that occur during the respiratory cycle. The heart rate gradually slows down with expiration and then gradually speeds up with inspiration. Sinus arrhythmia is of no clinical significance and does not require treatment unless it is associated with a bradycardic rate that causes symptoms.

Sinus Pause (Sinus Arrest and Sinus Exit Block)

Sinus pause is a broad term used to describe rhythms in which there is a sudden failure of the SA node to initiate or conduct an impulse. Two rhythms fall under this category: sinus arrest and sinus block. Sinus arrest and sinus exit block, two separate arrhythmias with different pathophysiologies (Figures 6.7 to 6.9 and Box 6.5), are discussed together because distinguishing between them is at times difficult and because their treatment and clinical significance are the same.

Both sinus arrest and sinus exit block originate in the sinus node and are characterized by a sudden pause in the sinus rhythm in which one or more beats (cardiac cycles) are missing, followed by a resumption of the basic rhythm after the pause. With sinus block, an electrical impulse is initiated by the SA node but is blocked as it exits the sinus node, preventing conduction of the impulse to the atria. Thus, SA exit block is a disorder of conductivity. Because the regularity of the sinus node discharge isn't interrupted (just blocked), the underlying rhythm will resume on time after the pause (see Figure 6.7). Sinus arrest is caused by a failure of the SA node to initiate an impulse and is therefore a disorder

of automaticity. This failure in the automaticity of the SA node upsets the timing of the sinus node discharge, and the underlying rhythm won't resume on time after the pause (see Figure 6.8). Once the underlying rhythm resumes after the pause (in both sinus block and sinus arrest), it is common for the rate to be slower for several cycles (rate suppression). Rate suppression is temporary, and after several cardiac cycles, the basic rate will return. An example of rate suppression is shown in Figure 6.9.

To differentiate between the two rhythms, mark the R-R interval of the underlying rhythm on an index card and measure the R-R interval across the strip and through the pause

box 6.5	Sinus Arrest and Sinus Exit Block: Identifying ECG Features
Rhythm:	Basic rhythm usually regular; there is a sudden pause in the basic rhythm (causing irregularity) with one or more missing beats; heart rate may slow down for several beats after pause (temporary rate suppression) but returns to basic rate.
Rate:	That of underlying rhythm, usually sinus
P waves:	Sinus P waves with basic rhythm; absent during pause
PR interval:	Normal (0.12 to 0.20 second) with basic rhythm; absent during pause
QRS complex:	Normal (0.10 second or less) with basic rhythm; absent during pause

Differentiating features

Sinus block:	Basic rhythm (R-R regularity) resumes on time after pause
Sinus arrest:	Basic rhythm (R-R regularity) doesn't resume on time after pause

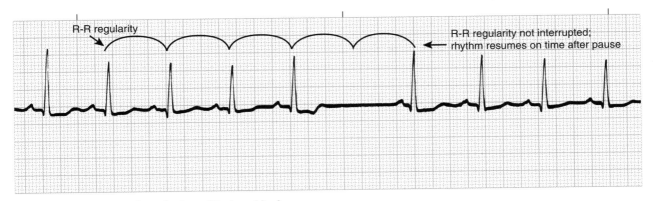

Figure 6.7   **Normal sinus rhythm with sinus block.**

Rhythm:	Basic rhythm regular; irregular during pause
Rate:	Basic rhythm 84 beats/minute
P waves:	Normal in basic rhythm; absent during pause
PR interval:	0.16 to 0.18 second in basic rhythm; absent during pause
QRS complex:	0.08 to 0.10 second in basic rhythm; absent during pause
Comment:	ST segment depression is present.

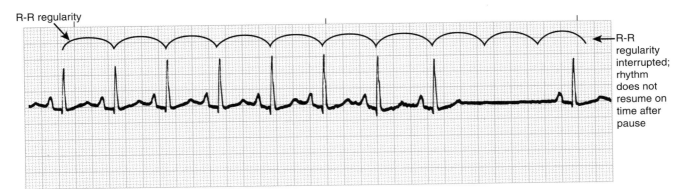

Figure 6.8   **Normal sinus rhythm with sinus arrest.**

Rhythm:	Basic rhythm regular; irregular during pause
Rate:	Basic rhythm 100 beats/minute
P waves:	Normal in basic rhythm; absent during pause
PR interval:	0.16 to 0.18 second in basic rhythm; absent during pause
QRS complex:	0.06 to 0.08 second in basic rhythm; absent during pause.

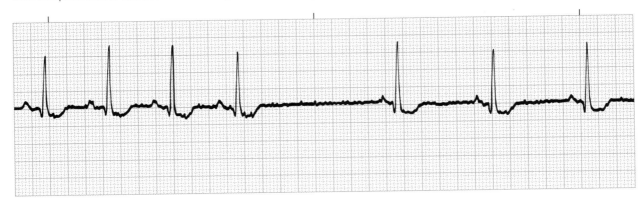

Figure 6.9   **Normal sinus rhythm with sinus arrest; rate suppression is present following pause.**

Rhythm:	Basic rhythm regular; irregular during pause
Rate:	Basic rhythm 84 beats/minute; rate slows to 56 beats/minute following pause (temporary rate suppression may occur following a pause in the basic rhythm)
P waves:	Sinus in basic rhythm; absent during pause
PR interval:	0.16 to 0.18 second in basic rhythm; absent during pause
QRS complex:	0.08 to 0.10 second in basic rhythm; absent during pause.

until the underlying rhythm resumes. If the right mark on the index card matches the R wave when the rhythm resumes, the event causing the pause is called sinus block. If the right mark on the index card does not match the R wave when the rhythm resumes, the event causing the pause is called sinus arrest. This can only be determined if the underlying rhythm is regular. If the underlying rhythm is irregular, as in sinus arrhythmia, it is impossible to distinguish sinus arrest from sinus exit block. In this case, the event causing the pause would best be interpreted using the broad term sinus pause, indicating that either rhythm could be present (Figure 6.10). From a clinical viewpoint, distinguishing between sinus arrest and sinus exit block usually isn't essential.

Sinus arrest or sinus exit block may occur with the following:
- Increased vagal tone
- Ischemic, inflammatory, or fibrotic disease of the SA node
- Damage to the SA node from myocardial infarction
- Drugs such as digitalis, beta-blockers, or calcium channel blockers

Pauses in the cardiac rhythm may cause several problems. If the heart misses a beat, blood doesn't flow during that time period, resulting in a lack of oxygen to the brain and body. Patients who have pauses may complain of feeling faint, dizzy, or light-headed or experience a syncopal episode (passing out). Frequent pauses would heighten these symptoms. Also, a pause in the rhythm provides an opportunity for pacemaker cells in other areas of the heart to take over control from the sinus node and become the dominant pacemaker of the heart. Any pacemaker site other than the SA node is called an ectopic pacemaker. Ectopic pacemaker sites in the atria, AV node, or ventricles may assume pacemaker control for one beat, for several beats, or as a continuous rhythm. If symptomatic, the rhythm is treated the same as in symptomatic sinus bradycardia. In addition, all medications that depress sinus node discharge or conduction should be stopped.

A **pull-out arrhythmia summary** of the sinus arrhythmias can be found in Table 6.1 at the back of the book. This may be used as a *quick guide to assist with rhythm interpretation*.

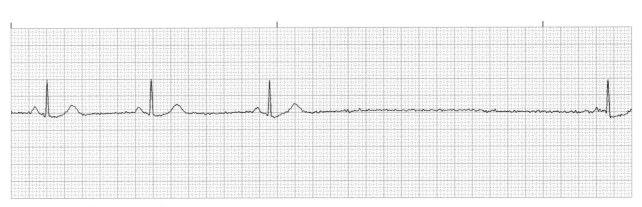

Figure 6.10   **Sinus arrhythmia with sinus pause.**

Rhythm:	Basic rhythm irregular
Rate:	60 beats/minute
P waves:	Normal in basic rhythm; absent during pause
PR interval:	0.14 to 0.16 second in basic rhythm; absent during pause
QRS complex:	0.04 second in basic rhythm; absent during pause
Comment:	Because of the irregularity of the basic rhythm, it is impossible to differentiate sinus arrest from sinus block. Therefore, the event causing the pause would best be interpreted using the broad term sinus pause, indicating that either event could be present.

Rhythm Strip Practice: Sinus Arrhythmias

Analyze the following rhythm strips by following the five basic steps:

- Determine *rhythm regularity*.
- Calculate *heart rate* (this usually refers to the ventricular rate, but if atrial differs, you need to calculate both).
- Identify and examine *P waves*.
- Measure *PR interval*.
- Measure *QRS complex*.

Interpret the rhythm by comparing this data with the ECG characteristics for each rhythm. All rhythm strips are lead II, a positive lead, unless otherwise noted. Check your answers with the answer key in the appendix.

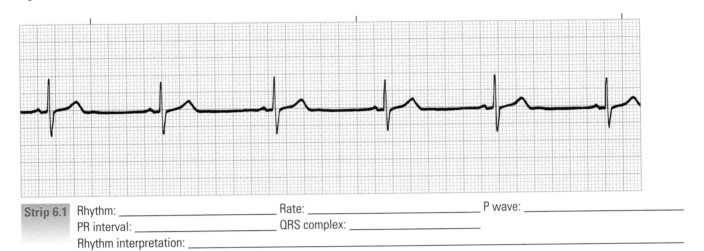

Strip 6.1   Rhythm: _____   Rate: _____   P wave: _____
PR interval: _____   QRS complex: _____
Rhythm interpretation: _____

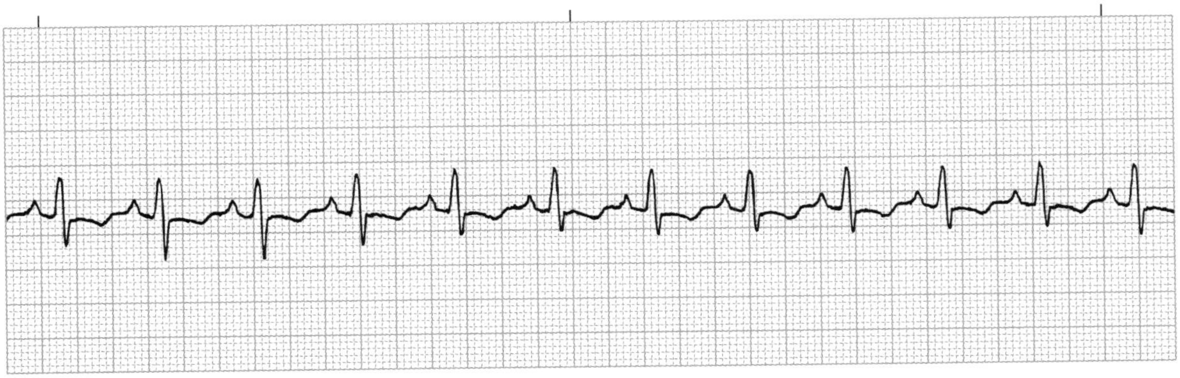

Strip 6.2   Rhythm: _____   Rate: _____   P wave: _____
PR interval: _____   QRS complex: _____
Rhythm interpretation: _____

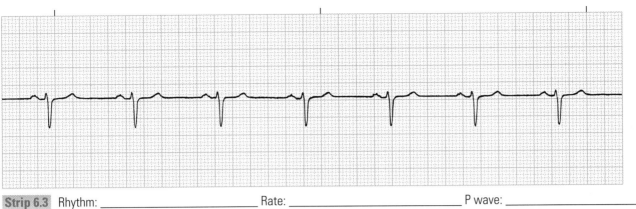

Strip 6.3 Rhythm: _____ Rate: _____ P wave: _____

PR interval: _____ QRS complex: _____

Rhythm interpretation: _____

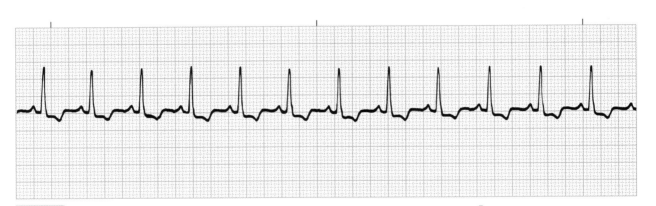

Strip 6.4 Rhythm: _____ Rate: _____ P wave: _____

PR interval: _____ QRS complex: _____

Rhythm interpretation: _____

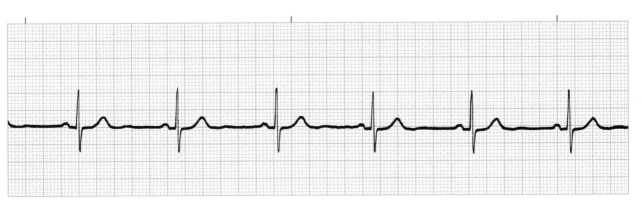

Strip 6.5 Rhythm: _____ Rate: _____ P wave: _____

PR interval: _____ QRS complex: _____

Rhythm interpretation: _____

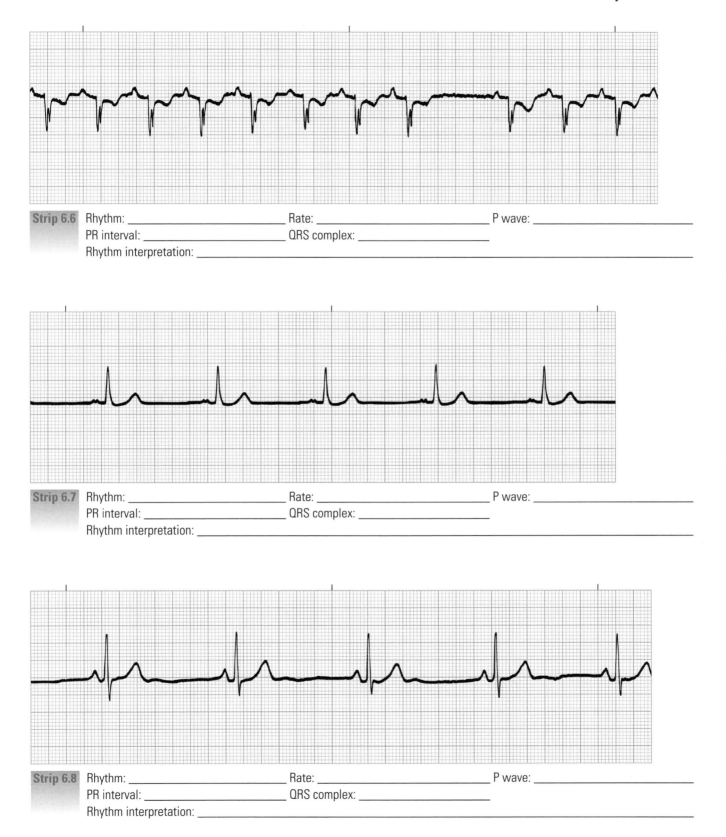

Strip 6.6   Rhythm: _____   Rate: _____   P wave: _____

PR interval: _____   QRS complex: _____

Rhythm interpretation: _____

Strip 6.7   Rhythm: _____   Rate: _____   P wave: _____

PR interval: _____   QRS complex: _____

Rhythm interpretation: _____

Strip 6.8   Rhythm: _____   Rate: _____   P wave: _____

PR interval: _____   QRS complex: _____

Rhythm interpretation: _____

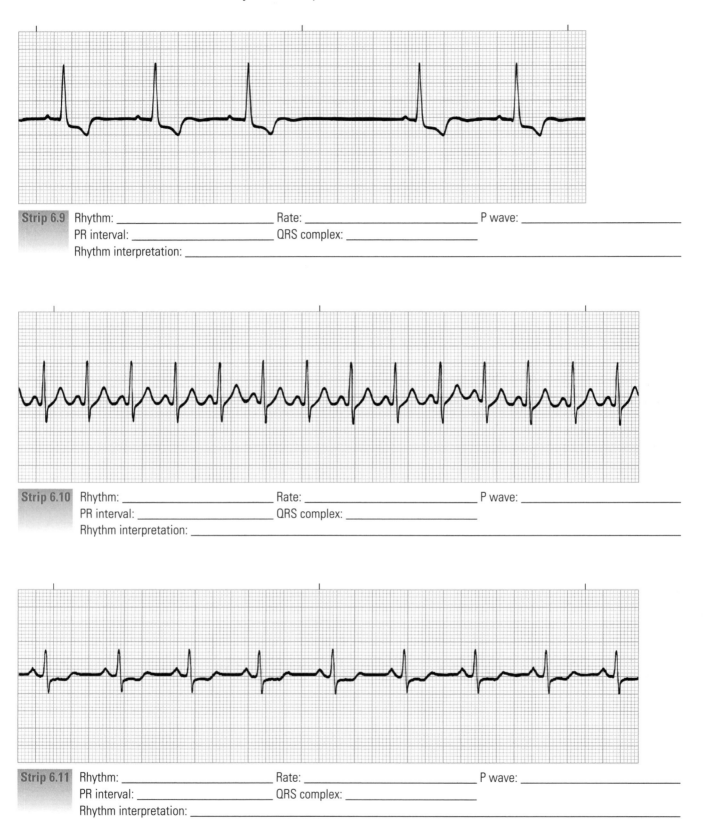

Strip 6.9 Rhythm: _____ Rate: _____ P wave: _____

PR interval: _____ QRS complex: _____

Rhythm interpretation: _____

Strip 6.10 Rhythm: _____ Rate: _____ P wave: _____

PR interval: _____ QRS complex: _____

Rhythm interpretation: _____

Strip 6.11 Rhythm: _____ Rate: _____ P wave: _____

PR interval: _____ QRS complex: _____

Rhythm interpretation: _____

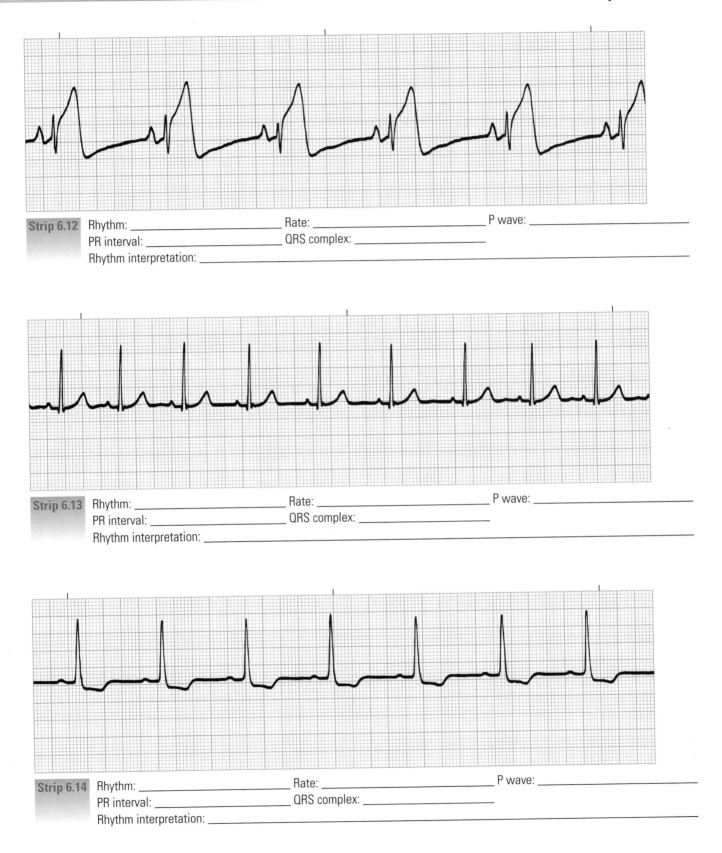

Strip 6.12 Rhythm: _____ Rate: _____ P wave: _____

PR interval: _____ QRS complex: _____

Rhythm interpretation: _____

Strip 6.13 Rhythm: _____ Rate: _____ P wave: _____

PR interval: _____ QRS complex: _____

Rhythm interpretation: _____

Strip 6.14 Rhythm: _____ Rate: _____ P wave: _____

PR interval: _____ QRS complex: _____

Rhythm interpretation: _____

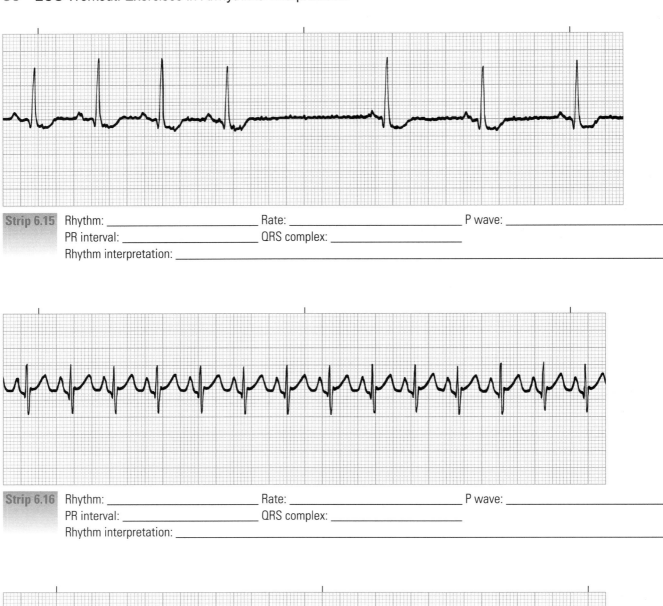

Strip 6.15 Rhythm: _____ Rate: _____ P wave: _____

PR interval: _____ QRS complex: _____

Rhythm interpretation: _____

Strip 6.16 Rhythm: _____ Rate: _____ P wave: _____

PR interval: _____ QRS complex: _____

Rhythm interpretation: _____

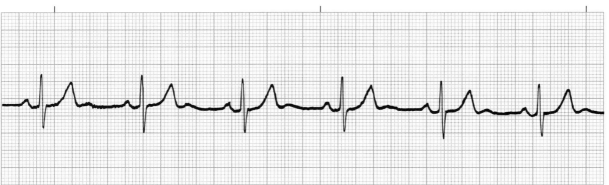

Strip 6.17 Rhythm: _____ Rate: _____ P wave: _____

PR interval: _____ QRS complex: _____

Rhythm interpretation: _____

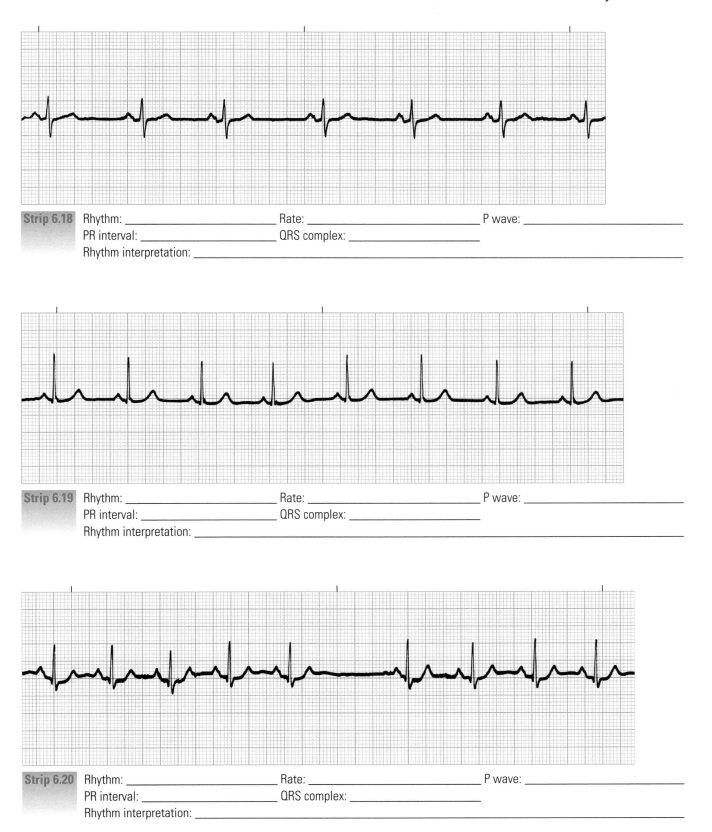

Strip 6.18 Rhythm: _____ Rate: _____ P wave: _____
PR interval: _____ QRS complex: _____
Rhythm interpretation: _____

Strip 6.19 Rhythm: _____ Rate: _____ P wave: _____
PR interval: _____ QRS complex: _____
Rhythm interpretation: _____

Strip 6.20 Rhythm: _____ Rate: _____ P wave: _____
PR interval: _____ QRS complex: _____
Rhythm interpretation: _____

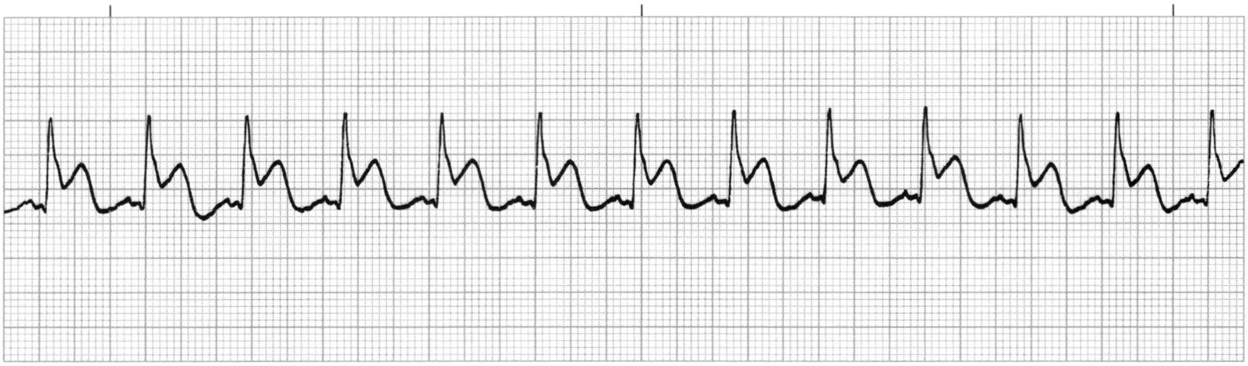

Strip 6.21 Rhythm: _____ Rate: _____ P wave: _____

PR interval: _____ QRS complex: _____

Rhythm interpretation: _____

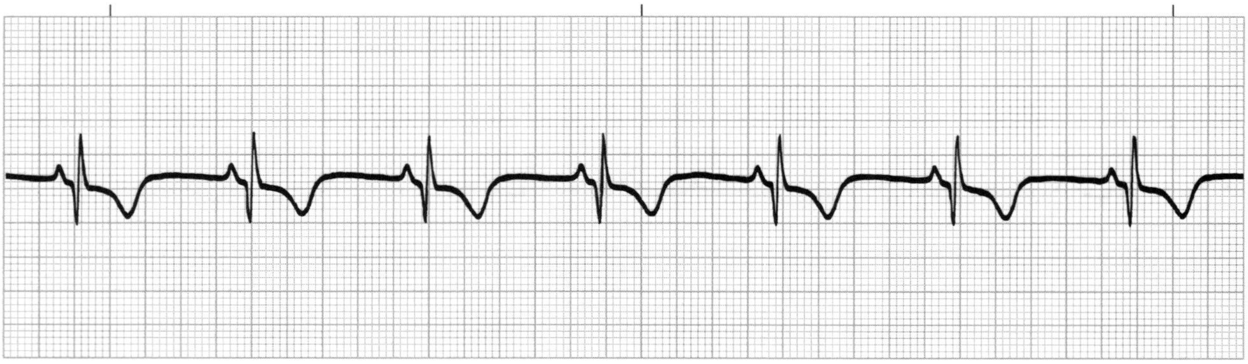

Strip 6.22 Rhythm: _____ Rate: _____ P wave: _____

PR interval: _____ QRS complex: _____

Rhythm interpretation: _____

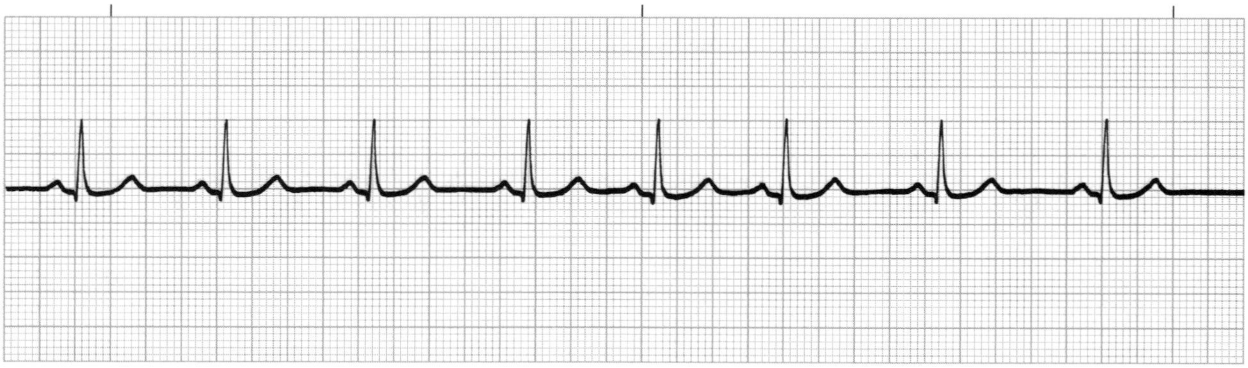

Strip 6.23 Rhythm: _____ Rate: _____ P wave: _____

PR interval: _____ QRS complex: _____

Rhythm interpretation: _____

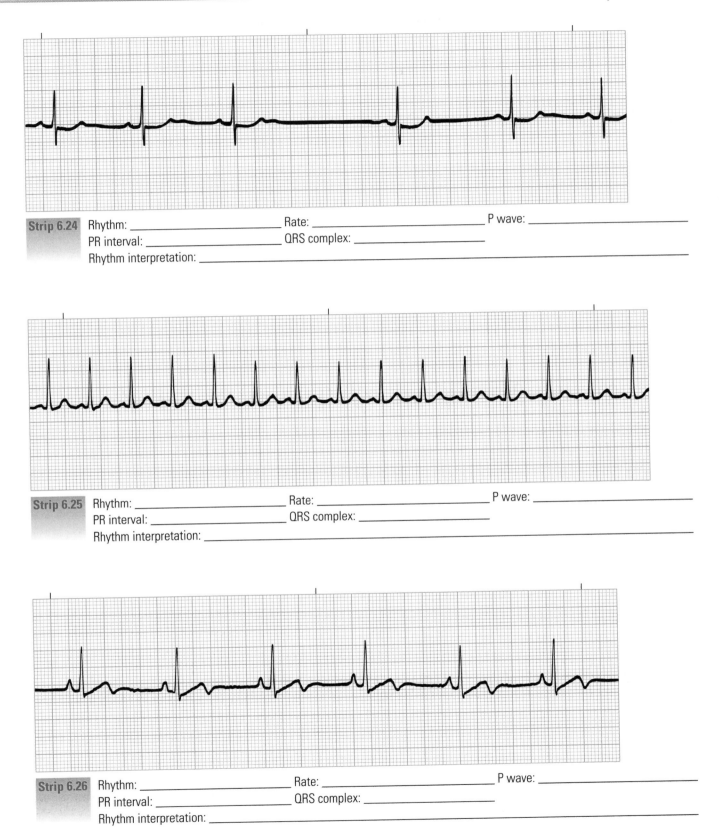

Strip 6.24 Rhythm: _____ Rate: _____ P wave: _____
PR interval: _____ QRS complex: _____
Rhythm interpretation: _____

Strip 6.25 Rhythm: _____ Rate: _____ P wave: _____
PR interval: _____ QRS complex: _____
Rhythm interpretation: _____

Strip 6.26 Rhythm: _____ Rate: _____ P wave: _____
PR interval: _____ QRS complex: _____
Rhythm interpretation: _____

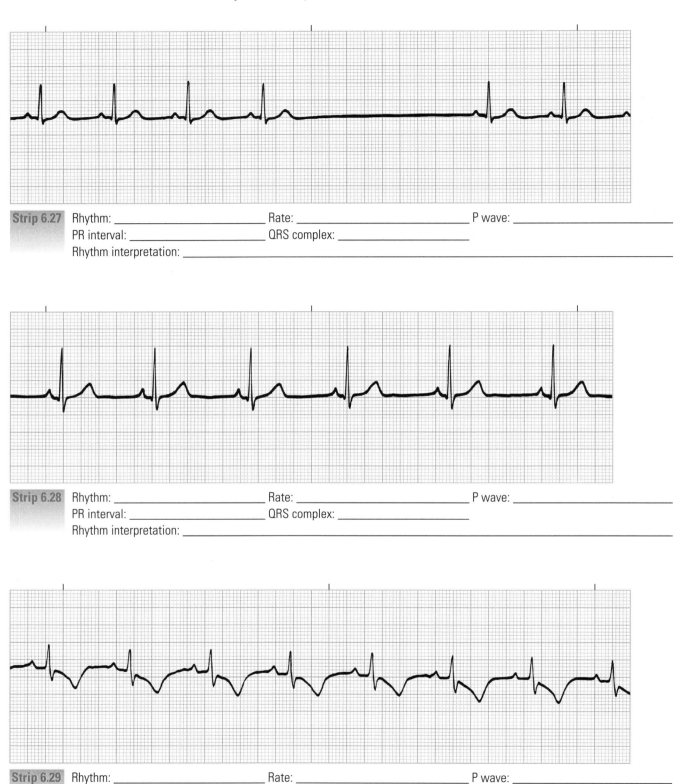

Strip 6.27 Rhythm: _____ Rate: _____ P wave: _____
PR interval: _____ QRS complex: _____
Rhythm interpretation: _____

Strip 6.28 Rhythm: _____ Rate: _____ P wave: _____
PR interval: _____ QRS complex: _____
Rhythm interpretation: _____

Strip 6.29 Rhythm: _____ Rate: _____ P wave: _____
PR interval: _____ QRS complex: _____
Rhythm interpretation: _____

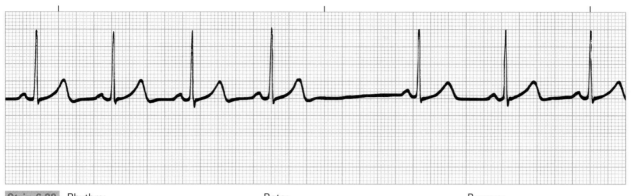

| Strip 6.30 | Rhythm: _____ Rate: _____ P wave: _____ |
| PR interval: _____ QRS complex: _____ |
| Rhythm interpretation: _____ |

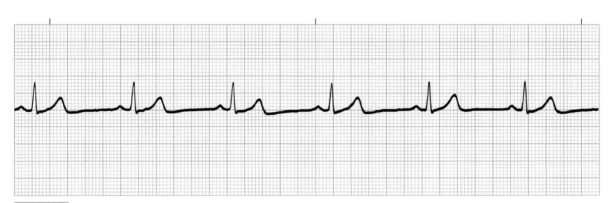

| Strip 6.31 | Rhythm: _____ Rate: _____ P wave: _____ |
| PR interval: _____ QRS complex: _____ |
| Rhythm interpretation: _____ |

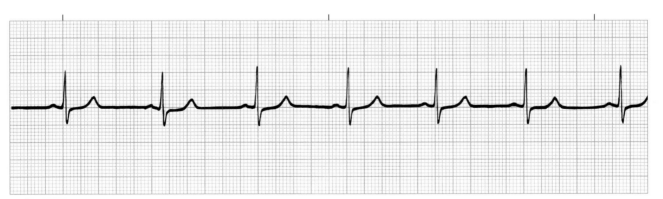

| Strip 6.32 | Rhythm: _____ Rate: _____ P wave: _____ |
| PR interval: _____ QRS complex: _____ |
| Rhythm interpretation: _____ |

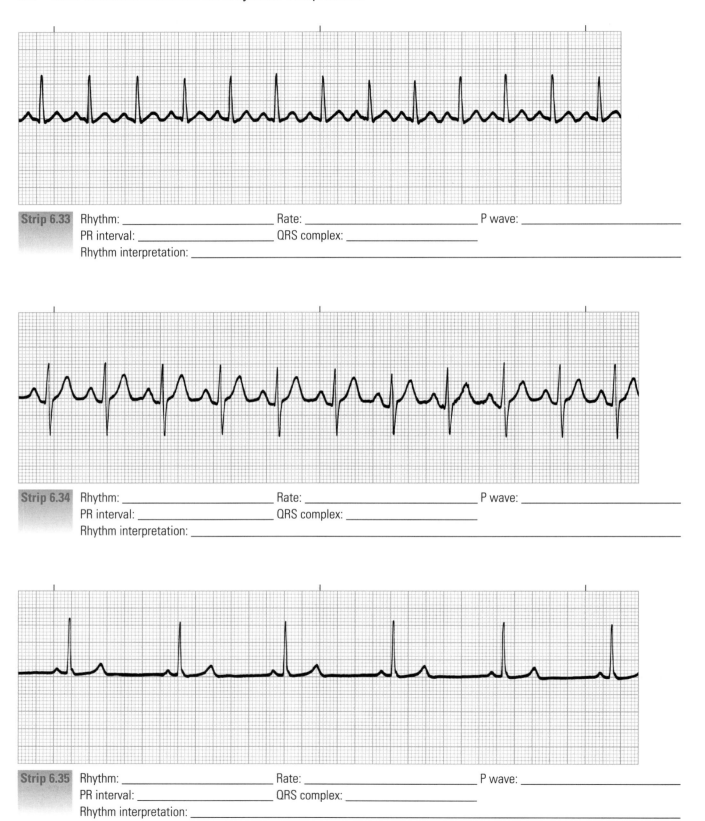

Strip 6.33 Rhythm: _____ Rate: _____ P wave: _____
PR interval: _____ QRS complex: _____
Rhythm interpretation: _____

Strip 6.34 Rhythm: _____ Rate: _____ P wave: _____
PR interval: _____ QRS complex: _____
Rhythm interpretation: _____

Strip 6.35 Rhythm: _____ Rate: _____ P wave: _____
PR interval: _____ QRS complex: _____
Rhythm interpretation: _____

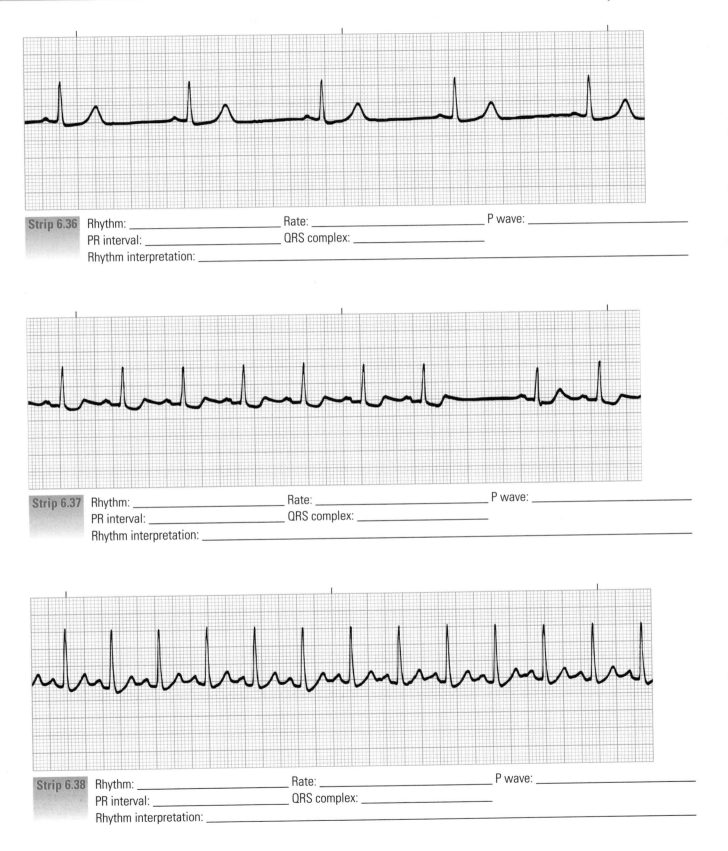

Strip 6.36 Rhythm: _____ Rate: _____ P wave: _____
PR interval: _____ QRS complex: _____
Rhythm interpretation: _____

Strip 6.37 Rhythm: _____ Rate: _____ P wave: _____
PR interval: _____ QRS complex: _____
Rhythm interpretation: _____

Strip 6.38 Rhythm: _____ Rate: _____ P wave: _____
PR interval: _____ QRS complex: _____
Rhythm interpretation: _____

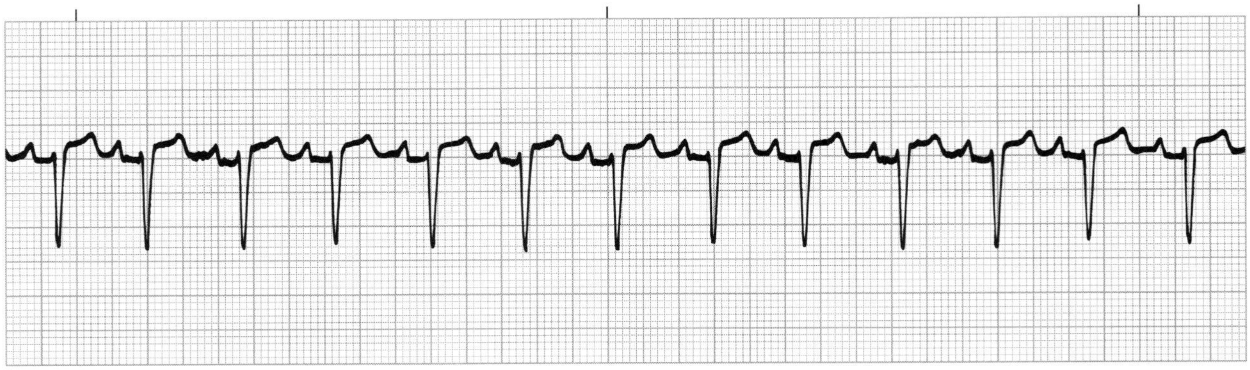

Strip 6.39 Rhythm: _____ Rate: _____ P wave: _____
PR interval: _____ QRS complex: _____
Rhythm interpretation: _____

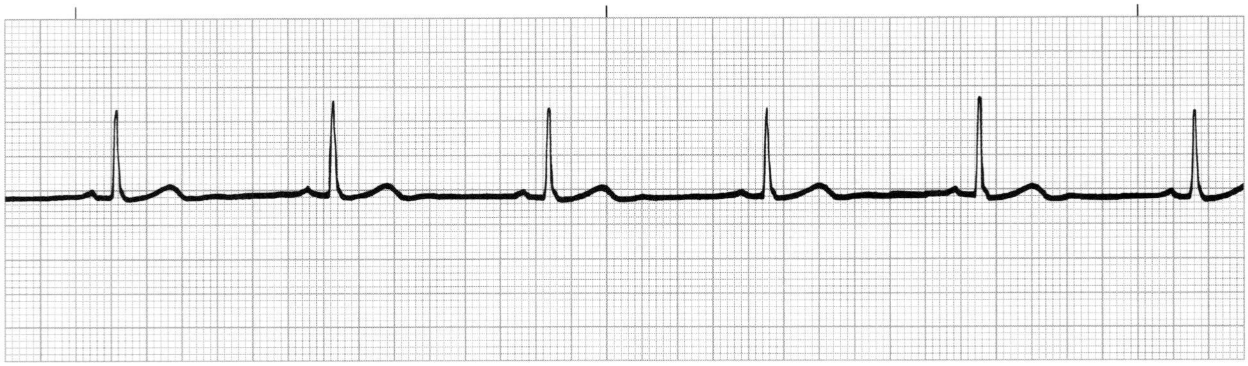

Strip 6.40 Rhythm: _____ Rate: _____ P wave: _____
PR interval: _____ QRS complex: _____
Rhythm interpretation: _____

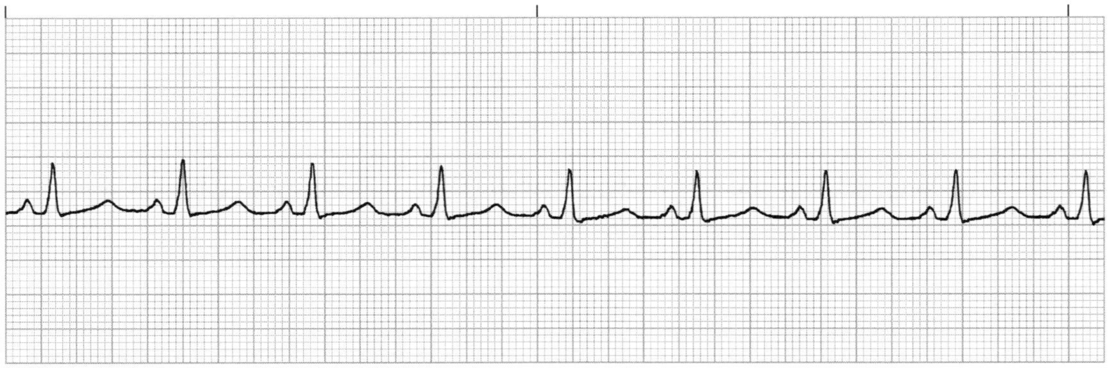

Strip 6.41 Rhythm: _____ Rate: _____ P wave: _____
PR interval: _____ QRS complex: _____
Rhythm interpretation: _____

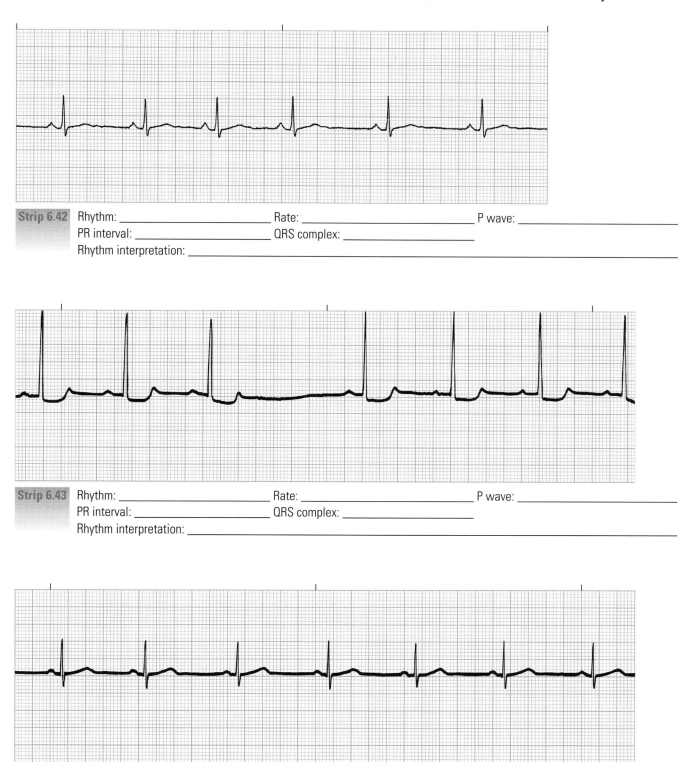

Strip 6.42 Rhythm: _____ Rate: _____ P wave: _____

PR interval: _____ QRS complex: _____

Rhythm interpretation: _____

Strip 6.43 Rhythm: _____ Rate: _____ P wave: _____

PR interval: _____ QRS complex: _____

Rhythm interpretation: _____

Strip 6.44 Rhythm: _____ Rate: _____ P wave: _____

PR interval: _____ QRS complex: _____

Rhythm interpretation: _____

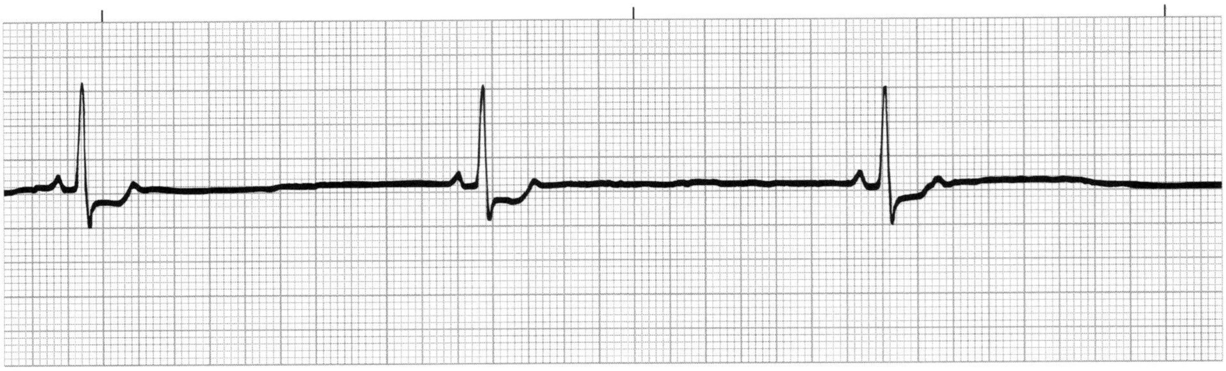

Strip 6.45   Rhythm: _____ Rate: _____ P wave: _____

PR interval: _____ QRS complex: _____

Rhythm interpretation: _____

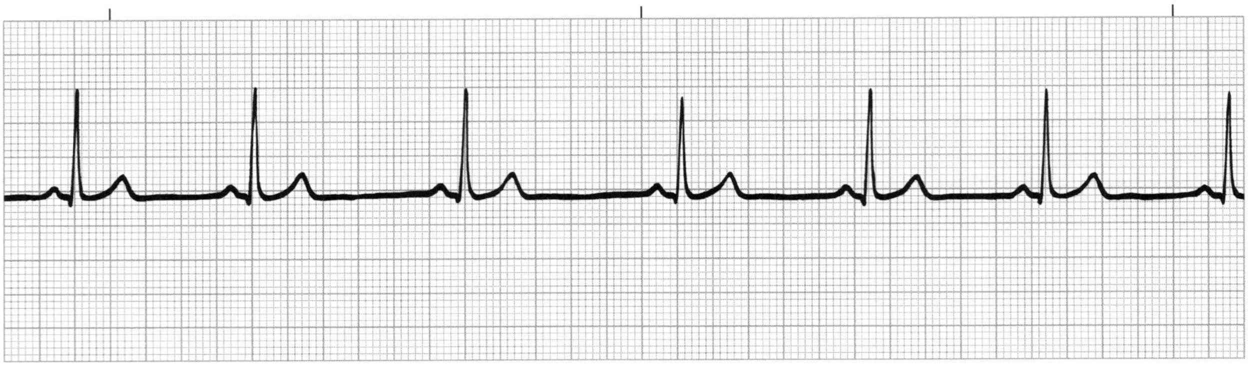

Strip 6.46   Rhythm: _____ Rate: _____ P wave: _____

PR interval: _____ QRS complex: _____

Rhythm interpretation: _____

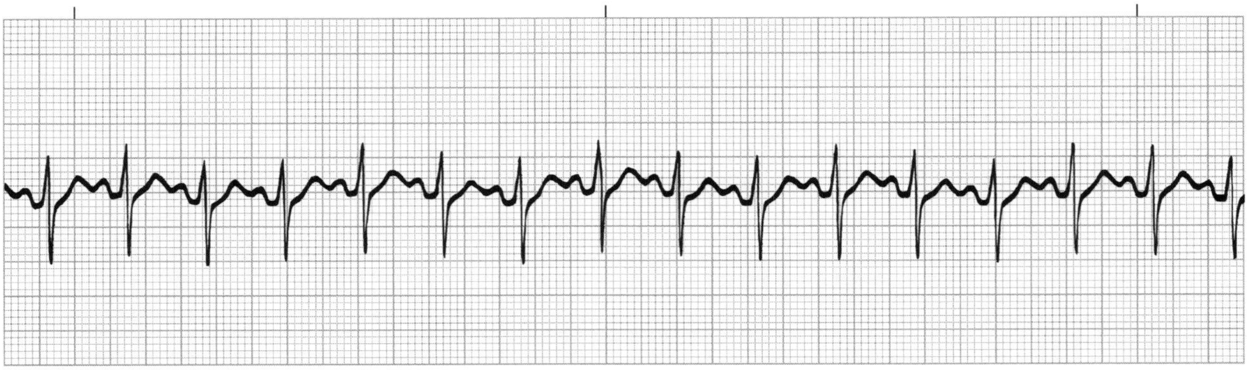

Strip 6.47   Rhythm: _____ Rate: _____ P wave: _____

PR interval: _____ QRS complex: _____

Rhythm interpretation: _____

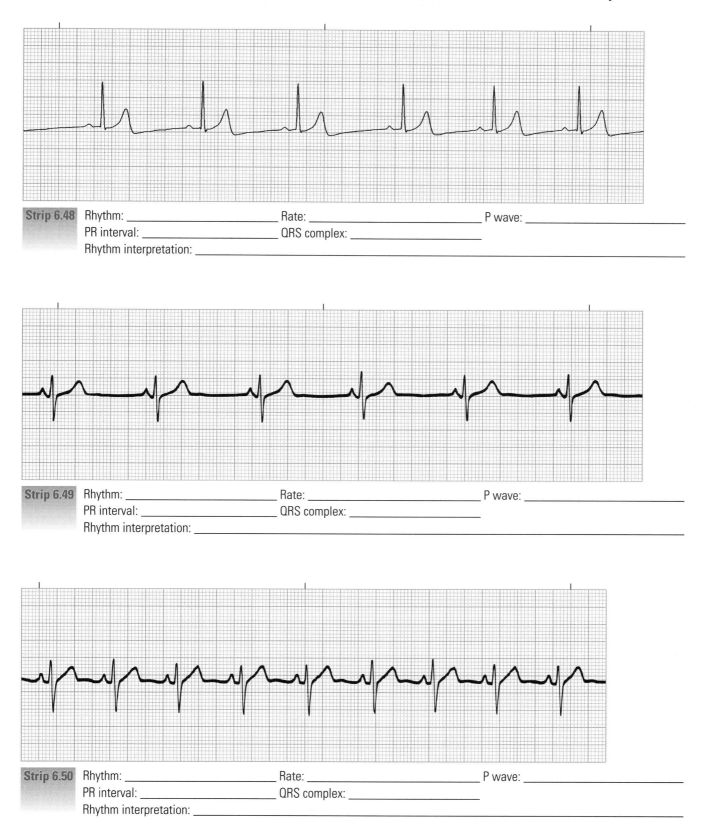

Strip 6.48 Rhythm: _____ Rate: _____ P wave: _____
PR interval: _____ QRS complex: _____
Rhythm interpretation: _____

Strip 6.49 Rhythm: _____ Rate: _____ P wave: _____
PR interval: _____ QRS complex: _____
Rhythm interpretation: _____

Strip 6.50 Rhythm: _____ Rate: _____ P wave: _____
PR interval: _____ QRS complex: _____
Rhythm interpretation: _____

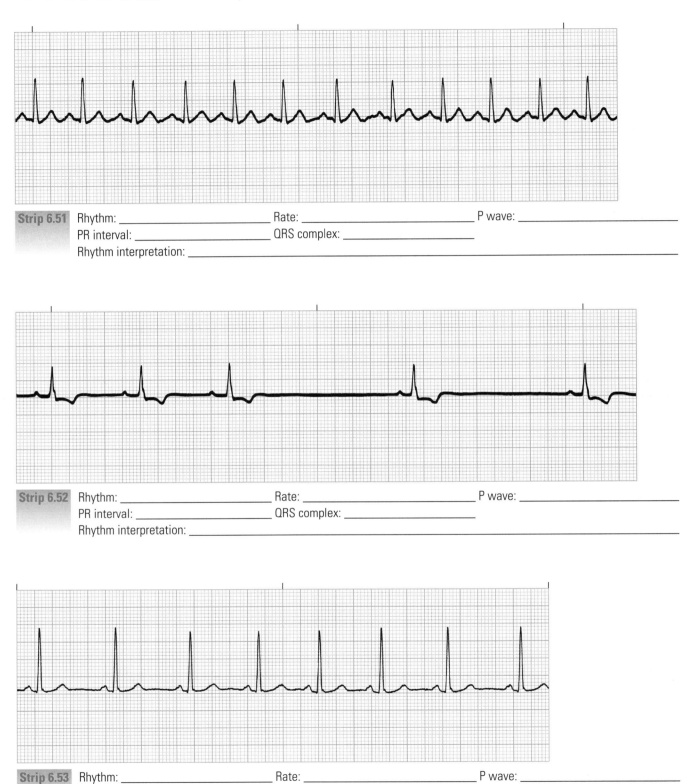

Strip 6.51	Rhythm: _____	Rate: _____	P wave: _____
	PR interval: _____	QRS complex: _____	
	Rhythm interpretation: _____		

Strip 6.52	Rhythm: _____	Rate: _____	P wave: _____
	PR interval: _____	QRS complex: _____	
	Rhythm interpretation: _____		

Strip 6.53	Rhythm: _____	Rate: _____	P wave: _____
	PR interval: _____	QRS complex: _____	
	Rhythm interpretation: _____		

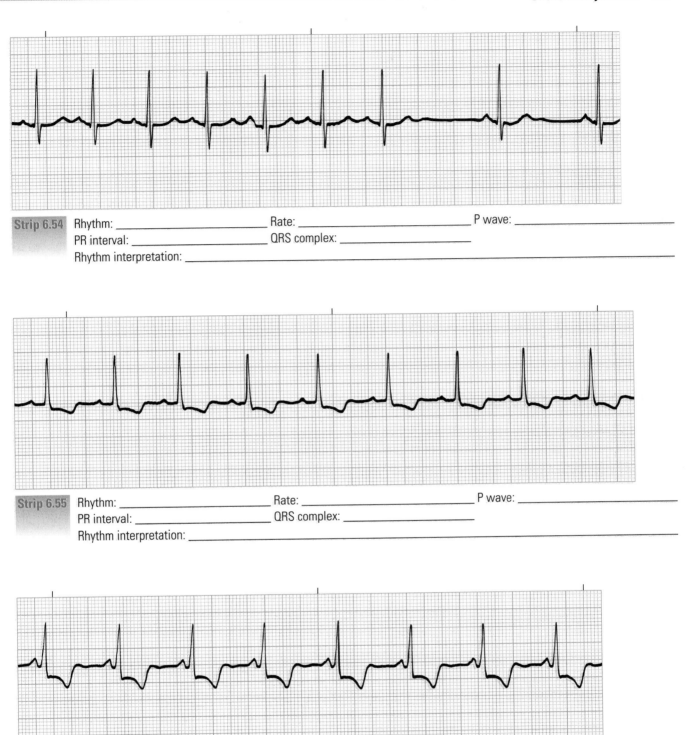

Strip 6.54 Rhythm: _____ Rate: _____ P wave: _____

PR interval: _____ QRS complex: _____

Rhythm interpretation: _____

Strip 6.55 Rhythm: _____ Rate: _____ P wave: _____

PR interval: _____ QRS complex: _____

Rhythm interpretation: _____

Strip 6.56 Rhythm: _____ Rate: _____ P wave: _____

PR interval: _____ QRS complex: _____

Rhythm interpretation: _____

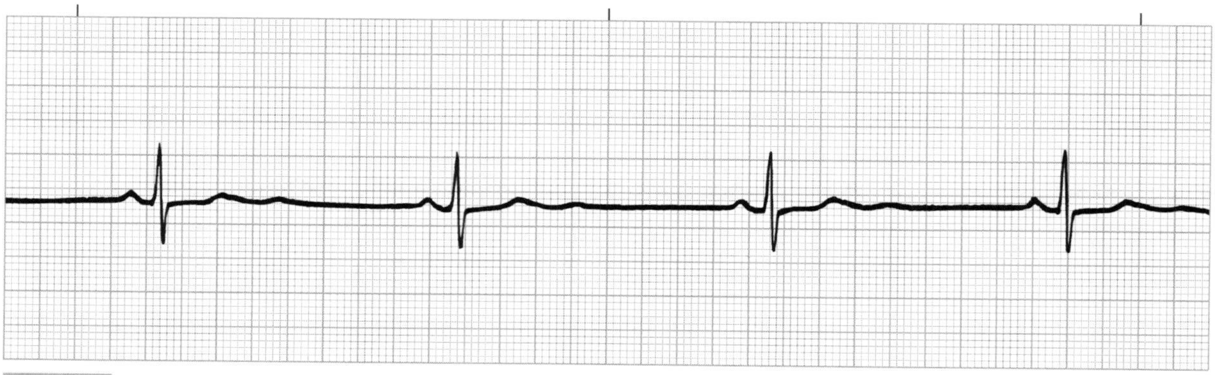

Strip 6.57 Rhythm: _____ Rate: _____ P wave: _____

PR interval: _____ QRS complex: _____

Rhythm interpretation: _____

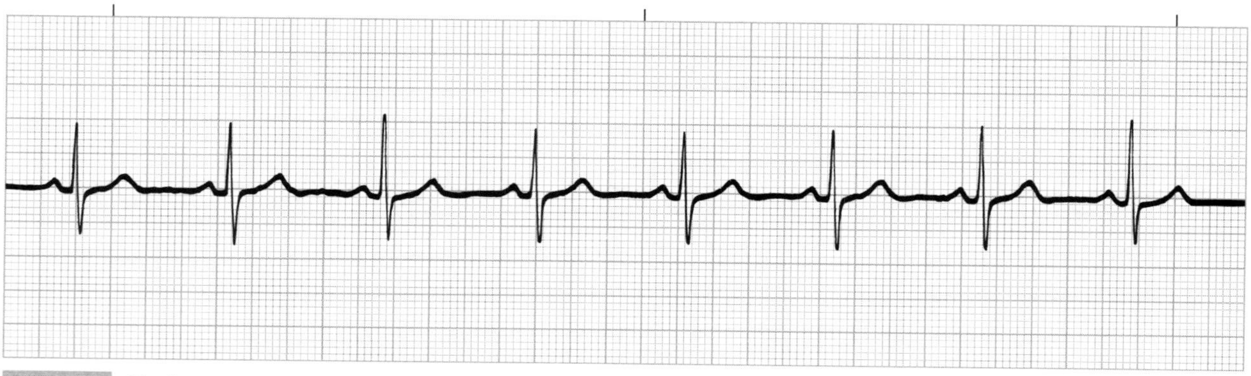

Strip 6.58 Rhythm: _____ Rate: _____ P wave: _____

PR interval: _____ QRS complex: _____

Rhythm interpretation: _____

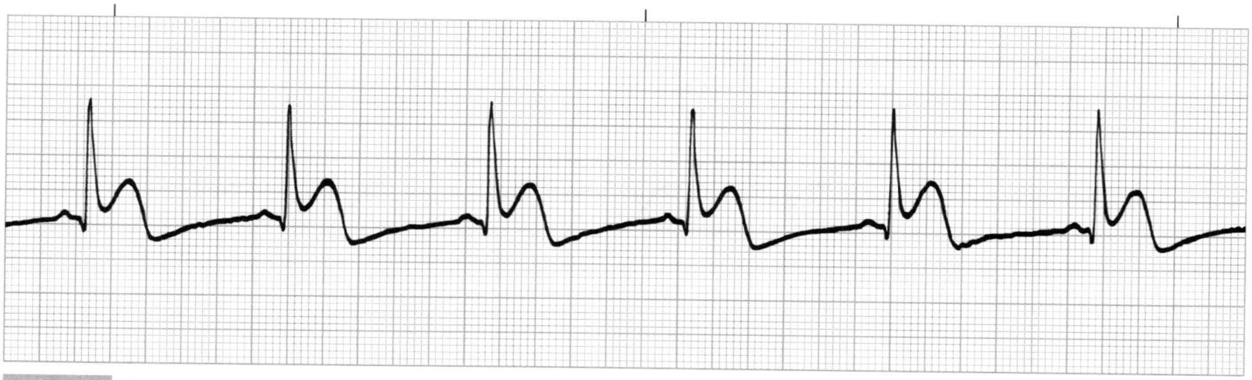

Strip 6.59 Rhythm: _____ Rate: _____ P wave: _____

PR interval: _____ QRS complex: _____

Rhythm interpretation: _____

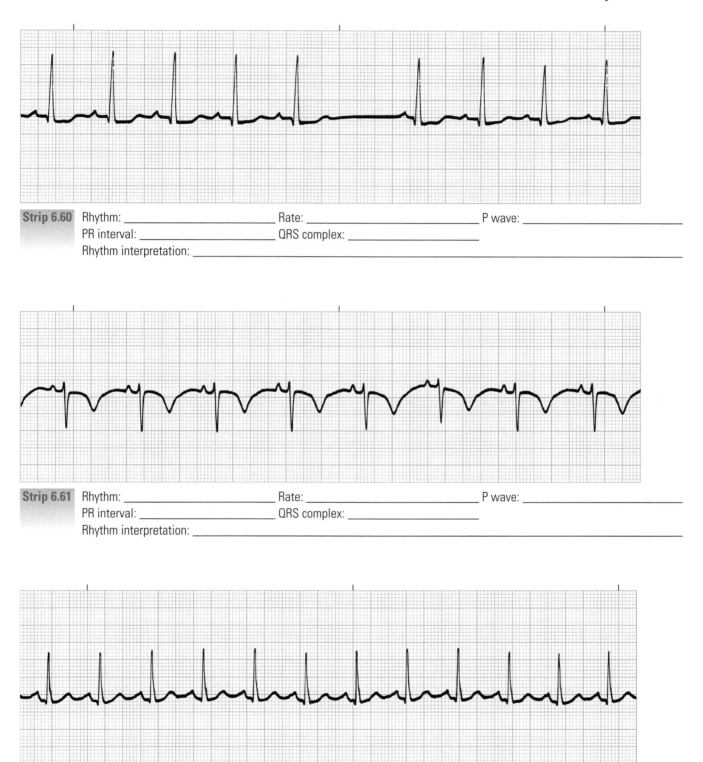

Strip 6.60 Rhythm: _____ Rate: _____ P wave: _____
PR interval: _____ QRS complex: _____
Rhythm interpretation: _____

Strip 6.61 Rhythm: _____ Rate: _____ P wave: _____
PR interval: _____ QRS complex: _____
Rhythm interpretation: _____

Strip 6.62 Rhythm: _____ Rate: _____ P wave: _____
PR interval: _____ QRS complex: _____
Rhythm interpretation: _____

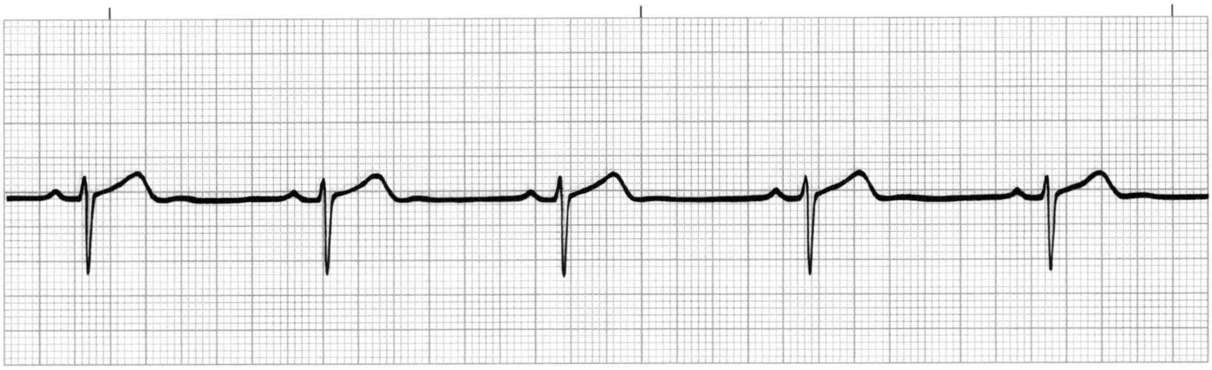

Strip 6.63 Rhythm: _____ Rate: _____ P wave: _____
PR interval: _____ QRS complex: _____
Rhythm interpretation: _____

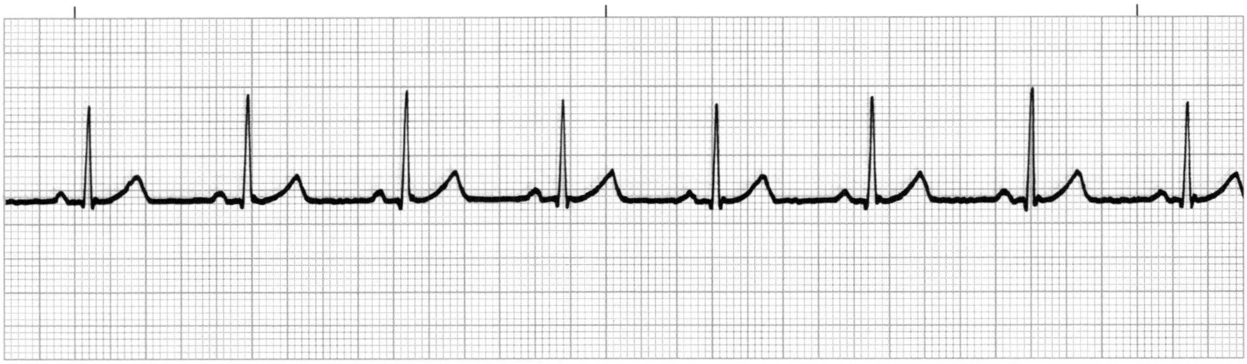

Strip 6.64 Rhythm: _____ Rate: _____ P wave: _____
PR interval: _____ QRS complex: _____
Rhythm interpretation: _____

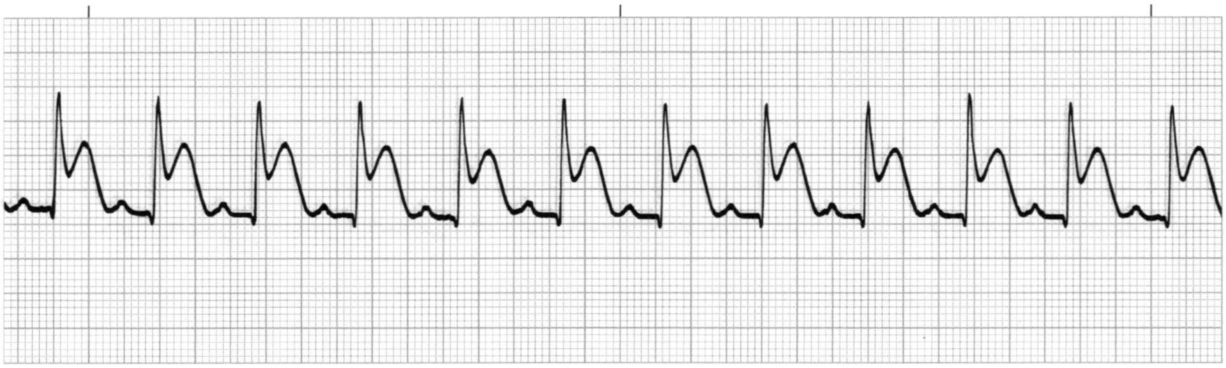

Strip 6.65 Rhythm: _____ Rate: _____ P wave: _____
PR interval: _____ QRS complex: _____
Rhythm interpretation: _____

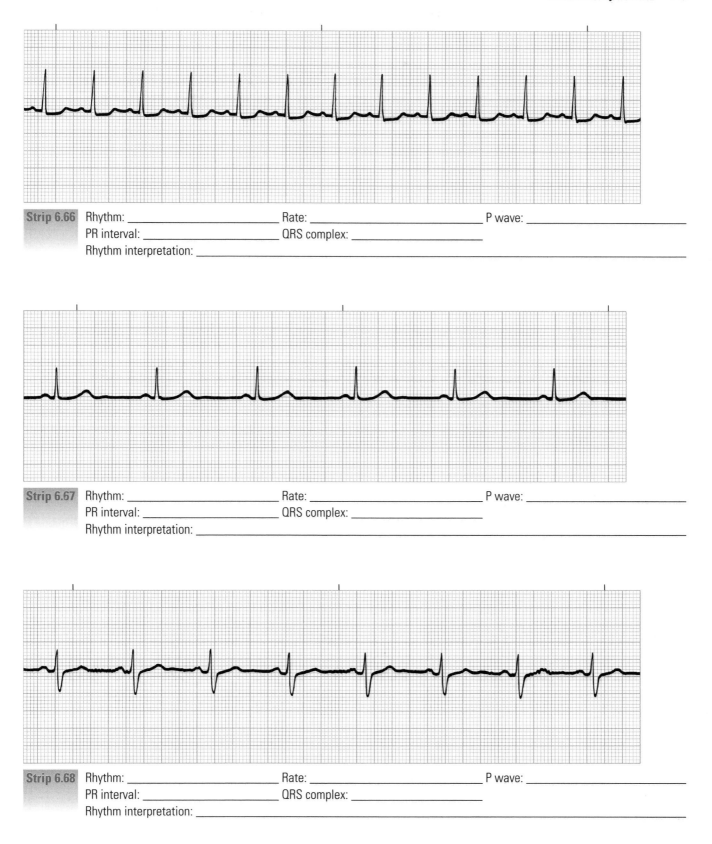

Strip 6.66   Rhythm: _____ Rate: _____ P wave: _____

PR interval: _____ QRS complex: _____

Rhythm interpretation: _____

Strip 6.67   Rhythm: _____ Rate: _____ P wave: _____

PR interval: _____ QRS complex: _____

Rhythm interpretation: _____

Strip 6.68   Rhythm: _____ Rate: _____ P wave: _____

PR interval: _____ QRS complex: _____

Rhythm interpretation: _____

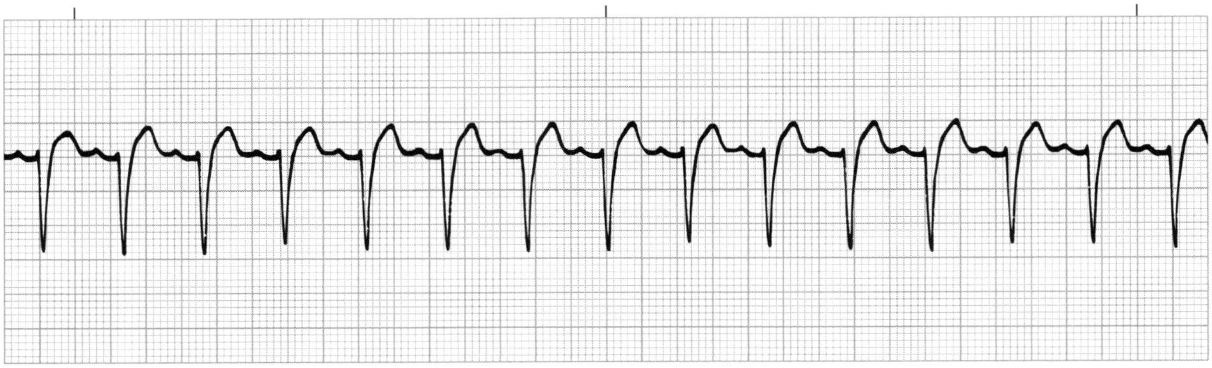

Strip 6.69 Rhythm: _____ Rate: _____ P wave: _____
PR interval: _____ QRS complex: _____
Rhythm interpretation: _____

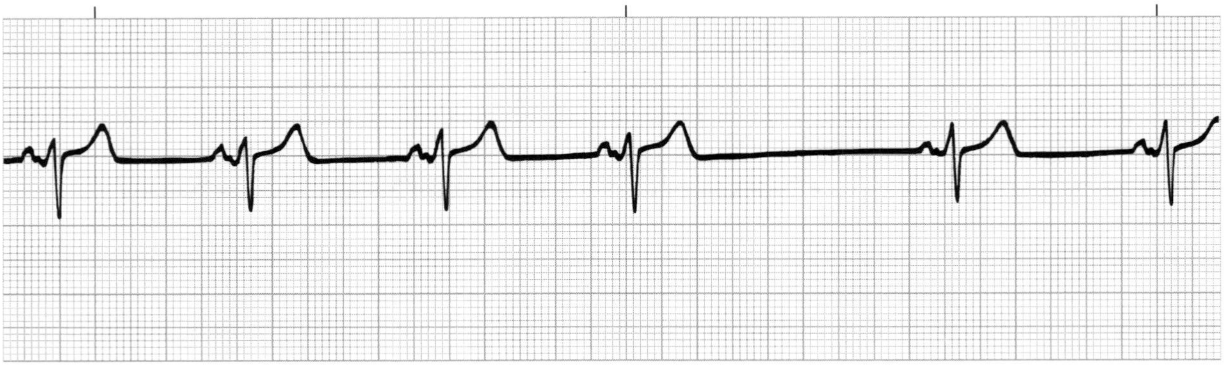

Strip 6.70 Rhythm: _____ Rate: _____ P wave: _____
PR interval: _____ QRS complex: _____
Rhythm interpretation: _____

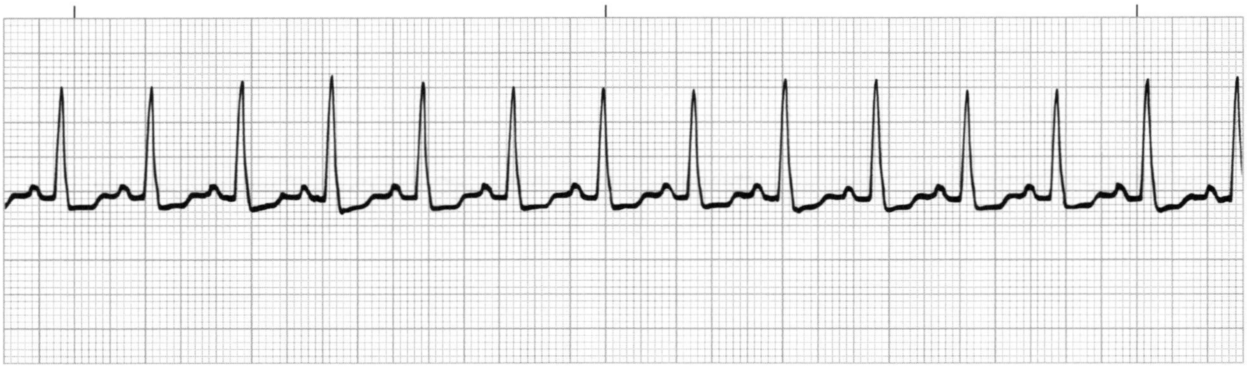

Strip 6.71 Rhythm: _____ Rate: _____ P wave: _____
PR interval: _____ QRS complex: _____
Rhythm interpretation: _____

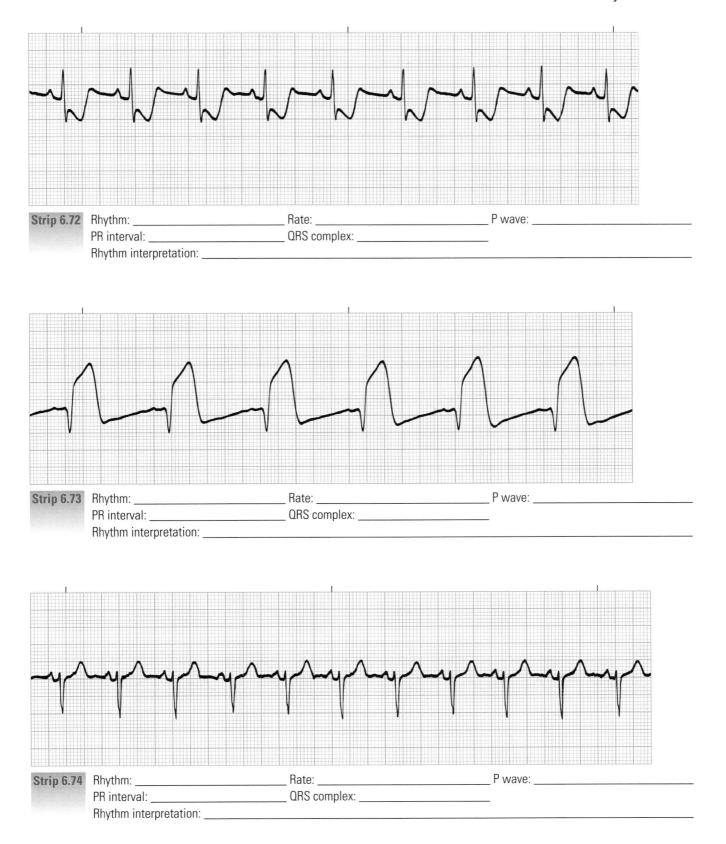

Strip 6.72 Rhythm: _____ Rate: _____ P wave: _____
PR interval: _____ QRS complex: _____
Rhythm interpretation: _____

Strip 6.73 Rhythm: _____ Rate: _____ P wave: _____
PR interval: _____ QRS complex: _____
Rhythm interpretation: _____

Strip 6.74 Rhythm: _____ Rate: _____ P wave: _____
PR interval: _____ QRS complex: _____
Rhythm interpretation: _____

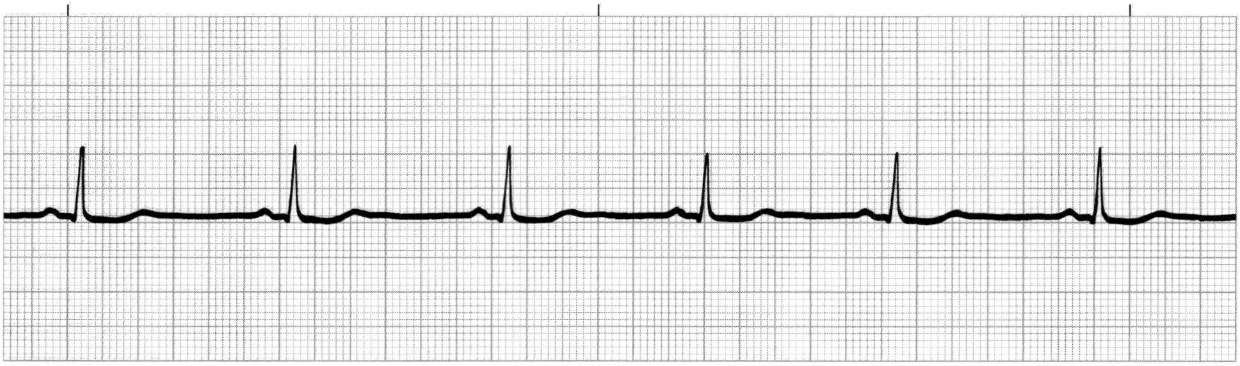

Strip 6.75 Rhythm: _____ Rate: _____ P wave: _____

PR interval: _____ QRS complex: _____

Rhythm interpretation: _____

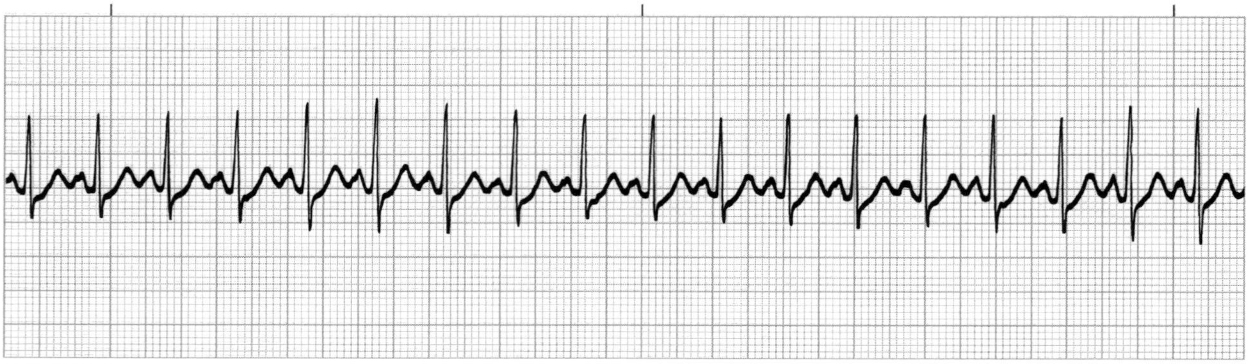

Strip 6.76 Rhythm: _____ Rate: _____ P wave: _____

PR interval: _____ QRS complex: _____

Rhythm interpretation: _____

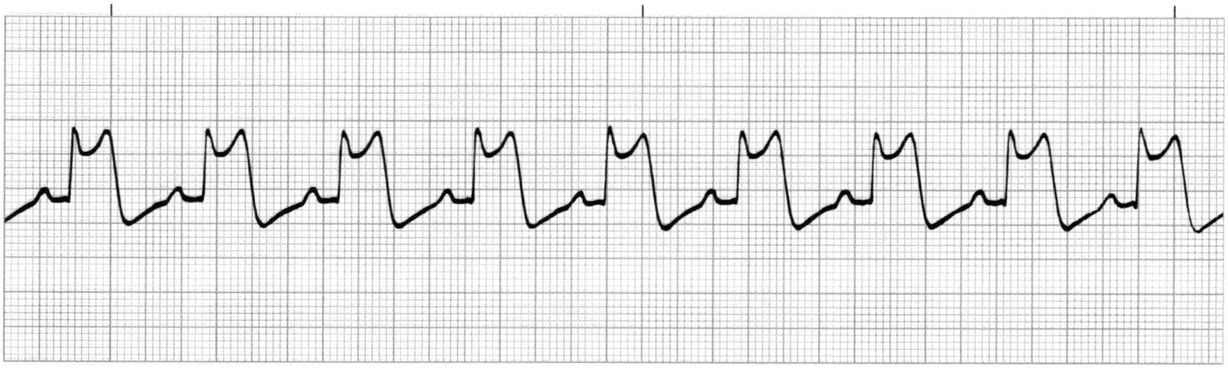

Strip 6.77 Rhythm: _____ Rate: _____ P wave: _____

PR interval: _____ QRS complex: _____

Rhythm interpretation: _____

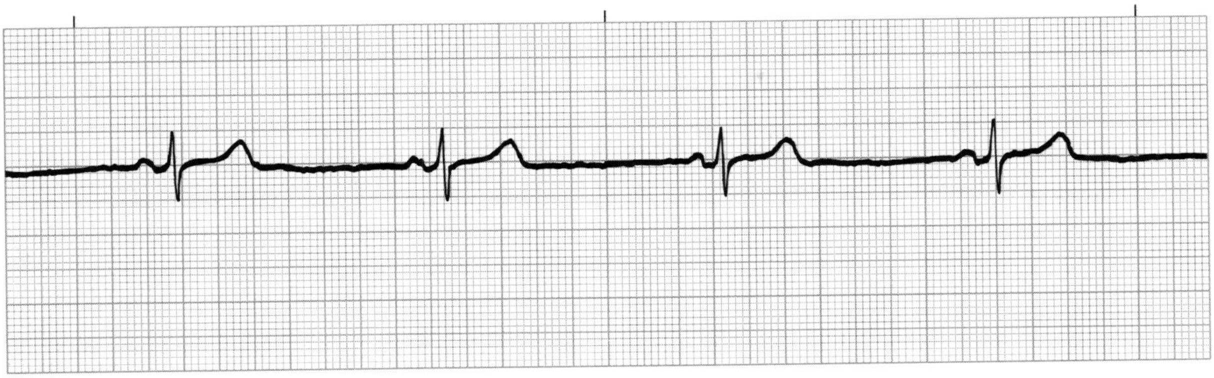

Strip 6.78 Rhythm: _____ Rate: _____ P wave: _____

PR interval: _____ QRS complex: _____

Rhythm interpretation: _____

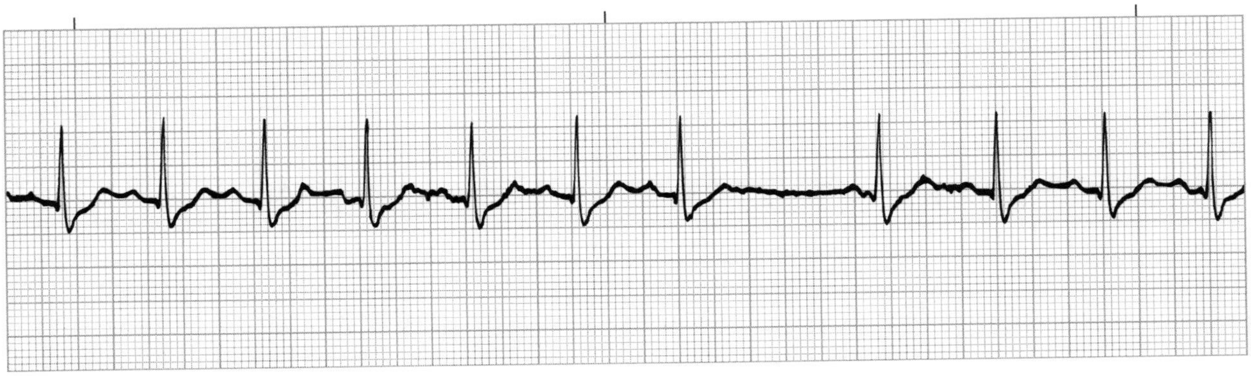

Strip 6.79 Rhythm: _____ Rate: _____ P wave: _____

PR interval: _____ QRS complex: _____

Rhythm interpretation: _____

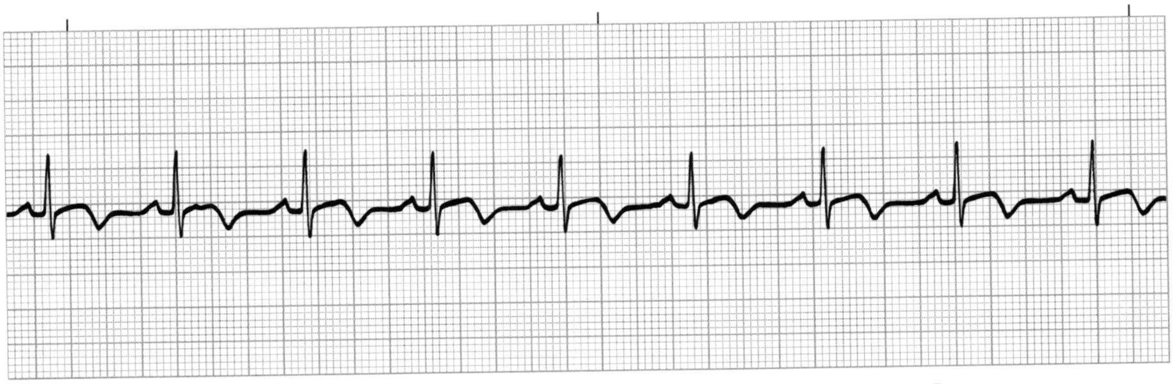

Strip 6.80 Rhythm: _____ Rate: _____ P wave: _____

PR interval: _____ QRS complex: _____

Rhythm interpretation: _____

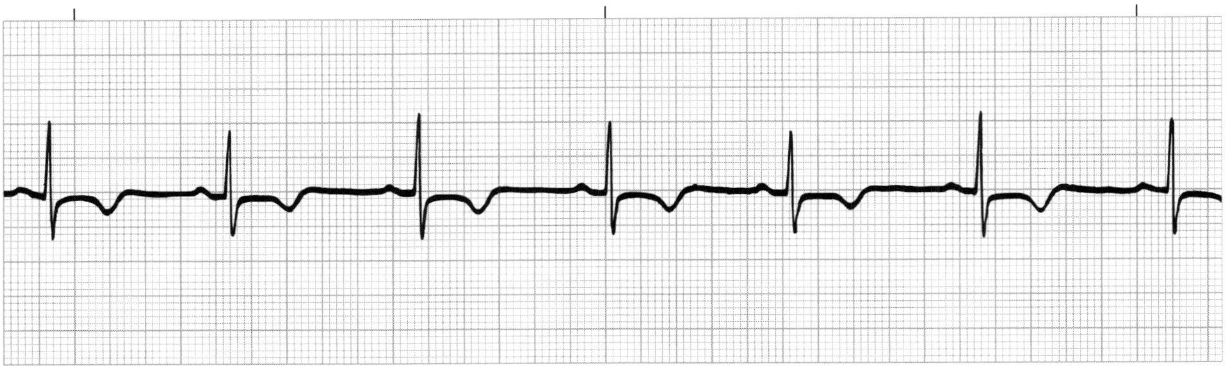

Strip 6.81 Rhythm: _____ Rate: _____ P wave: _____

PR interval: _____ QRS complex: _____

Rhythm interpretation: _____

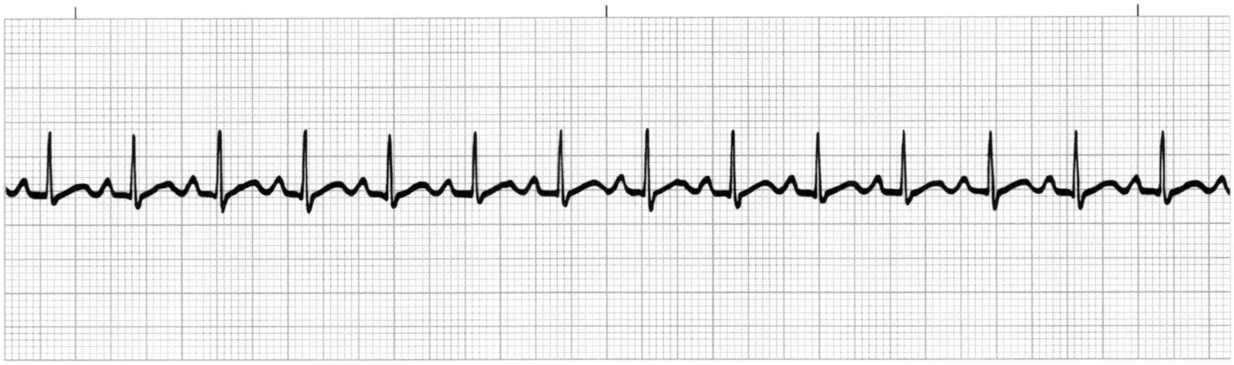

Strip 6.82 Rhythm: _____ Rate: _____ P wave: _____

PR interval: _____ QRS complex: _____

Rhythm interpretation: _____

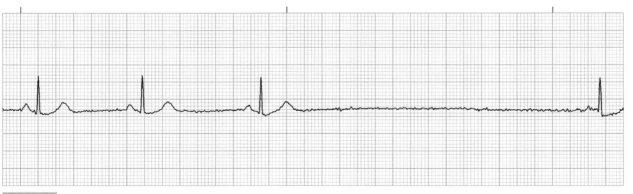

Strip 6.83 Rhythm: _____ Rate: _____ P wave: _____

PR interval: _____ QRS complex: _____

Rhythm interpretation: _____

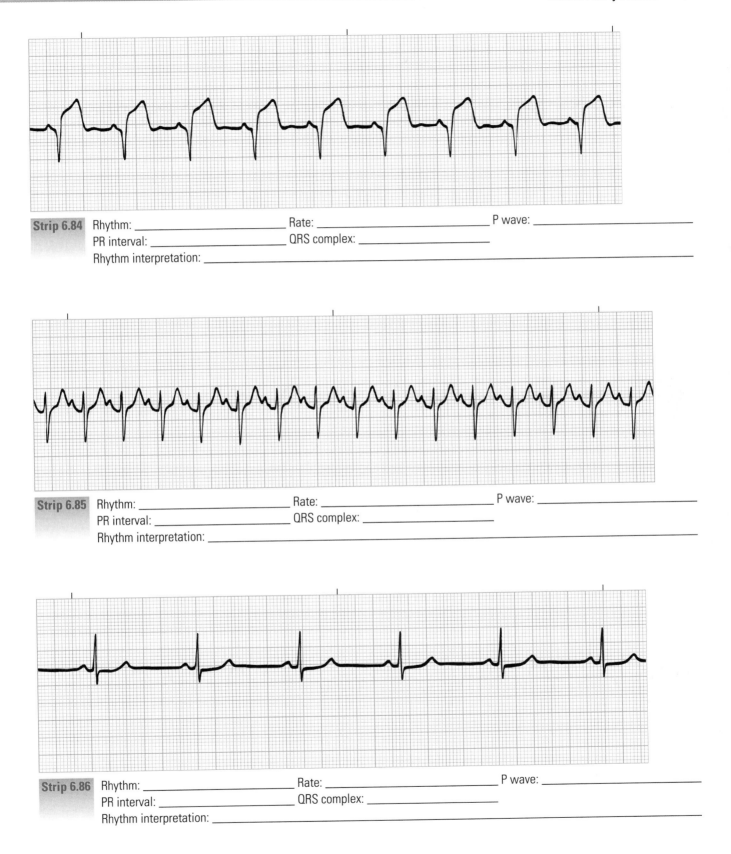

Strip 6.84 Rhythm: _____ Rate: _____ P wave: _____
PR interval: _____ QRS complex: _____
Rhythm interpretation: _____

Strip 6.85 Rhythm: _____ Rate: _____ P wave: _____
PR interval: _____ QRS complex: _____
Rhythm interpretation: _____

Strip 6.86 Rhythm: _____ Rate: _____ P wave: _____
PR interval: _____ QRS complex: _____
Rhythm interpretation: _____

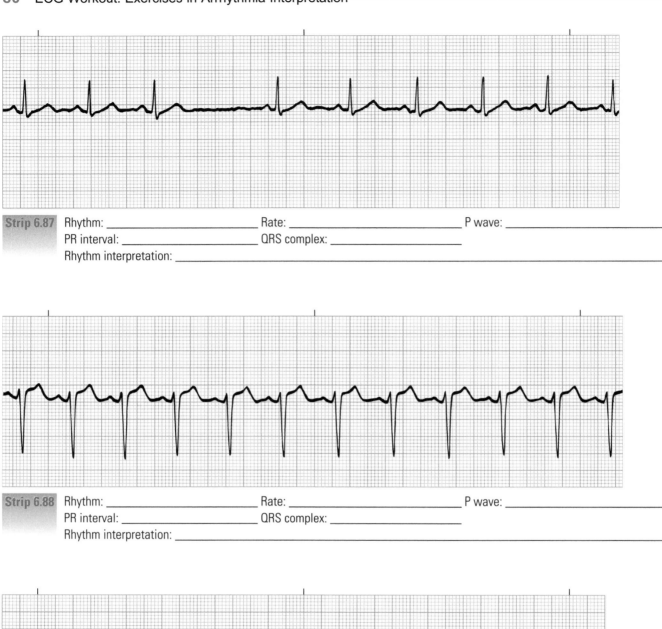

Strip 6.87 Rhythm: _____ Rate: _____ P wave: _____
PR interval: _____ QRS complex: _____
Rhythm interpretation: _____

Strip 6.88 Rhythm: _____ Rate: _____ P wave: _____
PR interval: _____ QRS complex: _____
Rhythm interpretation: _____

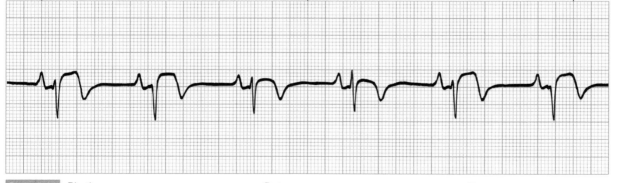

Strip 6.89 Rhythm: _____ Rate: _____ P wave: _____
PR interval: _____ QRS complex: _____
Rhythm interpretation: _____

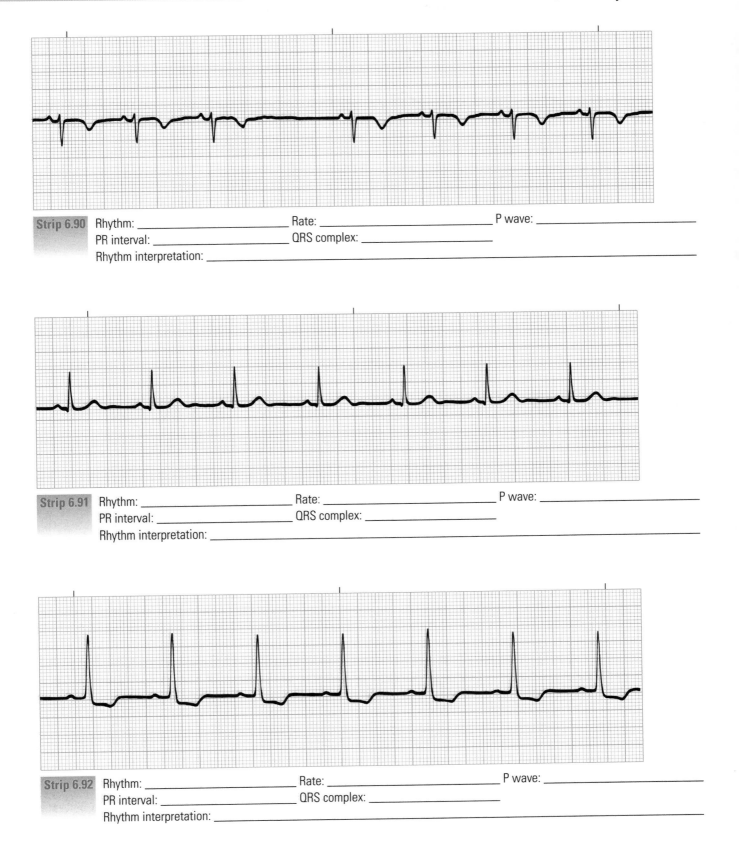

Strip 6.90 Rhythm: _____ Rate: _____ P wave: _____

PR interval: _____ QRS complex: _____

Rhythm interpretation: _____

Strip 6.91 Rhythm: _____ Rate: _____ P wave: _____

PR interval: _____ QRS complex: _____

Rhythm interpretation: _____

Strip 6.92 Rhythm: _____ Rate: _____ P wave: _____

PR interval: _____ QRS complex: _____

Rhythm interpretation: _____

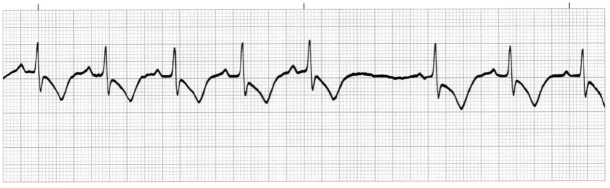

Strip 6.93 Rhythm: _____ Rate: _____ P wave: _____

PR interval: _____ QRS complex: _____

Rhythm interpretation: _____

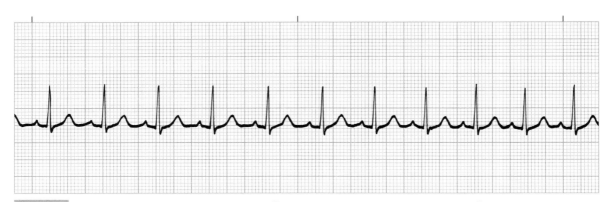

Strip 6.94 Rhythm: _____ Rate: _____ P wave: _____

PR interval: _____ QRS complex: _____

Rhythm interpretation: _____

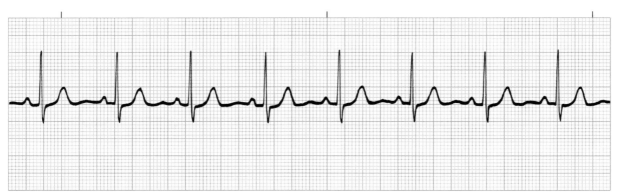

Strip 6.95 Rhythm: _____ Rate: _____ P wave: _____

PR interval: _____ QRS complex: _____

Rhythm interpretation: _____

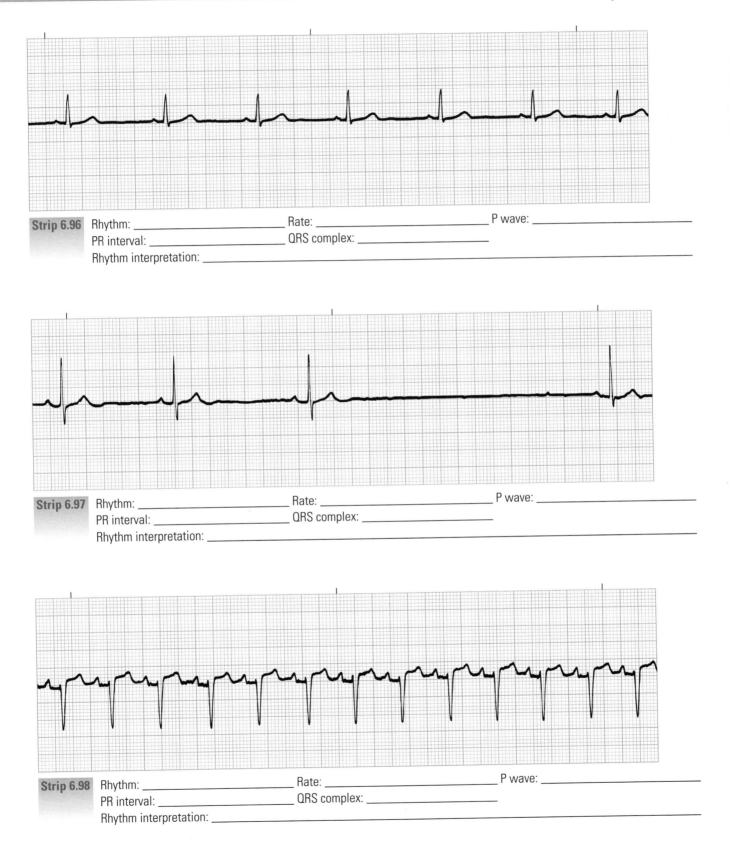

Strip 6.96 Rhythm: _____ Rate: _____ P wave: _____
PR interval: _____ QRS complex: _____
Rhythm interpretation: _____

Strip 6.97 Rhythm: _____ Rate: _____ P wave: _____
PR interval: _____ QRS complex: _____
Rhythm interpretation: _____

Strip 6.98 Rhythm: _____ Rate: _____ P wave: _____
PR interval: _____ QRS complex: _____
Rhythm interpretation: _____

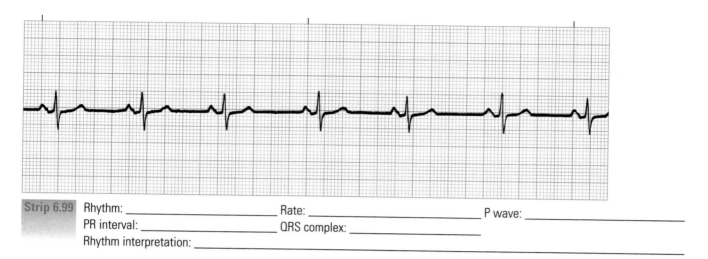

Rhythm: _____ Rate: _____ P wave: _____

PR interval: _____ QRS complex: _____

Rhythm interpretation: _____

seven

Atrial Arrhythmias

Mechanisms of Arrhythmias

Under certain circumstances, cardiac cells in any part of the heart may take on the role of pacemaker of the heart. Such a pacemaker is called an ectopic pacemaker (a pacemaker other than the sinus node). The result can be ectopic beats or rhythms. These rhythms are identified according to the location of the ectopic pacemaker (for example, atrial, junctional, or ventricular). The three basic mechanisms that are responsible for ectopic beats and rhythms are *altered automaticity*, *triggered activity*, and *reentry*:

- **Altered Automaticity**—Normally the automaticity of the sinus node exceeds that of all other parts of the conduction system, allowing it to control the heart rate and rhythm. Pacemaker cells in other areas of the heart also have the property of automaticity, including cells in the atria, atrioventricular (AV) junction, and the ventricles. The rates of these other pacemaker sites are slower. Therefore, they're suppressed by the sinus node under normal circumstances. Because the inherent firing rate of the pacemaker cells of the sinus node is faster than that of the other pacemaker sites, it is the dominant and primary pacemaker of the heart. An ectopic pacemaker site can take over the role of pacemaker either because it usurps control from the sinus node by accelerating its own automaticity (enhanced automaticity) or because the sinus node relinquishes its role by decreasing its automaticity. The rate of sinus node firing is altered by:
  1. *Changes in autonomic nerve activity (sympathetic and parasympathetic)*—Stimulation of the sympathetic nervous system releases norepinephrine, which increases heart rate. Stimulation of the parasympathetic nervous system releases acetylcholine, which decreases heart rate.
  2. *Circulating hormones*—Pacemaker activity is also altered by hormones. For example, an increase in thyroid hormone induces tachycardia and a decrease in thyroid hormone induces bradycardia.
  3. *Serum ion concentration*—Changes in the serum concentration of ions, particularly potassium, can cause changes in the SA node firing rate. An increase in serum potassium can cause bradycardia whereas a decrease in serum potassium can cause tachycardia.
  4. *Cellular hypoxia*—Cellular hypoxia (usually caused by ischemia) can cause bradycardia. Severe hypoxia can completely stop pacemaker activity.
  5. *Drugs*—Various drugs can also affect SA node activity. Some examples include digitalis, calcium-channel blockers, and beta-blockers.
- **Triggered Activity**—Triggered activity results from abnormal electrical impulses that occur during repolarization when cells are normally quiet. The ectopic pacemaker cells may depolarize more than once after stimulation by a single electrical impulse. Triggered activity may result in atrial, junctional, or ventricular beats occurring singly, in pairs, in runs (3 or more beats), or as a sustained ectopic rhythm. Causes of triggered activity include myocardial ischemia and injury, cellular hypoxia, excessive catecholamine stimulation, digitalis toxicity, and a prolonged QT interval.
- **Reentry**—Normally, an impulse spreads through the heart only once. With reentry, an impulse can travel through an area of myocardium, depolarize it, and then reenter that same area to depolarize it again. Reentry involves a circular movement of the impulse, which continues as long as it encounters receptive cells. Reentry (like triggered activity) may result in atrial, junctional, or ventricular beats occurring singly, in pairs, in runs, or as a sustained ectopic rhythm. Myocardial ischemia is a common cause of reentry. Another cause of the reentry mechanism is the presence of an accessory conduction pathway between the atria and ventricles.

Overview

Atrial arrhythmias (Figure 7.1) originate from ectopic sites in the atria. Ectopic P waves from the atria (Figure 7.2) differ in morphology (size, shape, or direction) from the normal sinus P waves. For example, in slower atrial rhythms (premature atrial contractions, wandering atrial pacemaker), the P wave may appear as a small, pointed, and upright waveform or a small squiggle that is barely visible, or it may be inverted. In faster atrial rhythms, the ectopic P wave is superimposed on the preceding T wave (atrial tachycardia); appears in a sawtooth pattern (atrial flutter); or is seen as a wavy baseline (atrial fibrillation).

Some atrial arrhythmias may be associated with rapid ventricular rates. Increases in heart rate decrease the length of time spent in diastole. If diastole is shortened, there is less time for coronary artery perfusion and less time for adequate ventricular filling. Thus, an excessively rapid heart rate may lead to myocardial ischemia and may compromise cardiac output.

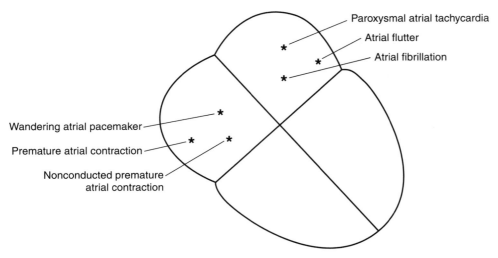

Figure 7.1 Atrial arrhythmias.

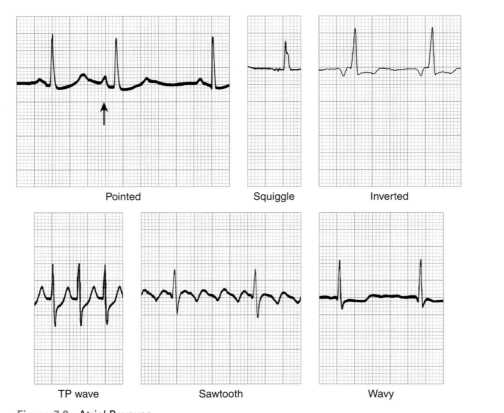

Figure 7.2 Atrial P waves.

Wandering Atrial Pacemaker

Wandering atrial pacemaker (WAP) (Figure 7.3 and Box 7.1) occurs when the pacemaker site shifts back and forth between the sinus node and ectopic atrial sites. The P-wave morphology will vary across the rhythm strip as the pacemaker "wanders" between the multiple sites. The ectopic P wave may appear as a small, pointed, and upright waveform or as a small squiggle that is barely visible, or it may be inverted if the impulse originates from a site in the lower atrium near the AV junction. Generally, at least three different P-wave morphologies should be identified before making the diagnosis of WAP.

The heart rate is usually normal, but may be slow. The rhythm may be regular or irregular (each impulse travels through the atria via a slightly different route). The PR interval is usually normal, but may be abnormal because of the different sites of impulse formation. The QRS complex is normal in duration. The distinguishing feature of this rhythm is the changing P-wave morphology across the rhythm strip.

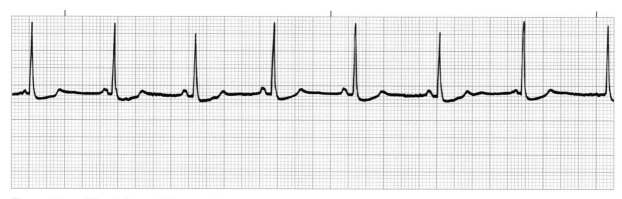

Figure 7.3   **Wandering atrial pacemaker.**

Rhythm:	Irregular
Rate:	60 beats/minute
P waves:	Vary in size, shape, across rhythm strip
PR interval:	0.08 to 0.12 second
QRS complex:	0.04 to 0.08 second.

---

box 7.1	**Wandering Atrial Pacemaker:** **Identifying ECG Features**
Rhythm:	Regular or irregular
Rate:	Usually normal (60 to 100 beats/minute) but may be slow (less than 60 beats/minute)
P waves:	Vary in size, shape, and direction across rhythm strip; one P wave precedes each QRS complex
PR interval:	Usually normal duration, but may be abnormal depending on changing pacemaker location
QRS complex:	Normal (0.10 second or less)

WAP is usually seen as a result of increased vagal effect on the SA node, slowing the sinus rate and allowing other pacemaker sites an opportunity to compete for control of the heart rate. WAP is also seen in the very young, in the very old, and in athletes, and can manifest itself during a person's normal sleep cycle. It may also be caused by the administration of digitalis.

WAP isn't clinically significant, and treatment is not indicated. If the heart rate is slow, medications should be reviewed and discontinued if possible. If the heart rate is slow and the patient is symptomatic, treatment of the rhythm is the same as for symptomatic sinus bradycardia.

When WAP is associated with a heart rate greater than 100 beats per minute, the rhythm is called *multifocal atrial tachycardia* (MAT) (Figure 7.4). MAT is a relatively infrequent arrhythmia and is most commonly observed with lung disorders such as chronic obstructive pulmonary disease (COPD).

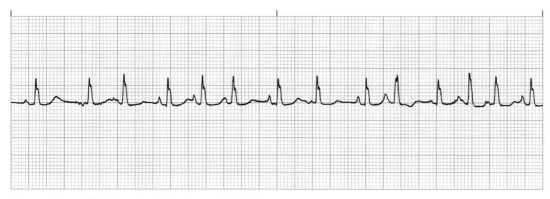

Figure 7.4   **Multifocal atrial tachycardia (MAT).**

Rhythm:	Irregular
Rate:	140 beats/minute
P waves:	Vary in size, shape, and direction across rhythm strip
PR interval:	0.08 to 0.12 second
QRS complex:	0.04 to 0.08 second.

Premature Atrial Contraction

A premature atrial contraction (PAC) (Figures 7.5 through 7.14 and Box 7.2) is an early beat originating from an ectopic pacemaker site in the atria. The early beat interrupts the regularity of the basic rhythm, which is usually a sinus rhythm. PACs may originate from a single ectopic site in the atria having the same appearance, or from multiple pacemaker sites in the atria having a different appearance. The premature beat occurs in addition to the underlying rhythm. A PAC is not an entire rhythm—it is a single beat. Therefore, it is important to identify the underlying rhythm along with the premature ectopic beat (for example, normal sinus rhythm [NSR] with a PAC). The premature beat is characterized by a premature, abnormal P wave followed by a normal duration QRS and a pause.

P-wave morphology differs from sinus beats and varies depending on the origin of the impulse in the atria. If the ectopic focus is in the vicinity of the SA node, the P wave may closely resemble the sinus P wave (see Figure 7.5). Its sole distinguishing feature may be its prematurity. As a rule, however, the P wave is different from the sinus P waves. In lead II (a positive lead) it's generally upright and pointed (see Figure 7.6), or it may be inverted (see Figure 7.7) if the pacemaker site is near the AV junction. If the premature beat occurs very early, the abnormal P wave can be found hidden in the preceding T wave, causing a distortion of the T-wave contour (see Figure 7.8). When P waves are not easily seen, it is important to compare the T waves preceding each PAC with those of the underlying rhythm. If the contour of the T wave preceding the PAC is different (taller or different in shape) from the underlying rhythm, there is a hidden P wave in it. This occurs commonly with PACs.

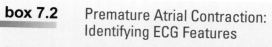

box 7.2	Premature Atrial Contraction: Identifying ECG Features
Rhythm:	Underlying rhythm usually regular; irregular with PACs
Rate:	That of underlying rhythm
P waves:	P wave associated with PAC is premature and abnormal in size, shape, and direction (commonly appears small, upright, and pointed; may be inverted); abnormal P wave commonly found hidden in preceding T wave, distorting the T-wave contour
PR interval:	Usually normal duration; not measurable if hidden in T wave
QRS complex:	Premature; normal duration (0.10 second or less)

The PR intervals of the PACs are usually normal, similar to those of the underlying rhythm. Occasionally the PR interval may be prolonged if the PAC is very early and finds the AV junction still partially refractory and unable to conduct at a normal rate (see Figure 7.9). The PR interval will be unmeasurable if the abnormal P wave is obscured in the preceding T wave (see Figure 7.8).

The QRS of the PAC usually resembles that of the underlying rhythm because the impulse is conducted normally through the bundle branches into the ventricles. The ventricles depolarize simultaneously, resulting in a normal duration QRS complex. If the PAC occurs very early, it is possible the bundle branches may not be repolarized sufficiently to conduct the premature electrical impulse normally. If the bundle branches are not sufficiently repolarized, the electrical impulse is conducted

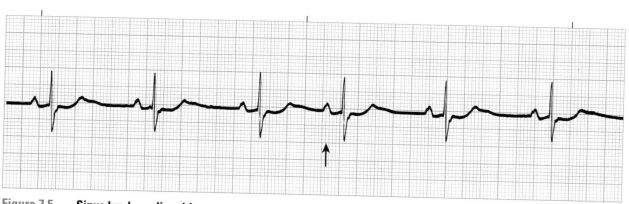

Figure 7.5   **Sinus bradycardia with premature atrial contraction (PAC).**

Rhythm:	Basic rhythm regular; irregular with PAC
Rate:	Basic rhythm rate 50 beats/minute
P waves:	Sinus P waves with basic rhythm; P wave associated with PAC is premature and closely resembles that of the sinus P waves in the underlying rhythm, indicating the ectopic atrial pacemaker site is close to the SA node.
PR interval:	0.20 second (basic rhythm and PAC)
QRS complex:	0.06 to 0.08 second (basic rhythm); 0.06 second (PAC).

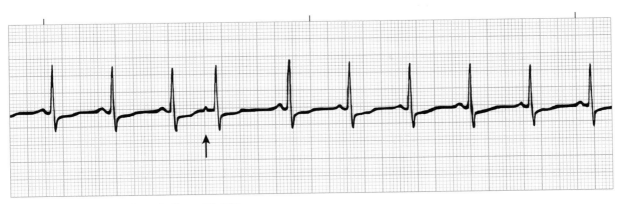

Figure 7.6   Normal sinus rhythm with PAC.

Rhythm: Basic rhythm regular; rhythm with PAC
Rate: Basic rhythm rate 88 beats/minute
P waves: Sinus P waves with basic rhythm; small, pointed P wave with PAC
PR interval: 0.12 to 0.16 second (basic rhythm); 0.12 second (PAC)
QRS complex: 0.08 second (basic rhythm and PAC).

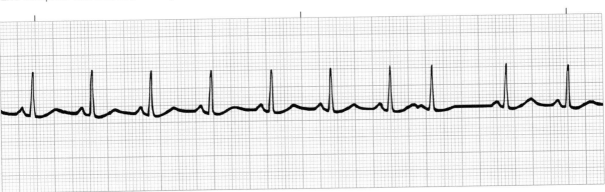

Figure 7.7   Normal sinus rhythm with premature atrial contraction.

Rhythm: Basic rhythm regular; irregular with PAC
Rate: Basic rhythm rate 88 beats/minute
P waves: Sinus P waves with basic rhythm; premature, inverted P wave with PAC
PR interval: 0.14 to 0.16 second (basic rhythm); 0.16 second (PAC)
QRS complex: 0.04 to 0.08 second (basic rhythm); 0.04 second (PAC).

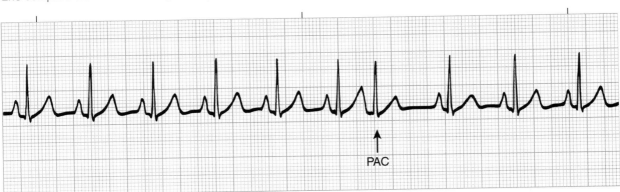

Figure 7.8   Normal sinus rhythm with premature atrial contraction.

Rhythm: Basic rhythm regular; irregular with PAC
Rate: Basic rhythm rate 84 beats/minute
P waves: Sinus P waves with basic rhythm; premature, abnormal P wave with PAC. The P wave of the PAC is hidden in the preceding T wave distorting the T-wave contour (T wave is taller and more pointed.)
PR interval: 0.12 to 0.14 second (basic rhythm)
QRS complex: 0.08 (basic rhythm); 0.04 second (PAC).

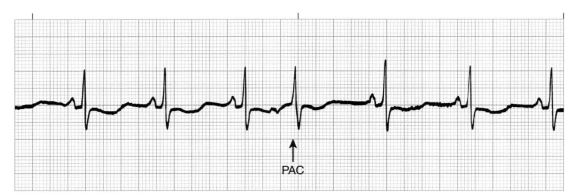

Figure 7.9 **Normal sinus rhythm 1 PAC with aberrant ventricular conduction.**

Rhythm: Basic rhythm regular; irregular with PAC
Rate: Basic rhythm rate 68 beats/minute
P waves: Sinus in basic rhythm; premature, abnormal P wave with PAC
PR interval: 0.16 to 0.20 second (basic rhythm); 0.24 second (PAC)
QRS complex: 0.08 to 0.10 second (basic rhythm); 0.12 second (PAC).

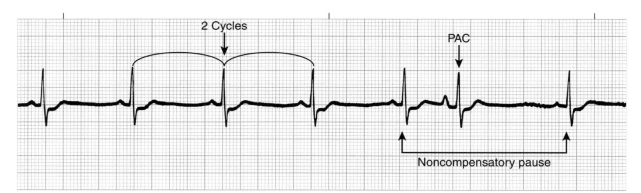

Figure 7.10 **Normal sinus rhythm premature atrial contraction.**

Rhythm: Basic rhythm regular; irregular with PAC
Rate: Basic rhythm rate 60 beats/minute
P waves: Sinus P waves with basic rhythm; premature, abnormal P wave with PAC
PR interval: 0.12 to 0.16 second (basic rhythm); 0.16 second (PAC)
QRS complex: 0.08 second (basic rhythm and PAC)
Comment: To determine the type of pause following premature beats, measure from the QRS preceding the premature beat to the QRS following the premature beat. If the measurement equals two R-R intervals, the pause is compensatory. If the measurement is less than two R-R intervals, the pause is noncompensatory. ST segment depression is present.

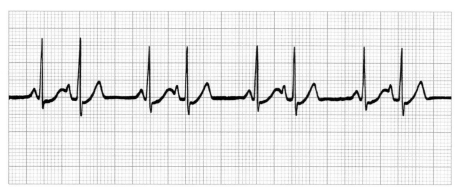

Figure 7.11 Bigeminal PACs.

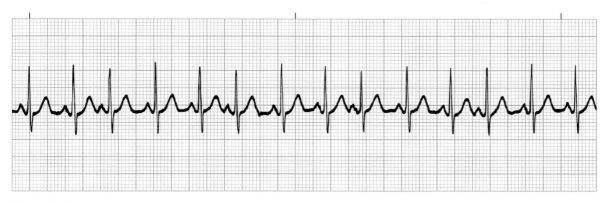

Figure 7.12   Trigeminal PACs.

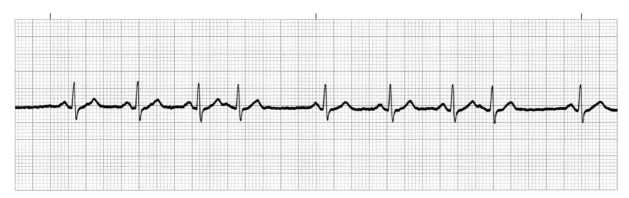

Figure 7.13   Quadrigeminal PACs.

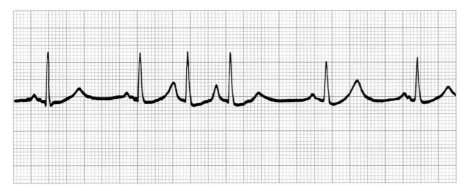

Figure 7.14   Paired PACs.

down one bundle branch (usually the left because it depolarizes quicker) and not conducted down the other. The left ventricle is depolarized first, followed by depolarization of the right ventricle (sequential depolarization). Sequential ventricular depolarization is slower, resulting in a wide QRS complex of 0.12 second or greater. A PAC

associated with a wide QRS complex is called a PAC with aberrancy, indicating that conduction through the ventricles is abnormal (aberrant). Figure 7.9 shows a PAC with aberrant ventricular conduction (QRS is wide) and a long PR interval, indicating that conduction through the AV node was also delayed. Aberrantly conducted PACs must be differentiated from a premature ventricular contraction [PVC]), especially if the abnormal P wave associated with the PAC is hidden in the preceding T wave. PVCs are discussed in Chapter 9.

The pause associated with the PAC is usually a *noncompensatory pause* (the measurement from the R wave before the premature beat to the R wave after the premature beat is less than two R-R intervals of the underlying regular rhythm (see Figure 7.10). This pause is called an incomplete pause because it doesn't equal two R-R intervals. Less commonly, the PAC may occur with a *compensatory pause* (a pause that is equal to two R-R intervals), but this is usually seen with the PVC. The compensatory pause is called a compete pause because it equals two R-R intervals. To differentiate between a complete pause and an incomplete pause, the underlying rhythm must be regular. Rarely, the PAC may occur with a pause that is longer than compensatory.

PACs may appear as a single beat (see Figure 7.10), as every other beat (bigeminal PACs, see Figure 7.11), as every third beat (trigeminal PACs, see Figure 7.12), as every fourth beat (quadrigeminal PACs, Figure 7.13), in pairs (also called couplets, see Figure 7.14), or in runs of three or more. Frequent PACs may initiate more serious atrial arrhythmias, such as paroxysmal atrial tachycardia (PAT), atrial flutter, or atrial fibrillation. Three or more beats of PACs in a row at a rate of 140 to 250 beats per minute constitute a run of PAT.

Premature atrial beats are common. They can occur in individuals with a normal heart or in those with heart disease. PACs may be seen with emotional stress (caused by an increase in sympathetic tone), or ingestion of certain substances such as alcohol, caffeine, or tobacco. Other causes include hypoxia, electrolyte imbalances, myocardial ischemia or injury, atrial enlargement, congestive heart failure, and the administration of certain drugs, such as epinephrine or norepinephrine that increase sympathetic tone. PACs may also occur without apparent cause.

Infrequent PACs require no treatment. Frequent PACs are treated by correcting the underlying cause: reducing stress; reducing or eliminating the consumption of alcohol, caffeine, or tobacco; administering oxygen; correcting electrolyte imbalances; treating congestive heart failure, or discontinuing certain drugs. If needed, frequent PACs may be treated with beta-blockers, calcium channel blockers, or antianxiety medications. Runs of PACs may require amiodarone to prevent more serious atrial arrhythmias from developing.

Occasionally an ectopic atrial beat will occur late instead of early. This beat is called an *atrial escape beat* (Figure 7.15). Atrial escape beats usually occur during a pause in the underlying rhythm (following sinus arrest or block, after premature beats, or during the pause associated with Mobitz I heart block). The pause in the rhythm allows an ectopic pacemaker site in the atria to assume control of the heartbeat. The morphologic characteristics of the late beat will be the same as the PAC. Escape beats act as an electrical backup to maintain the heart rate and require no treatment.

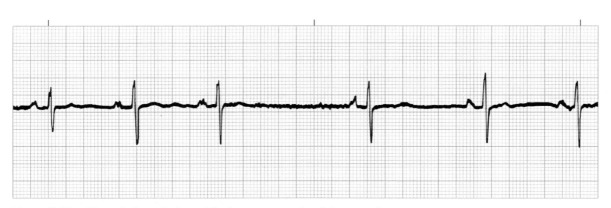

Figure 7.15   Normal sinus rhythm with sinus arrest and atrial escape beat.

Rhythm:	Basic rhythm regular; irregular during pause
Rate:	Basic rhythm rate 63 beats/minute—rate slows to 58 after pause owing to temporary rate suppression (common following pauses in the basic rhythm)
P waves:	Sinus P waves; P waves are notched in basic rhythm, which could be caused by left atrial enlargement; peaked P wave with escape beat
PR interval:	0.18 to 0.20 second basic rhythm and escape beat
QRS complex:	0.06 to 0.08 second (basic rhythm); 0.06 second (escape beat).

Nonconducted PAC

A nonconducted PAC (Figures 7.16 through 7.18 and Box 7.3) results when an ectopic atrial focus occurs so early that it finds the AV node refractory and the impulse isn't conducted to the ventricles. This results in a premature, abnormal P wave not accompanied by a QRS complex, but followed by a pause (Figure 7.16).

Like the conducted PAC, the P wave associated with the nonconducted PAC will be premature and abnormal in size, shape, or direction. The P wave is commonly found hidden in the preceding T wave, distorting the T-wave contour (see Figure 7.17), and the pause that follows is usually

box 7.3 Nonconducted PACs: Identifying ECG Features

Rhythm:	Underlying rhythm usually regular; irregular with nonconducted PACs
Rate:	That of underlying rhythm
P waves:	P wave associated with the nonconducted PAC is premature, and abnormal in size, shape, or direction; often found hidden in preceding T wave, distorting the T-wave contour
PR interval:	Absent with nonconducted PAC
QRS complex:	Absent with nonconducted PAC

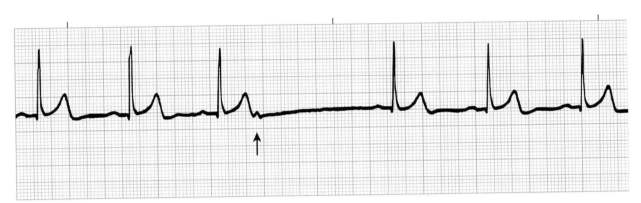

Figure 7.16   Normal sinus rhythm with nonconducted PAC.

Rhythm:	Basic rhythm regular; irregular with nonconducted PAC
Rate:	Basic rhythm rate 60 beats/minute; rate slows following nonconducted PAC; rate suppression can occur following a pause in the basic rhythm. After several cycles, the rate will return to the basic rhythm rate.
P waves:	Sinus P waves with basic rhythm; premature, abnormal P wave with nonconducted PAC
PR interval:	0.20 second with basic rhythm
QRS complex:	0.06 to 0.08 second with basic rhythm
Comment:	A U wave is present

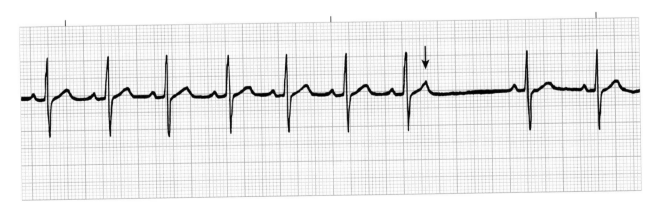

Figure 7.17   Normal sinus rhythm with nonconducted PAC.

Rhythm:	Basic rhythm regular; irregular with nonconducted PACs
Rate:	Basic rhythm rate 88 beats/minute
P waves:	Sinus P waves with basic rhythm; P wave of nonconducted PAC is premature, abnormal, and hidden in the preceding T wave (T wave is taller and more pointed than those of underlying rhythm)
PR interval:	0.16 to 0.18 second (basic rhythm); not present with nonconducted PAC
QRS complex:	0.06 to 0.08 (basic rhythm); not present with nonconducted PAC

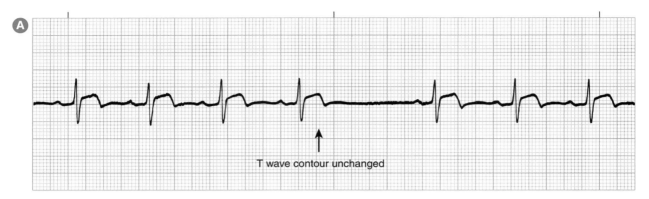

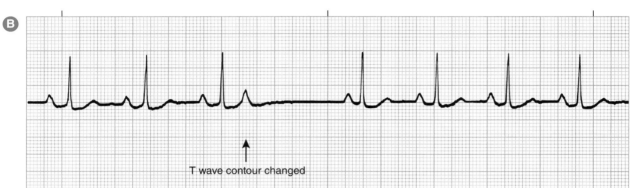

Figure 7.18   Differentiation of sinus arrest or block from the nonconducted premature atrial contraction (PAC).

A. Sinus arrest or block
   1. Sudden pause in the basic rhythm
   2. No P wave present
   3. T-wave contour occurring during pause remains unchanged
B. Nonconducted PAC
   1. Sudden pause in the basic rhythm
   2. Abnormal, premature P wave present and often found hidden in T wave
   3. T-wave contour occurring during pause will be different from the contours of the basic rhythm.

noncompensatory. The nonconducted PAC is the most common cause of unexpected pauses in a regular sinus rhythm.

The nonconducted PAC can be confused with sinus arrest or block (especially if the P wave of the PAC occurs early enough to be hidden in the preceding T wave). All three rhythms produce a sudden pause in the rhythm without QRS complexes. To differentiate between these rhythms, one must examine and compare T-wave contours (see Figure 7.18). The early, abnormal P wave of the nonconducted PAC will distort the preceding T wave. In sinus arrest or sinus block, no P wave is produced and the T-wave contour remains unchanged.

Nonconducted PACs have the same significance as do conducted PACs and may be treated in the same manner.

Paroxysmal Atrial Tachycardia

Paroxysmal atrial tachycardia (PAT) (Figures 7.19 through 7.21 and Box 7.4) originates in an ectopic pacemaker site in the atria producing a rapid, regular atrial rhythm between 140 and 250 beats per minute. Atrial tachycardia

is often precipitated by a PAC and commonly starts and stops abruptly, occurring in bursts or paroxysms (thus the name paroxysmal atrial tachycardia). The rhythm may be continuous (see Figure 7.19) or intermittent. By definition, three or more consecutive PACs (at a rate of 140 to 250 beats per minute) is considered to be atrial tachycardia (see Figure 7.20).

box 7.4	Atrial Tachycardia: Identifying ECG Features
Rhythm:	Regular
Rate:	140 to 250 beats/minute
P waves:	Abnormal (commonly pointed); usually hidden in preceding T wave, making T wave and P wave appear as one wave deflection (T-P wave); one P wave to each QRS complex unless AV block is present.
PR interval:	Usually not measurable
QRS complex:	Normal (0.10 second or less)

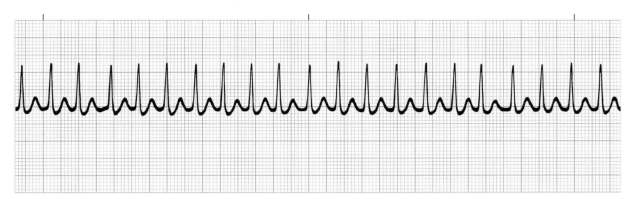

Figure 7.19 **Paroxysmal atrial tachycardia.**

Rhythm: Regular
Rate: 188
P waves: Hidden
PR interval: Not measurable
QRS complex: 0.04 to 0.08 second.

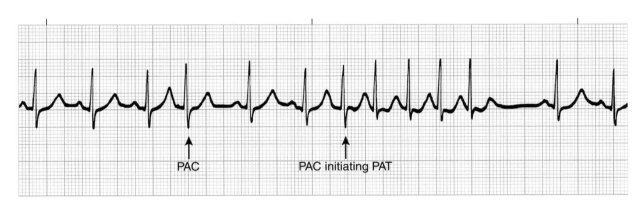

PAC   PAC initiating PAT

Figure 7.20 **Normal sinus rhythm with PAC and burst of PAT.**

Rhythm: Basic rhythm regular; irregular with PAC and burst of PAT
Rate: Basic rhythm rate 94 beats/minute; PAT rate (167)
P waves: Sinus P waves with basic rhythm; premature, pointed P waves with PAC and PAT (P waves are superimposed on preceding T waves)
PR interval: 0.16 second (basic rhythm)
QRS complex: 0.08 second (basic rhythm, PAC, and PAT)
Comment: A run of three or more consecutive PACs is considered PAT.

The P waves associated with PAT are abnormal (often pointed), but may be difficult to identify because they're usually hidden in the preceding T wave (the T and P wave appear as one deflection called the T-P wave). One P wave precedes each QRS complex, unless AV block is present. The PR interval is usually not measurable. The duration of the QRS complex is normal. Atrial tachycardia is characterized by regular, narrow QRS complexes, occurring at a rate of 140 to 250 beats per minute, and separated by the T-P wave.

This rhythm is usually caused by a single ectopic focus in the atria. The underlying mechanism of this rhythm can involve enhanced automaticity of atrial pacemaker cells, resulting in rapid firing of an ectopic atrial focus; an atrial reentry circuit in which an impulse travels rapidly and repeatedly around a circular pathway in the atria; or triggered activity during repolarization when ectopic atrial

impulses fire more than once in response to a single electrical stimulus.

Atrial tachycardia may occur in people with healthy hearts as well as those with diseased hearts. It is more common in women, but may occur in either sex. It is the most common arrhythmia in children. Atrial tachycardia has been associated with ingestion of substances such as caffeine, alcohol, or tobacco; anxiety; fatigue; electrolyte imbalances; lung disease; congenital heart disease; digitalis toxicity; atrial scarring following heart surgery; hyperthyroidism; and unknown causes.

During an episode of atrial tachycardia, many individuals can feel the *palpitations* (rapid heart rate), and this is a source of anxiety. When the ventricular rate is rapid, the ventricles are unable to fill completely during diastole, resulting in a significant reduction in cardiac output.

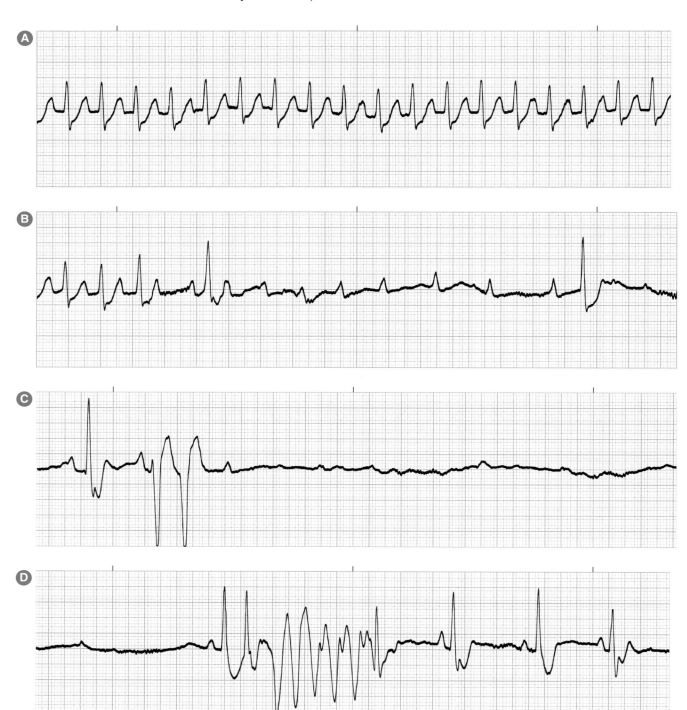

Figure 7.21   Continuous monitor tracing of a patient in PAT who received adenosine.

A. Strip shows PAT.

B. Strip shows PAT followed by a sinus beat, changing to P waves with no QRS complexes (ventricular standstill), followed by one normal duration QRS complex at end of strip.

C. Strip shows a sinus beat followed by paired PVCs changing again to ventricular standstill.

D. Strip shows a sinus beat, followed by a narrow QRS complex, changing to a 5-beat run of ventricular tachycardia, with conversion to NSR at end of strip.

In addition, a rapid heart rate increases myocardial oxygen requirements and cardiac workload. Treatment of atrial tachycardia is directed toward controlling the ventricular rate and converting the rhythm.

Priorities of treatment depend on the patient's tolerance of the rhythm. *Cardioversion* (synchronized electrical shock) is the initial treatment of choice in patients whose condition is unstable (systolic blood pressure less than 90 mm Hg; cool, clammy skin; reduced consciousness or cognitive function; reduced urine output; complaints of chest pain or dyspnea; or exhibits signs of heart failure). If the patient's condition is stable, sedation alone may terminate the rhythm or slow the heart rate. If sedation is unsuccessful, vagal maneuvers may terminate some episodes of PAT. Vagal maneuvers work by slowing the heart rate through increasing parasympathetic tone. Vagal maneuvers include coughing, bearing down (the Valsalva maneuver), squatting, breath-holding, carotid sinus pressure, stimulation of the gag reflex, and immersion of the face in ice water. If vagal maneuvers fail, administer a 6-mg bolus of adenosine IV rapidly over 1 to 2 seconds, followed by a rapid 10-mL flush of saline. If the initial dose is ineffective after 2 minutes, administer a 12-mg bolus of adenosine IV rapidly over 1 to 2 seconds, followed by a rapid 10-mL flush of saline. If the second dose is ineffective after 2 minutes, repeat a 12-mg dose of adenosine in the same manner. The administration of adenosine can cause some serious arrhythmias for a brief period of time (half-life of drug is 30 seconds) before conversion to NSR. The patient must be attached to a cardiac monitor with emergency drugs available. Figure 7.21 shows a continuous monitor tracing of a patient in PAT who received adenosine.

If the patient doesn't respond to vagal maneuvers or to the administration of three doses of adenosine, attempt rate control using a calcium channel blocker (such as diltiazem) or a beta-blocker. These drugs act primarily on AV nodal tissue, either to slow the ventricular response by blocking conduction through the AV node or to terminate the reentry mechanism that depends on conduction through the AV node. In the setting of significantly impaired left ventricular (LV) function (clinical evidence of congestive heart failure or moderately to severely reduced LV ejection fraction), caution should be exercised in administering drugs with negative inotropic effects. These include beta-blockers and calcium channel blockers, with the exception of diltiazem (a calcium channel blocker that exhibits less depression of contractility when compared with similar drugs).

When AV nodal agents are unsuccessful, cardioversion should be used to terminate the rhythm. Once the rhythm is terminated, antiarrhythmics may be effective in controlling the rhythm. For recurrent atrial tachycardia, radiofrequency catheter ablation of the ectopic focus or reentry circuit is successful in many cases.

Atrial Flutter

Atrial flutter (Figures 7.22 through 7.24 and Box 7.5) originates in an ectopic pacemaker site in the atria typically depolarizing at a rate between 250 and 400 beats per minute (the average rate is around 300 beats per minute). The atrial muscles respond to this rapid stimulation by producing V-shaped waveforms resembling the teeth of a saw. The sawtooth waveforms are called flutter waves (F waves). It is easier to count the number of flutter waves between QRS complexes if you put the tip of a pencil at the end of a QRS and count each downward "V" as a flutter wave, including the "V" going into the QRS complex (see Figure 7.22).

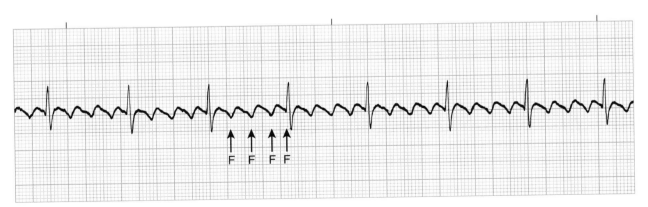

Figure 7.22   Atrial flutter with 4:1 AV conduction.

Rhythm:	Regular
Rate:	Atrial: 272 beats/minute
Ventricular:	68 beats/minute
	Note: If the ventricular rhythm is regular, multiply the number of flutter waves before each QRS by the ventricular rate to determine the atrial rate.
P waves:	Four flutter waves before each QRS (marked in the "V" of the sawtooth waves above)
PR interval:	Not measurable
QRS complex:	0.08 to 0.10 second.

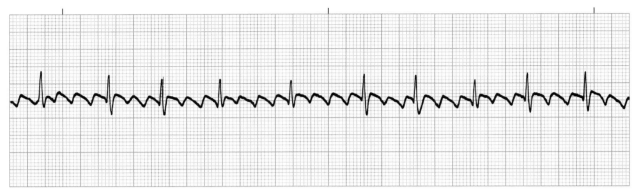

Figure 7.23   Atrial flutter with variable AV conduction.

Rhythm:	Irregular
Rate:	Atrial: 290 beats/minute
Ventricular:	90 beats/minute
	Note: If the ventricular rhythm is irregular, count the number of flutter waves in a 6-second strip and multiply by 10 to obtain atrial rate.
P waves:	Flutter waves before each QRS in varying ratios
PR interval:	Not measurable
QRS complex:	0.08 second.

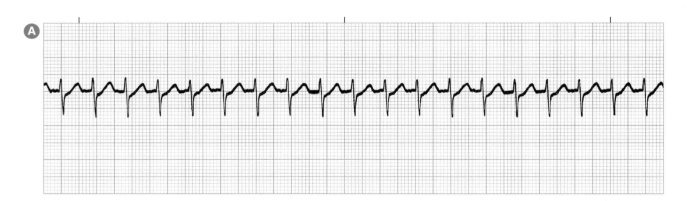

Figure 7.24   Comparison of atrial flutter with 2:1 AV conduction and paroxysmal atrial tachycardia (PAT).

A. The rhythm shows PAT. This strip shows the T-P wave (the T and P waves appear as one deflection). An isoelectric line is present after the T-P wave.

B. The rhythm shows atrial flutter with 2:1 AV conduction. This strip shows two flutter (sawtooth) waves before each QRS complex. There is no isoelectric line.

---

box 7.5	Atrial Flutter: Identifying ECG Features
Rhythm:	Regular to irregular (depends on AV conduction ratios)
Rate:	Atrial rate: 250 to 400 beats/minute Ventricular rate: Varies with number of impulses conducted through AV node (will be less than the atrial rate)
P waves:	Sawtooth deflections called flutter waves (F waves) affecting entire baseline
PR interval:	Not measurable
QRS complex:	Normal (0.10 second or less)

The flutter waves affect the whole baseline to such a degree that there is no isoelectric line between the F waves, and the T wave is partially or completely obscured by the flutter waves. Atrial flutter is primarily recognized by this sawtooth baseline. The PR interval is not measurable. The QRS complexes are normal.

Although the atria can tolerate the extremely high heart rate reasonably well, the lower chambers (ventricles) cannot. Fortunately, the AV node is present to slow down and diminish the number of impulses that pass through to the ventricles. The AV node conducts the impulses in various ratios. For example, the AV node might allow every second impulse to travel through the AV junction to the ventricles, resulting in a 2:1 AV conduction ratio (a 2:1 conduction ratio indicates that for every two flutter waves, only one is followed by a QRS complex). Even ratios (2:1, 4:1) are more common than odd ratios (3:1, 5:1). If the conduction ratio remains constant (for example, 2:1), the ventricular rhythm will be regular and the rhythm is described as atrial flutter with 2:1 AV conduction. If the conduction ratio varies (for example, from 4:1 to 3:1 to 5:1), the ventricular rhythm will be irregular, and the rhythm is described as atrial flutter with variable AV conduction. Conduction ratios are shown in Figures 7.22 and 7.23. In atrial flutter, the ventricular rate is slower than the atrial rate, with the rate depending on the number of impulses conducted through the AV node to the ventricles.

Because atrial flutter usually occurs at a rate of 300 beats/minute and the AV node usually blocks at least half of these impulses, a ventricular rate of 150 beats per minute is common (a 2:1 AV conduction ratio). Atrial flutter with 2:1 AV conduction may be difficult to differentiate from atrial tachycardia, especially if the heart rate in both rhythms is around 150 beats per minute. These two arrhythmias can be differentiated by closely examining the baseline. In atrial tachycardia, an isoelectric line can usually be seen, whereas in atrial flutter the isoelectric line is absent. A comparison of atrial flutter with 2:1 AV conduction and PAT is shown in Figure 7.24.

Atrial flutter typically originates from the right atrium and most often involves a large reentry circuit that travels around the area of the tricuspid valve. This type of atrial flutter is referred to as typical atrial flutter. Less commonly, atrial flutter can result from circuits in other areas of the right or left atrium (atypical atrial flutter). Atrial flutter is more common in men than women.

Atrial flutter is rarely seen in patients with normal hearts. This rhythm may be seen in patients with heart failure; decreased blood flow to the heart related to ischemia; cardiomyopathy; abnormalities of the heart valves, especially the mitral and tricuspid valves; septal defects of the heart; and following heart surgery. It is also seen in hypertension, hyperthyroidism, pulmonary embolism, older age, and chronic lung disease such as COPD. Substances that may contribute to development of atrial flutter include alcohol (especially binge drinking) and stimulants such as cocaine, amphetamines, diet pills, cold medicines, and caffeine. In a few people, no underlying cause is ever found.

Like PAT, the ventricular rate in atrial flutter may be rapid, increasing myocardial oxygen requirements and cardiac workload and decreasing cardiac output. In addition, the atria do not contract strongly enough to empty all the blood from the atrial chambers into the ventricles. This results in a loss of the atrial kick, which further decreases cardiac output. Over time, some blood in the atria may stagnate and mural thrombi (clots in the atrial chambers) may form. Pieces of the clot may break off, leading to a risk of systemic or pulmonary emboli.

Priorities of treatment include controlling the ventricular rate, assessing anticoagulation needs, and restoring sinus rhythm. As with PAT, controlling the ventricular rate should be attempted first using a calcium channel blocker (such as diltiazem) or a beta-blocker, using caution in those patients with impaired LV function. Before attempting conversion of the rhythm, it's essential to know the approximate onset of the arrhythmia. If atrial flutter has been present less than 48 hours, it's safe to convert the rhythm with cardioversion or amiodarone. If atrial flutter has been present for more than 48 hours (or the onset is unknown), pulmonary or systemic embolization with conversion to sinus rhythm is a risk unless the patient has been adequately anticoagulated. In this situation, attempts to convert the rhythm with cardioversion or an antiarrhythmic should be delayed until the patient is adequately anticoagulated.

One method of anticoagulation involves placing the patient on an oral anticoagulant at home for several weeks and then admitting the patient to the hospital for a transesophageal echocardiogram (TEE). If the TEE is negative for atrial clots, the patient can safely have the rhythm electrically cardioverted. The patient is then discharged home on an oral anticoagulant for several more weeks. Some physicians prefer a quicker approach, using IV heparin or subcutaneous Lovenox in a hospital setting. If the TEE is negative for mural thrombi, cardioversion may be attempted within 24 hours. The patient is discharged home on an oral anticoagulant for several weeks.

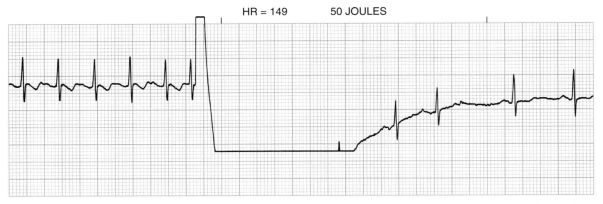

Figure 7.25   Cardioversion of atrial flutter with 2:1 atrioventricular conduction to normal sinus rhythm using 50 J electrical energy.

Unstable atrial flutter should be treated immediately with cardioversion, regardless of the duration of the arrhythmia. Figure 7.25 is an example of atrial flutter converting to sinus rhythm after cardioversion.

Atrial flutter is considerably more sensitive to cardioversion than atrial fibrillation, and usually requires a lower energy shock. Some cardiologists recommend an initial synchronized shock with 100 J, because it is nearly always successful in converting atrial flutter. When cardioversion is successful, the rate of recurrence is high even if the individual is taking a drug to prevent recurrence. Radiofrequency catheter ablation of the flutter reentry circuit is becoming the treatment of choice for recurrent atrial flutter. During the ablation procedure, a catheter is advanced through veins into the right atrium. Radiofrequency energy is delivered through the catheter to cauterize ("burn") a small area of cardiac muscle, creating a scar that disrupts the reentry circuit. The procedure is typically done under conscious sedation, and the patient can usually go home the same day or after a brief overnight stay.

Atrial Fibrillation

Atrial fibrillation (Figures 7.26 through 7.28 and Box 7.6) is a rapid and highly irregular heart rhythm caused by chaotic electrical impulses that arise from multiple ectopic sites in the atria, depolarizing at a rate greater than 400 beats per minute. These impulses are so rapid that they cause the atria to quiver instead of contracting regularly, producing irregular, wavy deflections. These deflections are called fibrillatory waves (f waves). If the waves are large, they're described as coarse fibrillatory waves and if small they're called fine fibrillatory waves. As in atrial flutter, the wavy deflections seen in atrial fibrillation affect the whole baseline. In atrial fibrillation, an actual atrial rate is not measurable. The PR interval is also not measurable. The QRS complex is normal. Because the atrial impulses occur irregularly, the ventricular response will be irregular also. Atrial fibrillation is primarily recognized by the wavy baseline between QRS complexes and the grossly irregular ventricular rhythm (see Figure 7.26). If the ventricular rate is very rapid, the

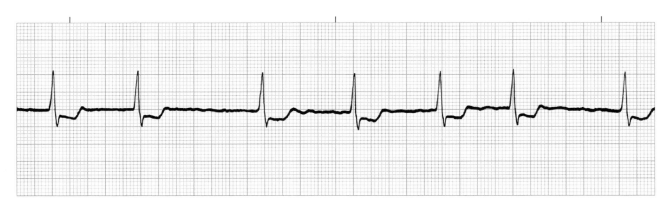

Figure 7.26   Atrial fibrillation (controlled rate).

Rhythm:	Irregular
Rate:	Atrial: Not measurable
Ventricular:	50 beats/minute
P waves:	Fibrillatory waves present
PR interval:	Not measurable
QRS complex:	0.10 second.

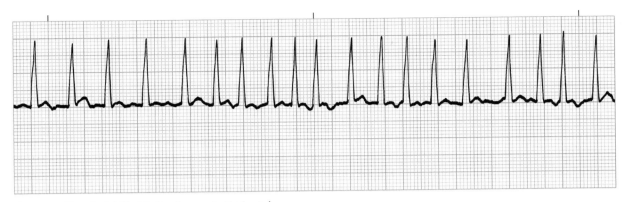

Figure 7.27   Atrial fibrillation (uncontrolled rate).

Rhythm: Irregular
Rate: Atrial: not measurable
Ventricular: 170 beats/minute
P waves: Fibrillatory waves present
PR interval: Not measurable
QRS complex: 0.08 second.

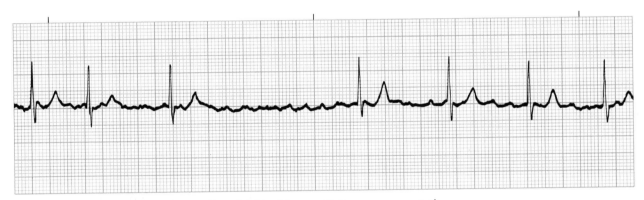

Figure 7.28   Atrial fib-flutter (basically atrial fib with some flutter waves present).

Rhythm: Irregular
Rate: Atrial: Not measurable
Ventricular: 50 beats/minute
P waves: Fibrillatory and flutter waves present
PR interval: Not measurable
QRS complex: 0.06 to 0.08 second
Note: In atrial flutter you can count an atrial rate. In atrial fibrillation you cannot count an atrial rate. In a mixed rhythm (atrial fib-flutter), if you cannot count an atrial rate across the strip the rhythm is basically atrial fibrillation (with some flutter waves mixed in).

ventricular rhythm becomes somewhat more regular (see Figure 7.27). Flutter waves are sometimes seen mixed with the fibrillatory waves. This mixed rhythm is commonly called atrial fib-flutter (basically atrial fib with some flutter waves present). Atrial fib-flutter is shown in Figure 7.28).

As in atrial flutter, the AV node blocks most of the impulses from entering the ventricles, thus protecting the ventricles from excessive rates. The ventricular rate is slower than the atrial rate and depends on the number of impulses conducted through the AV node to the ventricles. When the ventricular rate is less than 100 beats per minute, the rhythm is called controlled atrial fibrillation. When

the ventricular rate is greater than 100 beats per minute, the rhythm is called uncontrolled atrial fibrillation or atrial fibrillation with a rapid ventricular response.

Atrial fibrillation is the most common rhythm seen next to sinus rhythm. Atrial fibrillation may occur in episodes or be permanent (chronic) in nature. The prevalence of atrial fibrillation increases with age. Atrial fibrillation can occur in healthy individuals or in those with heart disease. In healthy individuals, the rhythm is usually temporary and may be associated with emotional stress or excessive alcohol consumption ("holiday heart syndrome"). In many patients, this type of atrial fibrillation spontaneously

box 7.6   Atrial Fibrillation: Identifying ECG Features

Rhythm: Grossly irregular (unless the ventricular rate is very rapid, in which case the rhythm becomes more regular.)

Rate: Atrial rate: 400 beats/minute or more; not measurable on surface ECG
Ventricular rate: Varies with number of impulses conducted through AV node to the ventricles (will be less than the atrial rate)

P waves: Irregular wave deflections called fibrillatory waves (f waves) affecting entire baseline

PR interval: Not measurable

QRS complex: Normal (0.10 second or less)

reverts to sinus rhythm or is easily converted with drug therapy alone. Other conditions commonly associated with atrial fibrillation include coronary artery disease, hypertension, valvular heart disease, congestive heart failure, and pulmonary disease. It is also common after cardiac surgery.

The clinical consequences of atrial fibrillation are similar to those of atrial flutter. The ventricular rate may be rapid, increasing myocardial oxygen demands and cardiac workload and decreasing cardiac output. Because the atria quiver rather than contract effectively, the atrial kick is lost, which can further reduce cardiac output. Decreased cardiac output is especially marked in patients with underlying cardiac impairment and in the elderly, who appear to be more dependent on atrial contraction for filling of the ventricles. The noncontracting atria cause blood to pool in the atrial chambers, increasing the potential for thrombus formation. Dislodgment of atrial clots may lead to pulmonary or systemic embolization.

Treatment of atrial fibrillation includes controlling the heart rate, providing anticoagulation as a prophylaxis for thromboembolism, and returning the atria to a sinus rhythm. The treatment protocols for atrial fibrillation are the same as those for atrial flutter. Rate control should be achieved first, using a calcium channel blocker, such

as diltiazem, or a beta-blocker using caution in individuals with impaired LV function. If the rhythm is less than 48 hours old, cardioversion or an antiarrhythmic such as amiodarone can be used in an attempt to restore the rhythm to a sinus rhythm. If atrial fibrillation has been present for more than 48 hours, the patient must be adequately anticoagulated (refer to anticoagulation protocols for atrial flutter) before attempts are made to restore sinus rhythm using cardioversion or an antiarrhythmic.

Unstable atrial fibrillation should be cardioverted immediately, regardless of the duration of the arrhythmia. Patients with chronic atrial fibrillation (present for months or years) may not convert to sinus rhythm with any therapy. Treatment of these patients should be directed at controlling the ventricular rate and providing anticoagulation.

Some individuals may be candidates for radiofrequency catheter ablation. Cardiac arrhythmias can be caused by a small, localized area somewhere within the heart that produces an electrical disruption of the normal heart rhythm. For those arrhythmias, ablation simply requires locating that small abnormal area and cauterizing it. The electrical disruptions associated with atrial fibrillation are much more extensive, essentially encompassing most of the left and right atria, making ablation of atrial fibrillation a challenge. In recent years, electrophysiologists (heart rhythm doctors) have had more success ablating atrial fibrillation by aiming their efforts at destroying the "triggers" of the arrhythmia. PACs often trigger atrial fibrillation. Studies have shown that in up to 90% of patients with atrial fibrillation, the PACs that trigger the arrhythmia arise from specific areas within the left atrium. Ablation is accomplished by delivering radiofrequency energy through a catheter to cauterize a small area of cardiac muscle, producing a scar that disrupts the trigger causing the arrhythmia. Ablation works best in patients with episodes of atrial fibrillation rather than chronic atrial fibrillation.

Cardioversion of atrial fibrillation to a sinus rhythm is shown in Figure 7.29. A **pull-out arrhythmia summary** of the atrial arrhythmias can be found in Table 7.1 at the back of the book. This may be used as a *quick guide to assist with rhythm interpretation.*

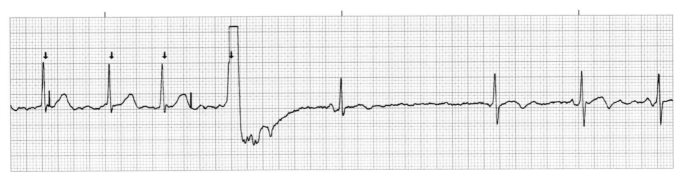

Figure 7.29   Cardioversion of atrial fibrillation to sinus rhythm; junctional escape beat (discussed in Chapter 8) follows the initial sinus beat.

RHYTHM STRIP PRACTICE: ATRIAL ARRHYTHMIAS

Analyze the following rhythm strips by following the five basic steps:

- Determine **rhythm regularity**.
- Calculate **heart rate** (this usually refers to the ventricular rate but, if atrial rate differs, you need to calculate both).
- Identify and examine **P waves**.
- Measure the **PR interval**.
- Measure the **QRS complex**.

Interpret the rhythm by comparing these data with the ECG characteristics for each rhythm. All rhythm strips are lead II, a positive lead, unless otherwise noted. Check your answers with the answer key in the appendix.

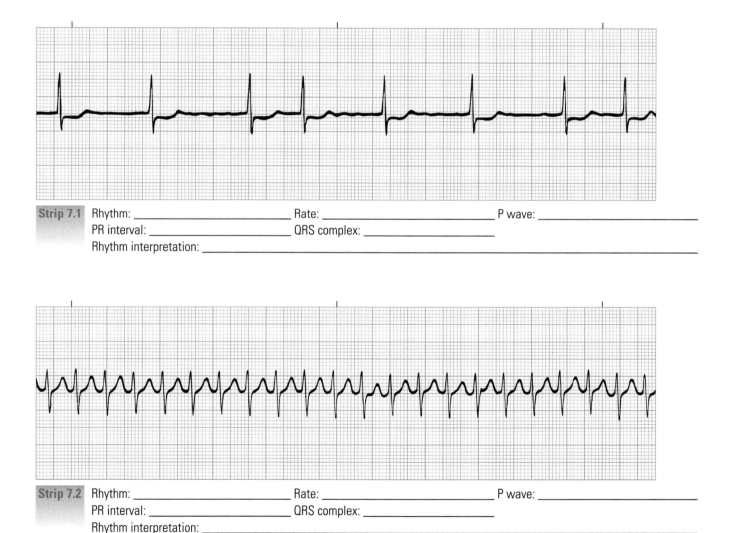

Strip 7.1 Rhythm: _____ Rate: _____ P wave: _____

PR interval: _____ QRS complex: _____

Rhythm interpretation: _____

Strip 7.2 Rhythm: _____ Rate: _____ P wave: _____

PR interval: _____ QRS complex: _____

Rhythm interpretation: _____

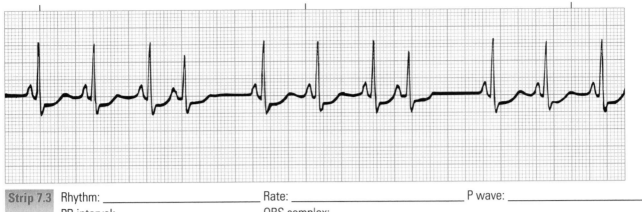

Strip 7.3 Rhythm: _____ Rate: _____ P wave: _____

PR interval: _____ QRS complex: _____

Rhythm interpretation: _____

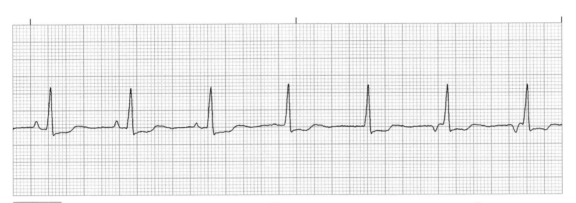

Strip 7.4 Rhythm: _____ Rate: _____ P wave: _____

PR interval: _____ QRS complex: _____

Rhythm interpretation: _____

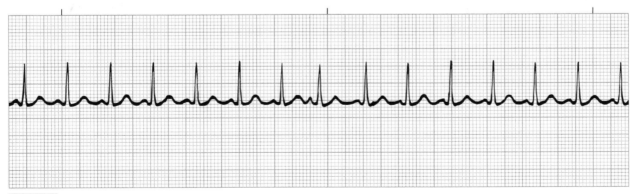

Strip 7.5 Rhythm: _____ Rate: _____ P wave: _____

PR interval: _____ QRS complex: _____

Rhythm interpretation: _____

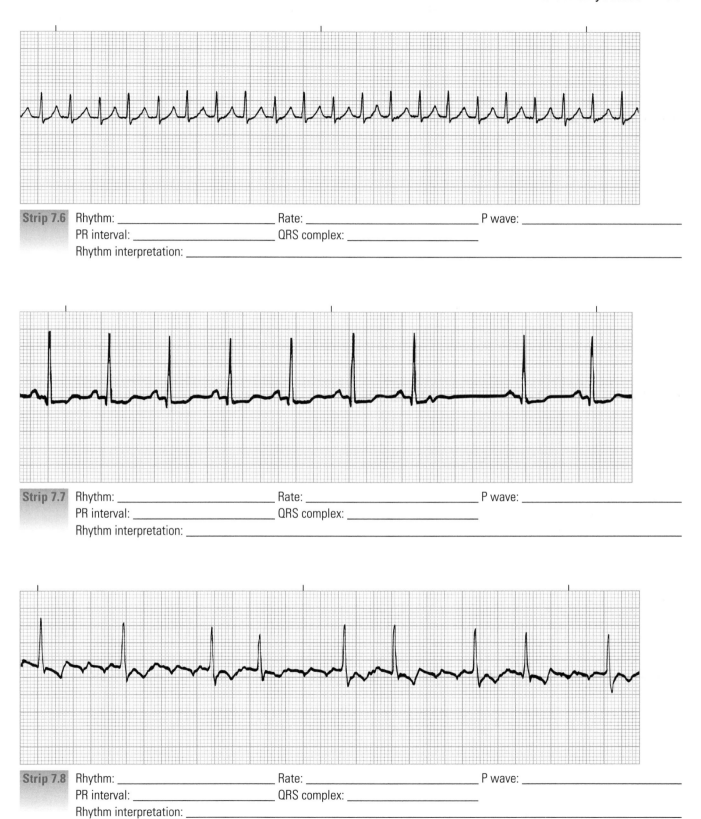

Strip 7.6   Rhythm: _____ Rate: _____ P wave: _____

PR interval: _____ QRS complex: _____

Rhythm interpretation: _____

Strip 7.7   Rhythm: _____ Rate: _____ P wave: _____

PR interval: _____ QRS complex: _____

Rhythm interpretation: _____

Strip 7.8   Rhythm: _____ Rate: _____ P wave: _____

PR interval: _____ QRS complex: _____

Rhythm interpretation: _____

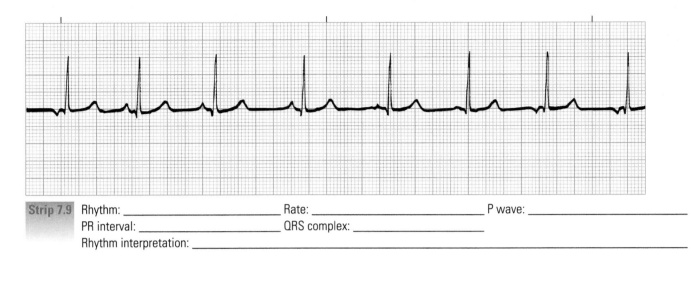

Strip 7.9   Rhythm: _____ Rate: _____ P wave: _____

PR interval: _____ QRS complex: _____

Rhythm interpretation: _____

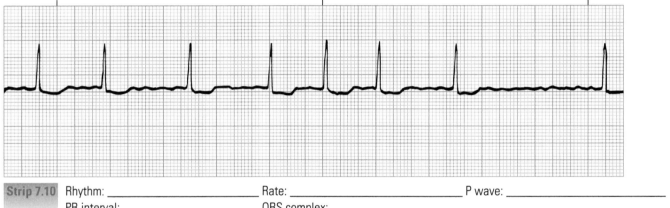

Strip 7.10   Rhythm: _____ Rate: _____ P wave: _____

PR interval: _____ QRS complex: _____

Rhythm interpretation: _____

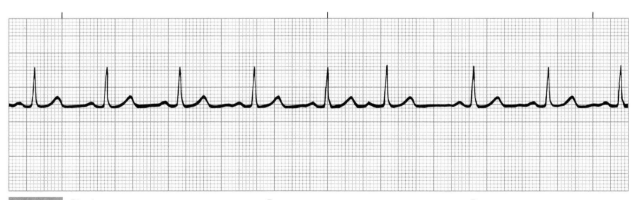

Strip 7.11   Rhythm: _____ Rate: _____ P wave: _____

PR interval: _____ QRS complex: _____

Rhythm interpretation: _____

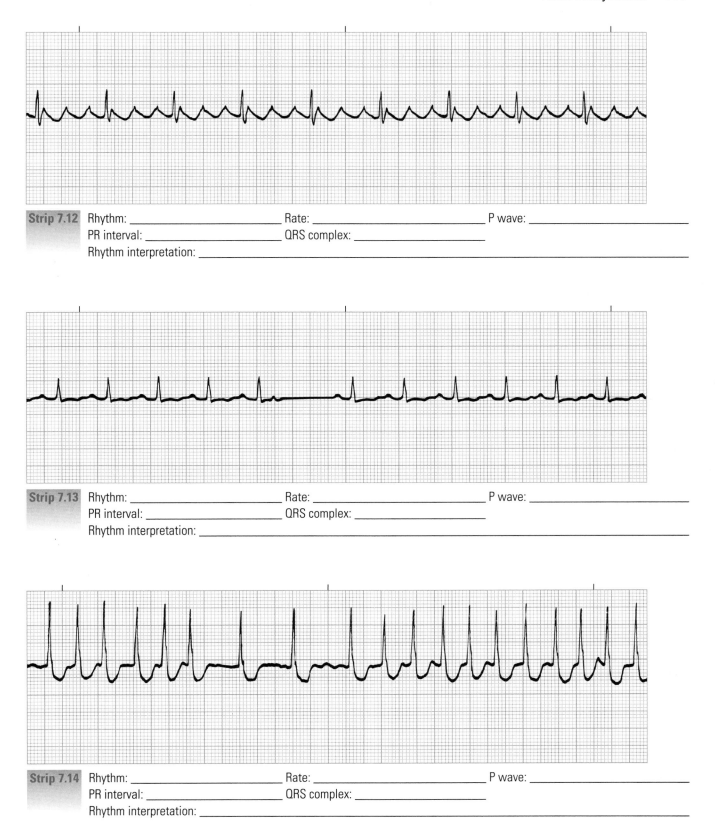

Strip 7.12   Rhythm: _____ Rate: _____ P wave: _____
PR interval: _____ QRS complex: _____
Rhythm interpretation: _____

Strip 7.13   Rhythm: _____ Rate: _____ P wave: _____
PR interval: _____ QRS complex: _____
Rhythm interpretation: _____

Strip 7.14   Rhythm: _____ Rate: _____ P wave: _____
PR interval: _____ QRS complex: _____
Rhythm interpretation: _____

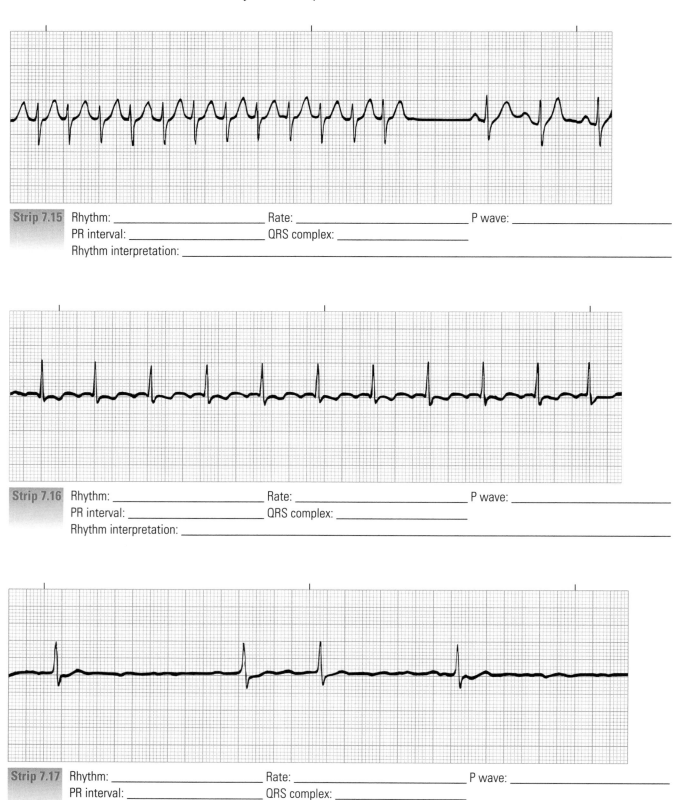

Strip 7.15 Rhythm: _____ Rate: _____ P wave: _____
PR interval: _____ QRS complex: _____
Rhythm interpretation: _____

Strip 7.16 Rhythm: _____ Rate: _____ P wave: _____
PR interval: _____ QRS complex: _____
Rhythm interpretation: _____

Strip 7.17 Rhythm: _____ Rate: _____ P wave: _____
PR interval: _____ QRS complex: _____
Rhythm interpretation: _____

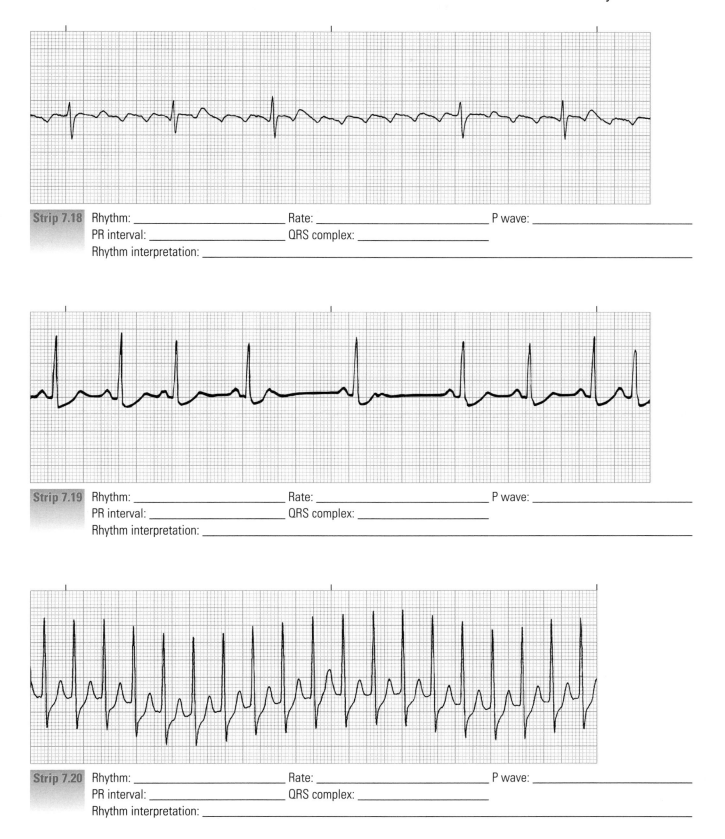

Strip 7.18 Rhythm: _____ Rate: _____ P wave: _____
PR interval: _____ QRS complex: _____
Rhythm interpretation: _____

Strip 7.19 Rhythm: _____ Rate: _____ P wave: _____
PR interval: _____ QRS complex: _____
Rhythm interpretation: _____

Strip 7.20 Rhythm: _____ Rate: _____ P wave: _____
PR interval: _____ QRS complex: _____
Rhythm interpretation: _____

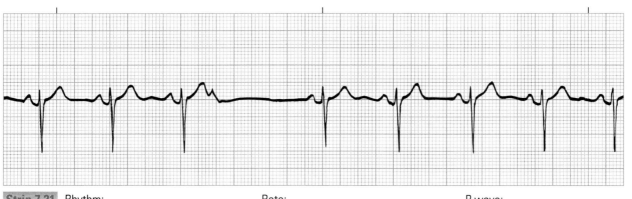

Strip 7.21 Rhythm: _____ Rate: _____ P wave: _____

PR interval: _____ QRS complex: _____

Rhythm interpretation: _____

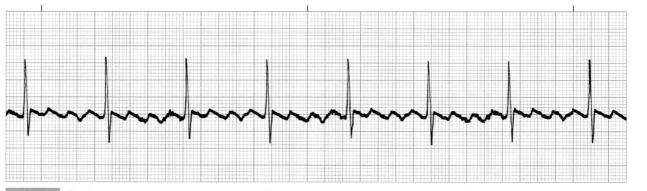

Strip 7.22 Rhythm: _____ Rate: _____ P wave: _____

PR interval: _____ QRS complex: _____

Rhythm interpretation: _____

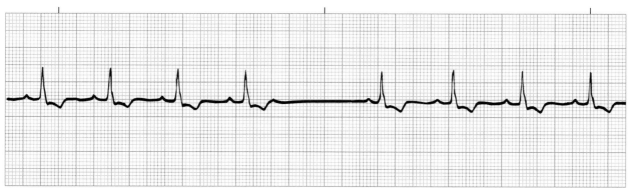

Strip 7.23 Rhythm: _____ Rate: _____ P wave: _____

PR interval: _____ QRS complex: _____

Rhythm interpretation: _____

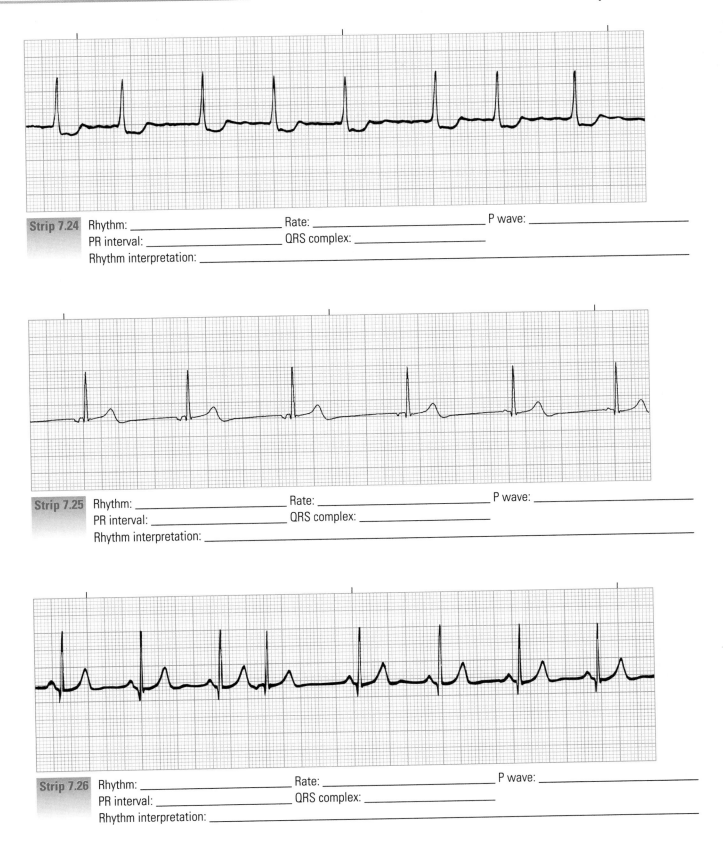

Strip 7.24 Rhythm: _____ Rate: _____ P wave: _____

PR interval: _____ QRS complex: _____

Rhythm interpretation: _____

Strip 7.25 Rhythm: _____ Rate: _____ P wave: _____

PR interval: _____ QRS complex: _____

Rhythm interpretation: _____

Strip 7.26 Rhythm: _____ Rate: _____ P wave: _____

PR interval: _____ QRS complex: _____

Rhythm interpretation: _____

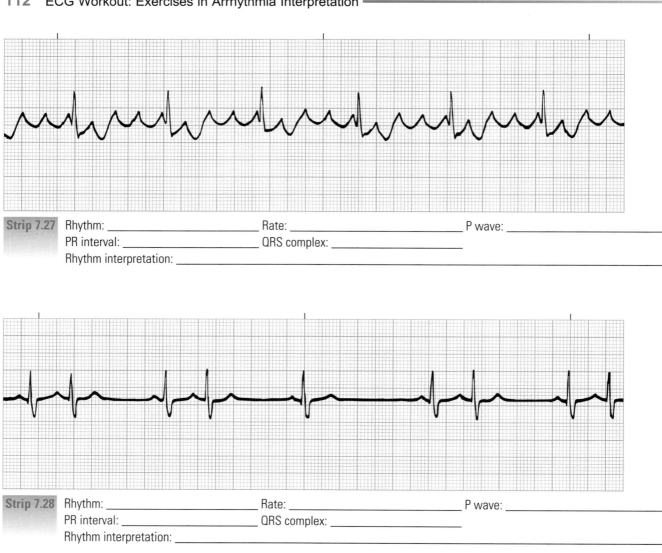

Strip 7.27 Rhythm: _____ Rate: _____ P wave: _____
PR interval: _____ QRS complex: _____
Rhythm interpretation: _____

Strip 7.28 Rhythm: _____ Rate: _____ P wave: _____
PR interval: _____ QRS complex: _____
Rhythm interpretation: _____

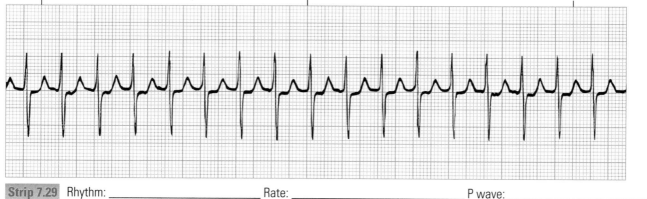

Strip 7.29 Rhythm: _____ Rate: _____ P wave: _____
PR interval: _____ QRS complex: _____
Rhythm interpretation: _____

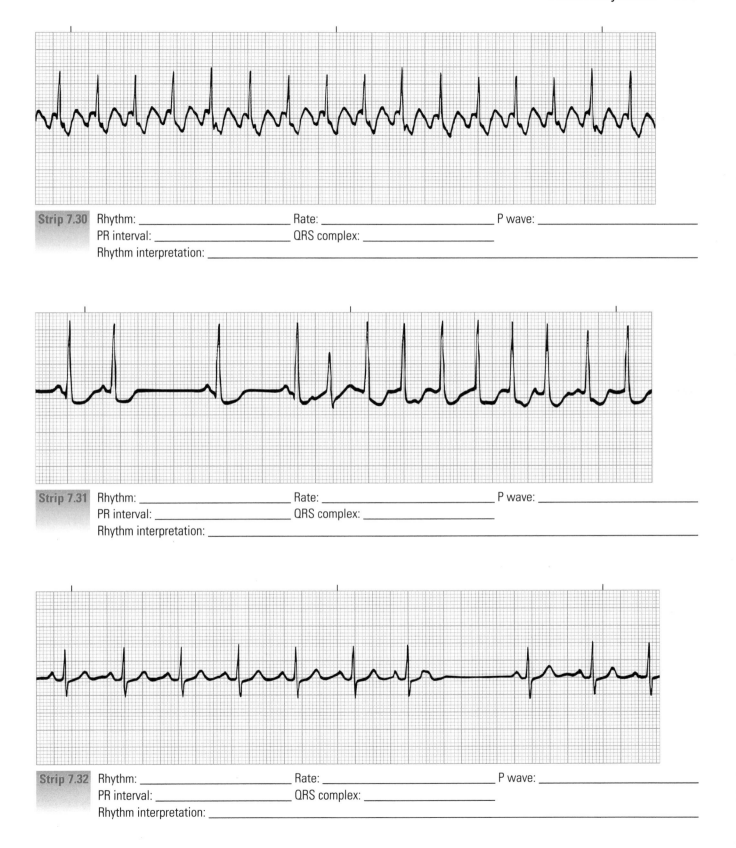

Strip 7.30 Rhythm: _____ Rate: _____ P wave: _____

PR interval: _____ QRS complex: _____

Rhythm interpretation: _____

Strip 7.31 Rhythm: _____ Rate: _____ P wave: _____

PR interval: _____ QRS complex: _____

Rhythm interpretation: _____

Strip 7.32 Rhythm: _____ Rate: _____ P wave: _____

PR interval: _____ QRS complex: _____

Rhythm interpretation: _____

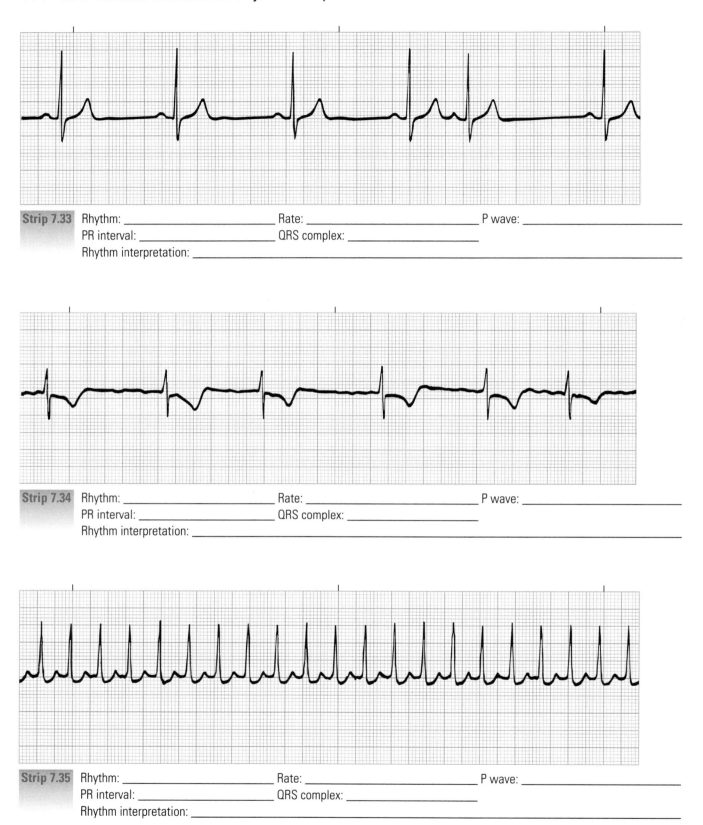

Strip 7.33 Rhythm: _____ Rate: _____ P wave: _____
PR interval: _____ QRS complex: _____
Rhythm interpretation: _____

Strip 7.34 Rhythm: _____ Rate: _____ P wave: _____
PR interval: _____ QRS complex: _____
Rhythm interpretation: _____

Strip 7.35 Rhythm: _____ Rate: _____ P wave: _____
PR interval: _____ QRS complex: _____
Rhythm interpretation: _____

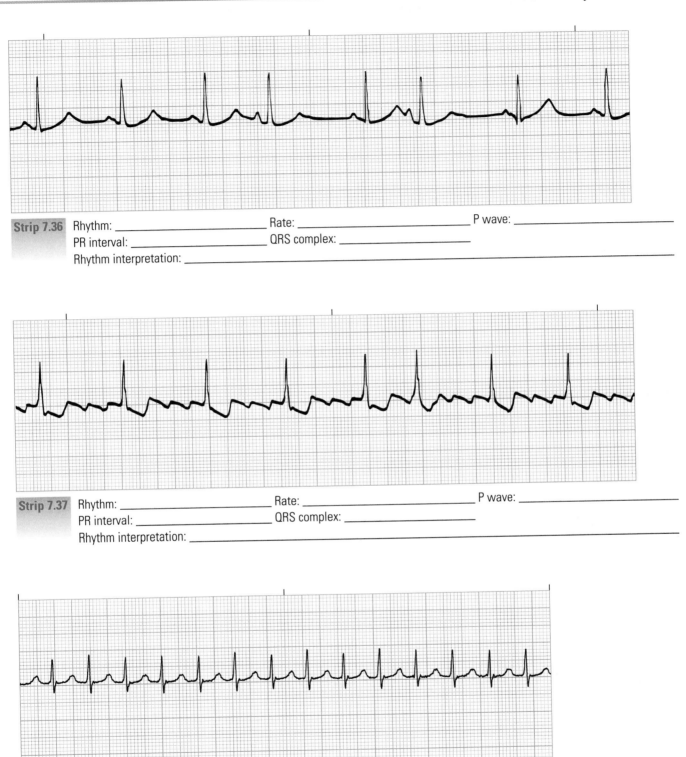

Strip 7.36 Rhythm: _____ Rate: _____ P wave: _____
PR interval: _____ QRS complex: _____
Rhythm interpretation: _____

Strip 7.37 Rhythm: _____ Rate: _____ P wave: _____
PR interval: _____ QRS complex: _____
Rhythm interpretation: _____

Strip 7.38 Rhythm: _____ Rate: _____ P wave: _____
PR interval: _____ QRS complex: _____
Rhythm interpretation: _____

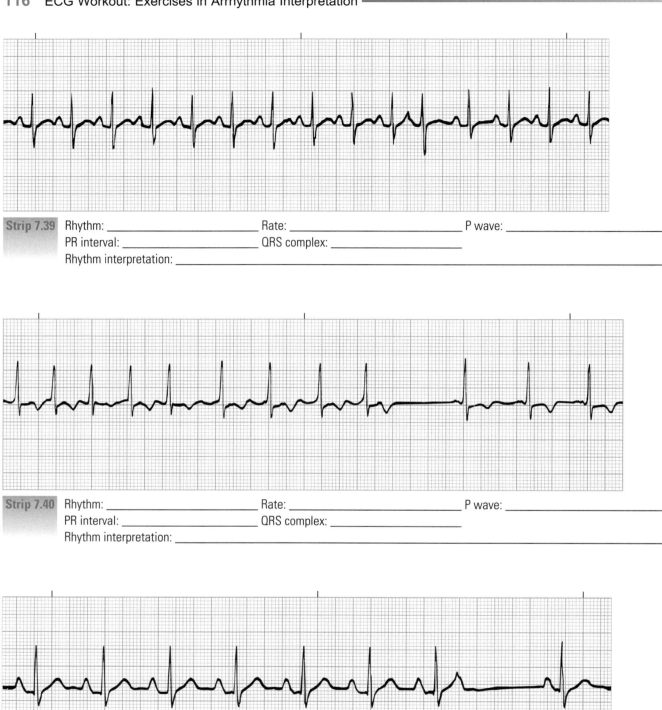

Strip 7.39 Rhythm: _____ Rate: _____ P wave: _____
PR interval: _____ QRS complex: _____
Rhythm interpretation: _____

Strip 7.40 Rhythm: _____ Rate: _____ P wave: _____
PR interval: _____ QRS complex: _____
Rhythm interpretation: _____

Strip 7.41 Rhythm: _____ Rate: _____ P wave: _____
PR interval: _____ QRS complex: _____
Rhythm interpretation: _____

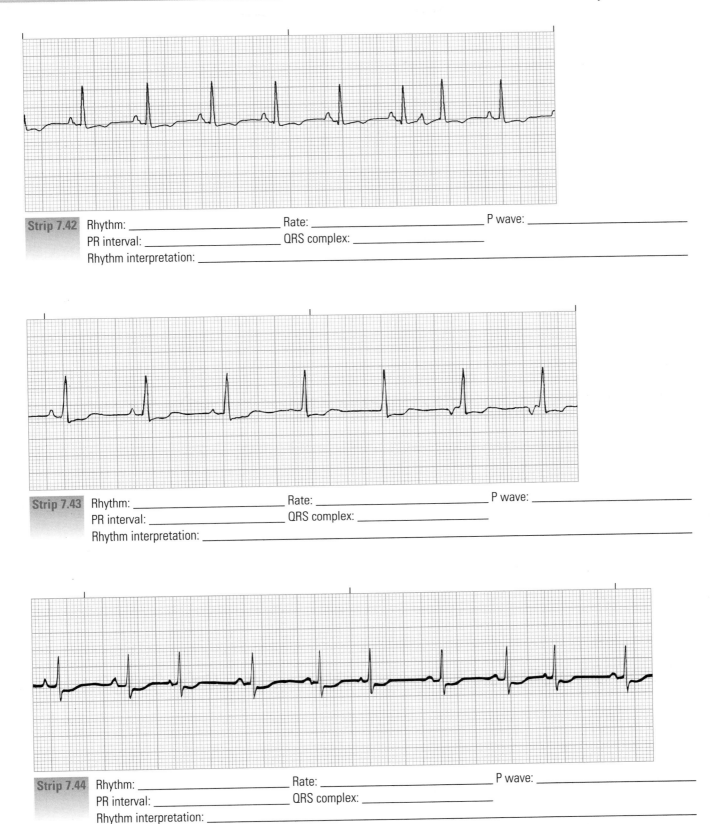

Strip 7.42 Rhythm: _____ Rate: _____ P wave: _____

PR interval: _____ QRS complex: _____

Rhythm interpretation: _____

Strip 7.43 Rhythm: _____ Rate: _____ P wave: _____

PR interval: _____ QRS complex: _____

Rhythm interpretation: _____

Strip 7.44 Rhythm: _____ Rate: _____ P wave: _____

PR interval: _____ QRS complex: _____

Rhythm interpretation: _____

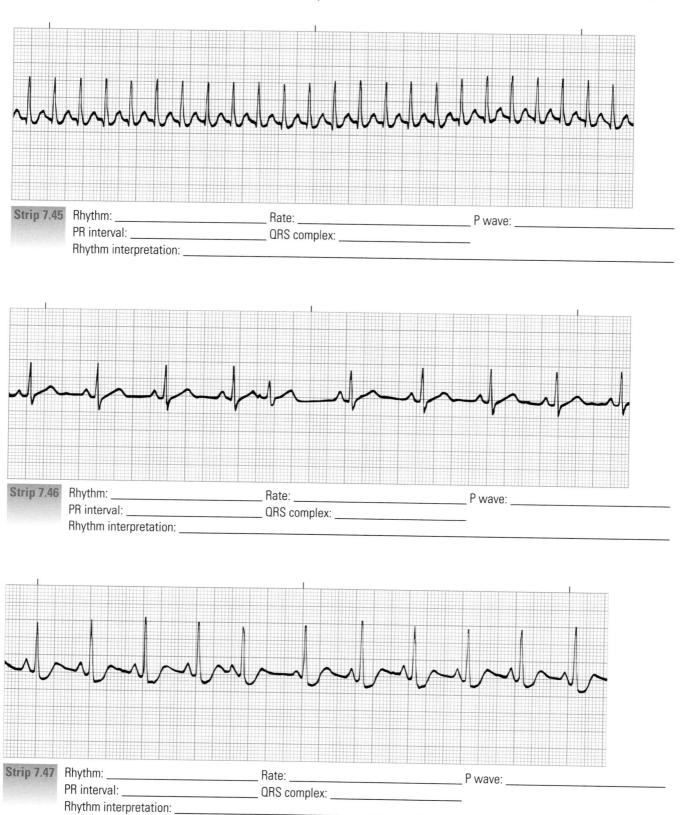

Strip 7.45 Rhythm: _____ Rate: _____ P wave: _____
PR interval: _____ QRS complex: _____
Rhythm interpretation: _____

Strip 7.46 Rhythm: _____ Rate: _____ P wave: _____
PR interval: _____ QRS complex: _____
Rhythm interpretation: _____

Strip 7.47 Rhythm: _____ Rate: _____ P wave: _____
PR interval: _____ QRS complex: _____
Rhythm interpretation: _____

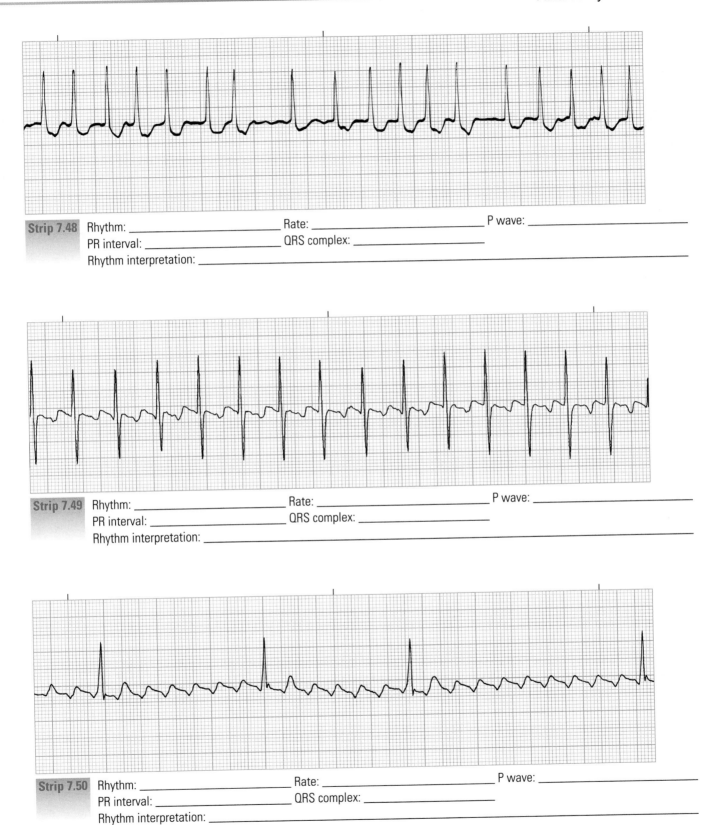

Strip 7.48 Rhythm: _____   Rate: _____   P wave: _____
PR interval: _____   QRS complex: _____
Rhythm interpretation: _____

Strip 7.49 Rhythm: _____   Rate: _____   P wave: _____
PR interval: _____   QRS complex: _____
Rhythm interpretation: _____

Strip 7.50 Rhythm: _____   Rate: _____   P wave: _____
PR interval: _____   QRS complex: _____
Rhythm interpretation: _____

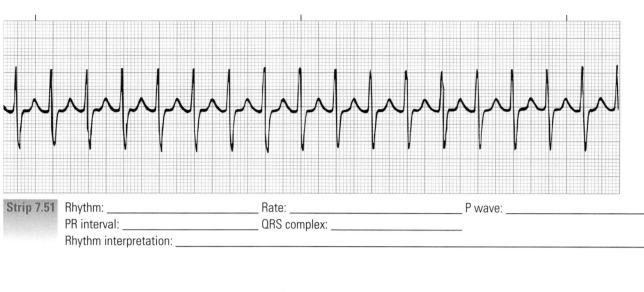

Strip 7.51 Rhythm: _____ Rate: _____ P wave: _____
PR interval: _____ QRS complex: _____
Rhythm interpretation: _____

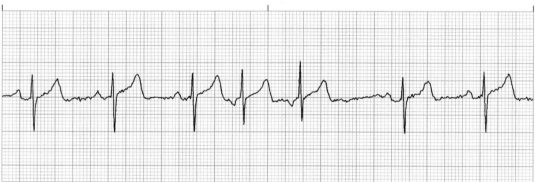

Strip 7.52 Rhythm: _____ Rate: _____ P wave: _____
PR interval: _____ QRS complex: _____
Rhythm interpretation: _____

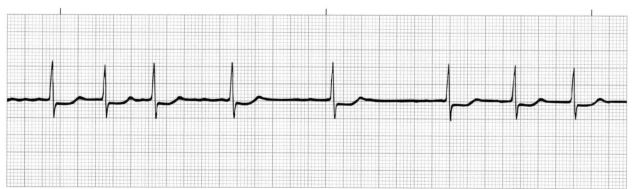

Strip 7.53 Rhythm: _____ Rate: _____ P wave: _____
PR interval: _____ QRS complex: _____
Rhythm interpretation: _____

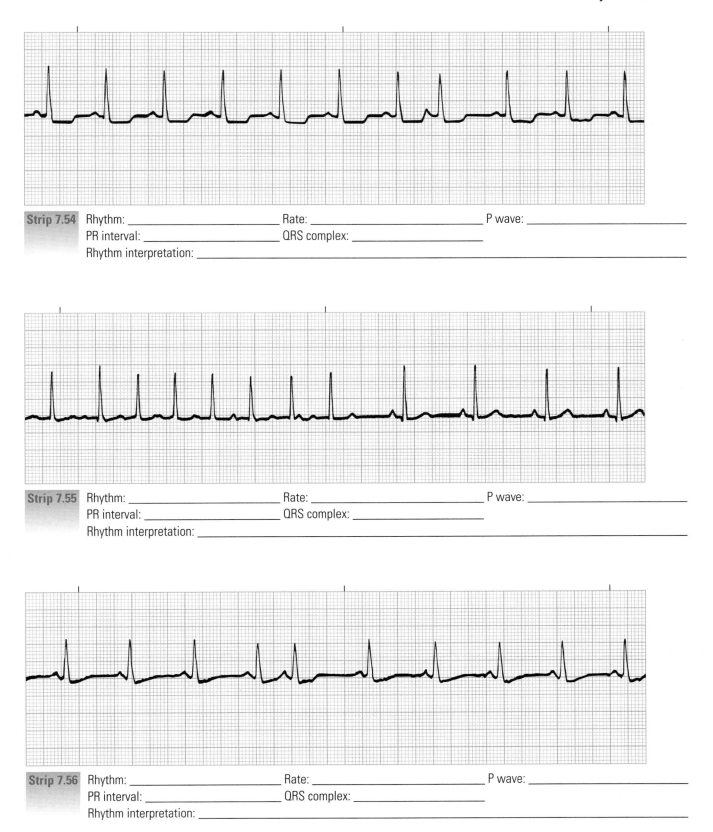

Strip 7.54 Rhythm: _____ Rate: _____ P wave: _____
PR interval: _____ QRS complex: _____
Rhythm interpretation: _____

Strip 7.55 Rhythm: _____ Rate: _____ P wave: _____
PR interval: _____ QRS complex: _____
Rhythm interpretation: _____

Strip 7.56 Rhythm: _____ Rate: _____ P wave: _____
PR interval: _____ QRS complex: _____
Rhythm interpretation: _____

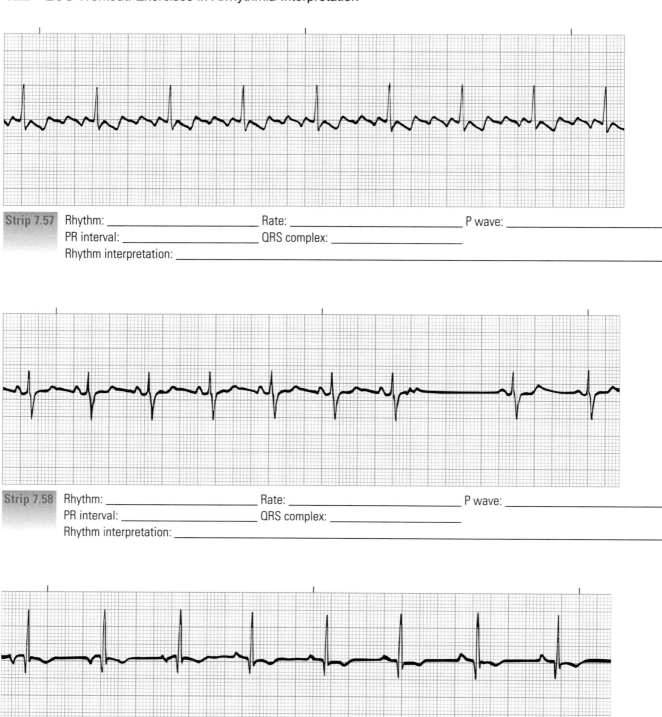

Strip 7.57   Rhythm: _____ Rate: _____ P wave: _____
PR interval: _____ QRS complex: _____
Rhythm interpretation: _____

Strip 7.58   Rhythm: _____ Rate: _____ P wave: _____
PR interval: _____ QRS complex: _____
Rhythm interpretation: _____

Strip 7.59   Rhythm: _____ Rate: _____ P wave: _____
PR interval: _____ QRS complex: _____
Rhythm interpretation: _____

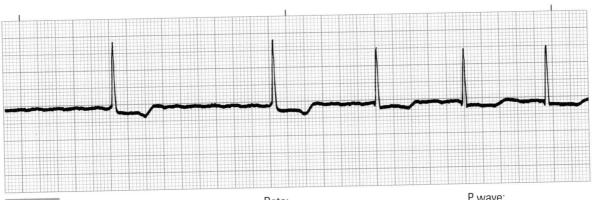

Strip 7.60 Rhythm: _____ Rate: _____ P wave: _____

PR interval: _____ QRS complex: _____

Rhythm interpretation: _____

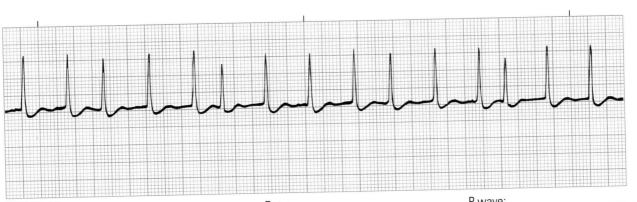

Strip 7.61 Rhythm: _____ Rate: _____ P wave: _____

PR interval: _____ QRS complex: _____

Rhythm interpretation: _____

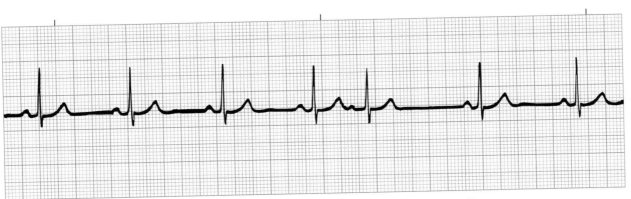

Strip 7.62 Rhythm: _____ Rate: _____ P wave: _____

PR interval: _____ QRS complex: _____

Rhythm interpretation: _____

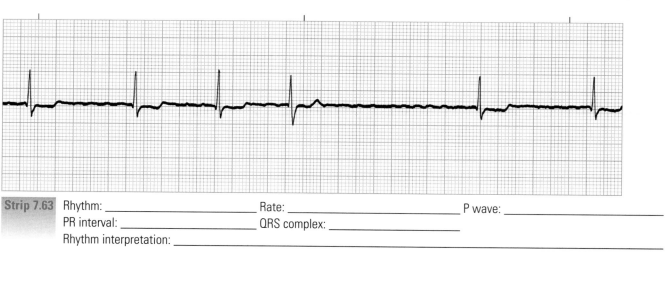

Strip 7.63 Rhythm: _____ Rate: _____ P wave: _____

PR interval: _____ QRS complex: _____

Rhythm interpretation: _____

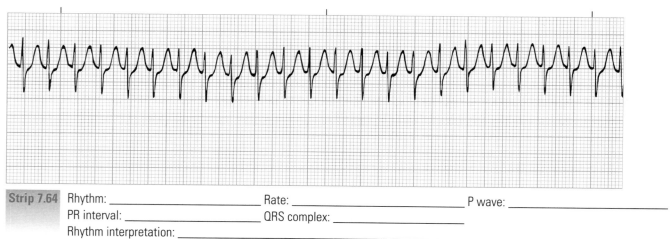

Strip 7.64 Rhythm: _____ Rate: _____ P wave: _____

PR interval: _____ QRS complex: _____

Rhythm interpretation: _____

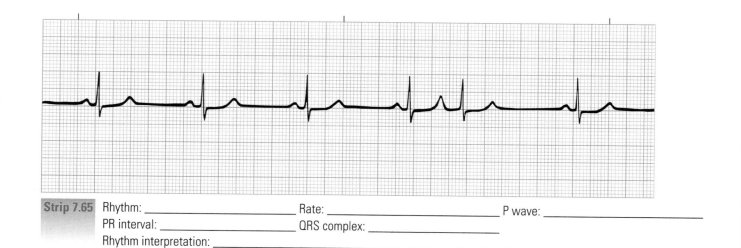

Strip 7.65 Rhythm: _____ Rate: _____ P wave: _____

PR interval: _____ QRS complex: _____

Rhythm interpretation: _____

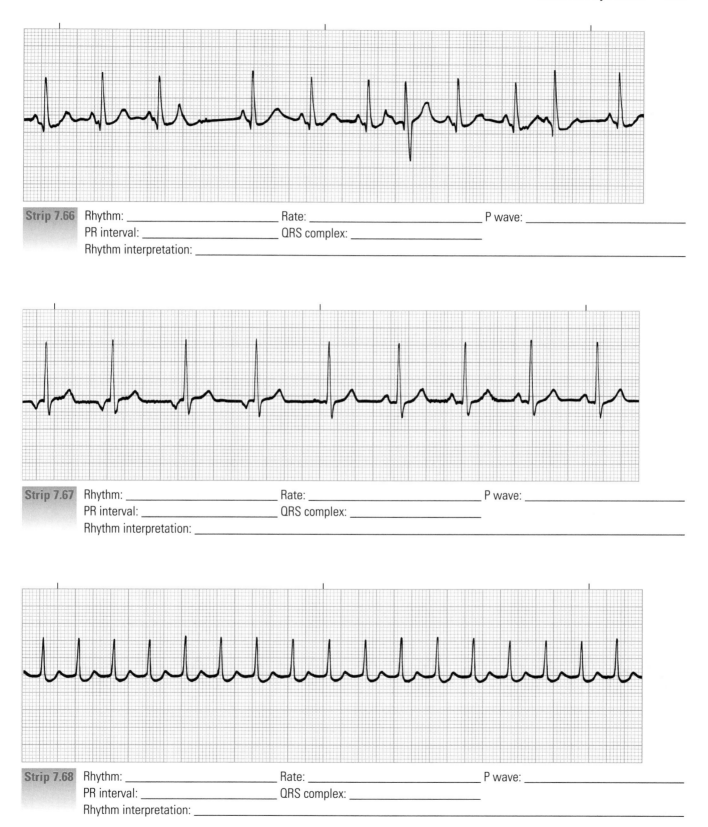

Strip 7.66 Rhythm: _____ Rate: _____ P wave: _____
PR interval: _____ QRS complex: _____
Rhythm interpretation: _____

Strip 7.67 Rhythm: _____ Rate: _____ P wave: _____
PR interval: _____ QRS complex: _____
Rhythm interpretation: _____

Strip 7.68 Rhythm: _____ Rate: _____ P wave: _____
PR interval: _____ QRS complex: _____
Rhythm interpretation: _____

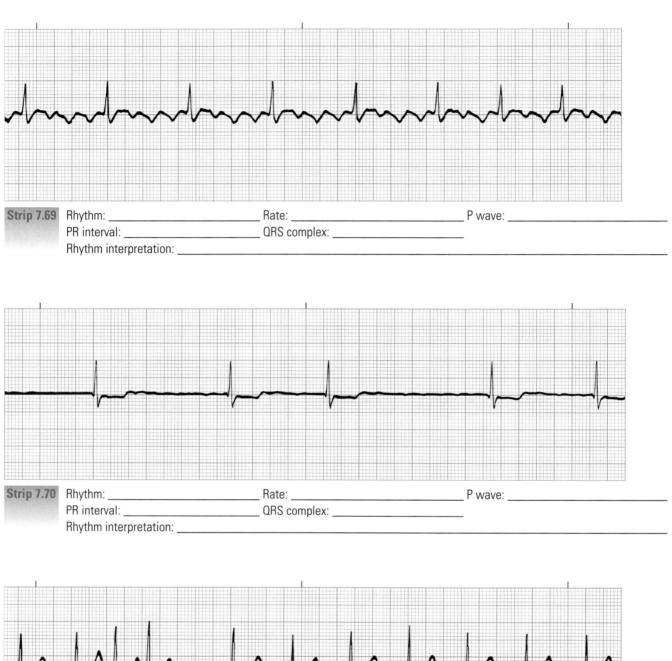

Strip 7.69 Rhythm: _____ Rate: _____ P wave: _____
PR interval: _____ QRS complex: _____
Rhythm interpretation: _____

Strip 7.70 Rhythm: _____ Rate: _____ P wave: _____
PR interval: _____ QRS complex: _____
Rhythm interpretation: _____

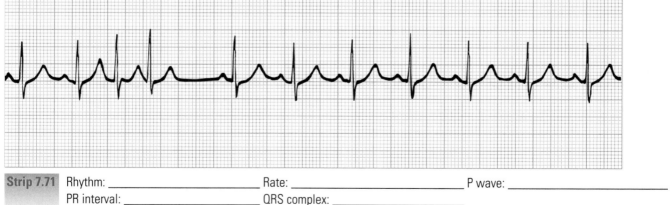

Strip 7.71 Rhythm: _____ Rate: _____ P wave: _____
PR interval: _____ QRS complex: _____
Rhythm interpretation: _____

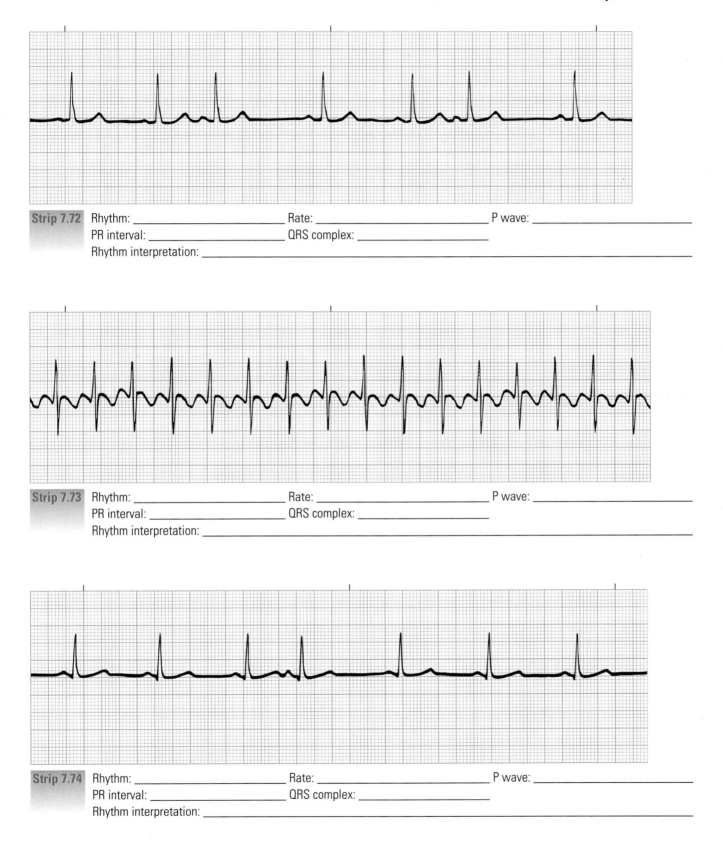

Strip 7.72 Rhythm: _____ Rate: _____ P wave: _____
PR interval: _____ QRS complex: _____
Rhythm interpretation: _____

Strip 7.73 Rhythm: _____ Rate: _____ P wave: _____
PR interval: _____ QRS complex: _____
Rhythm interpretation: _____

Strip 7.74 Rhythm: _____ Rate: _____ P wave: _____
PR interval: _____ QRS complex: _____
Rhythm interpretation: _____

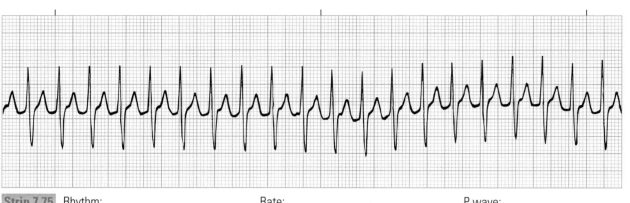

Strip 7.75 Rhythm: _____ Rate: _____ P wave: _____
PR interval: _____ QRS complex: _____
Rhythm interpretation: _____

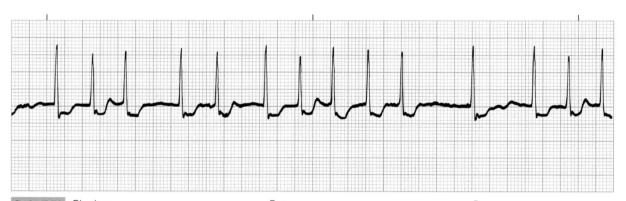

Strip 7.76 Rhythm: _____ Rate: _____ P wave: _____
PR interval: _____ QRS complex: _____
Rhythm interpretation: _____

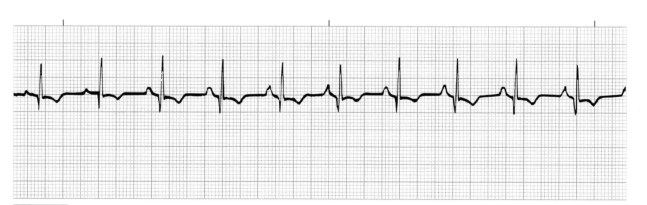

Strip 7.77 Rhythm: _____ Rate: _____ P wave: _____
PR interval: _____ QRS complex: _____
Rhythm interpretation: _____

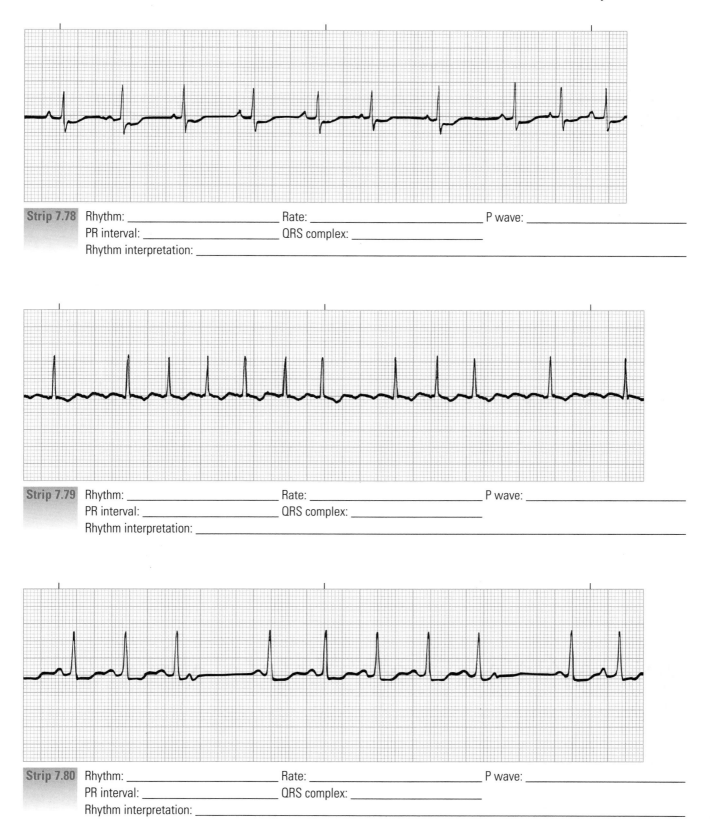

Strip 7.78 Rhythm: _____ Rate: _____ P wave: _____
PR interval: _____ QRS complex: _____
Rhythm interpretation: _____

Strip 7.79 Rhythm: _____ Rate: _____ P wave: _____
PR interval: _____ QRS complex: _____
Rhythm interpretation: _____

Strip 7.80 Rhythm: _____ Rate: _____ P wave: _____
PR interval: _____ QRS complex: _____
Rhythm interpretation: _____

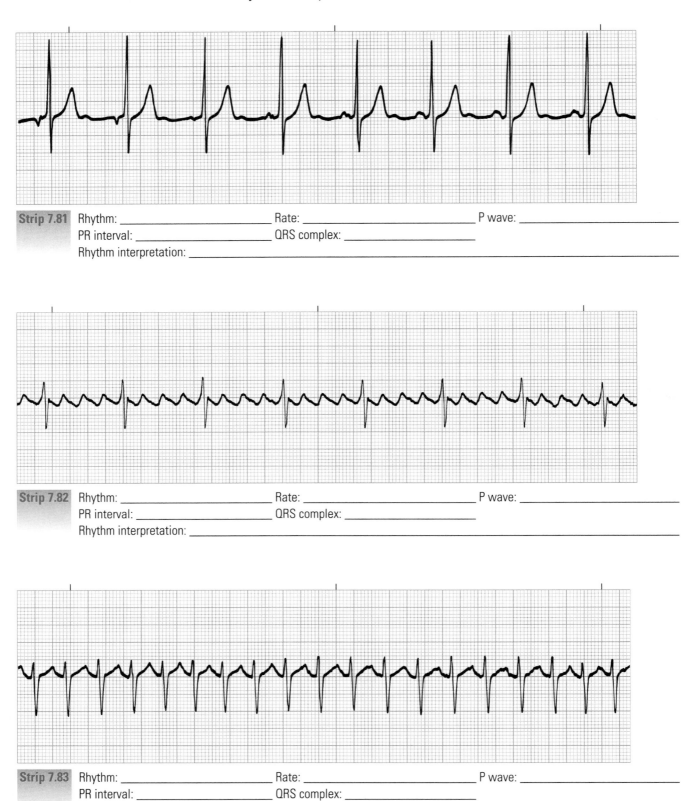

Strip 7.81 Rhythm: _____ Rate: _____ P wave: _____
PR interval: _____ QRS complex: _____
Rhythm interpretation: _____

Strip 7.82 Rhythm: _____ Rate: _____ P wave: _____
PR interval: _____ QRS complex: _____
Rhythm interpretation: _____

Strip 7.83 Rhythm: _____ Rate: _____ P wave: _____
PR interval: _____ QRS complex: _____
Rhythm interpretation: _____

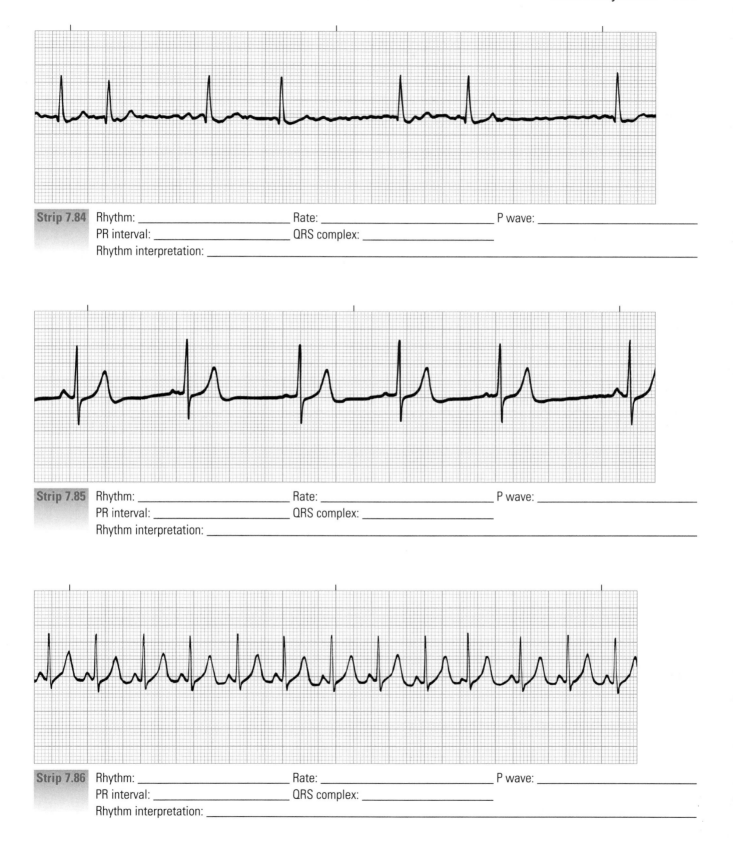

Strip 7.84 Rhythm: _____ Rate: _____ P wave: _____
PR interval: _____ QRS complex: _____
Rhythm interpretation: _____

Strip 7.85 Rhythm: _____ Rate: _____ P wave: _____
PR interval: _____ QRS complex: _____
Rhythm interpretation: _____

Strip 7.86 Rhythm: _____ Rate: _____ P wave: _____
PR interval: _____ QRS complex: _____
Rhythm interpretation: _____

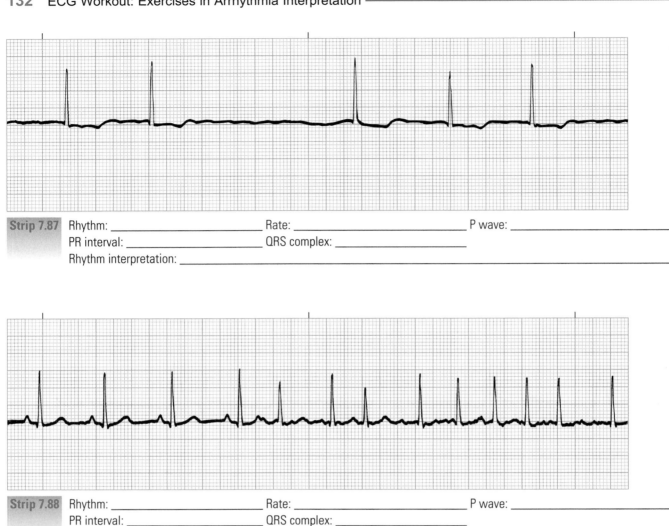

Strip 7.87   Rhythm: _____ Rate: _____ P wave: _____

PR interval: _____ QRS complex: _____

Rhythm interpretation: _____

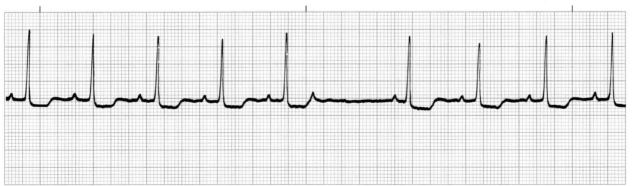

Strip 7.88   Rhythm: _____ Rate: _____ P wave: _____

PR interval: _____ QRS complex: _____

Rhythm interpretation: _____

Strip 7.89   Rhythm: _____ Rate: _____ P wave: _____

PR interval: _____ QRS complex: _____

Rhythm interpretation: _____

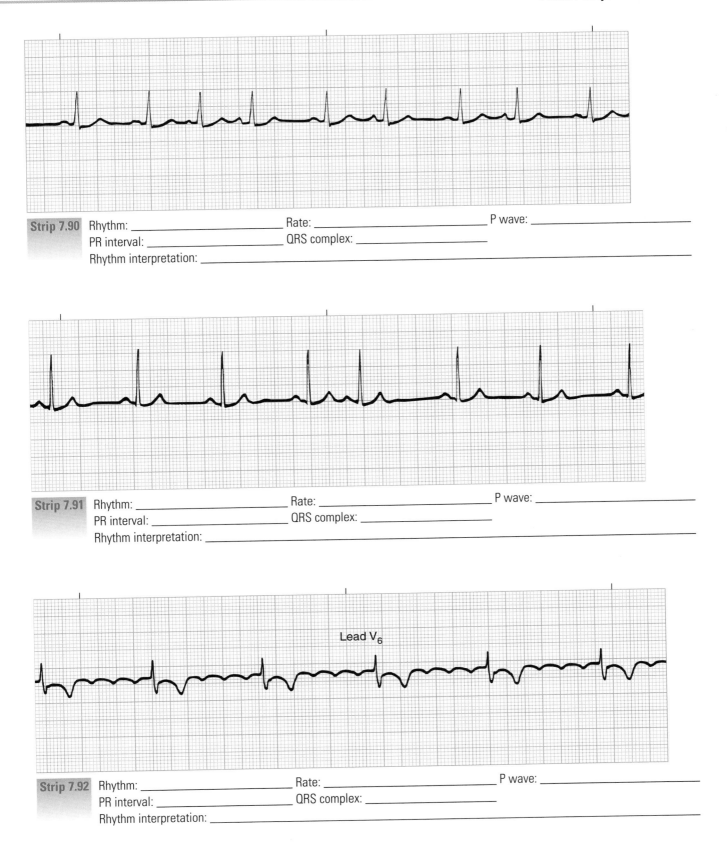

Strip 7.90 Rhythm: _____ Rate: _____ P wave: _____

PR interval: _____ QRS complex: _____

Rhythm interpretation: _____

Strip 7.91 Rhythm: _____ Rate: _____ P wave: _____

PR interval: _____ QRS complex: _____

Rhythm interpretation: _____

Lead V$_6$

Strip 7.92 Rhythm: _____ Rate: _____ P wave: _____

PR interval: _____ QRS complex: _____

Rhythm interpretation: _____

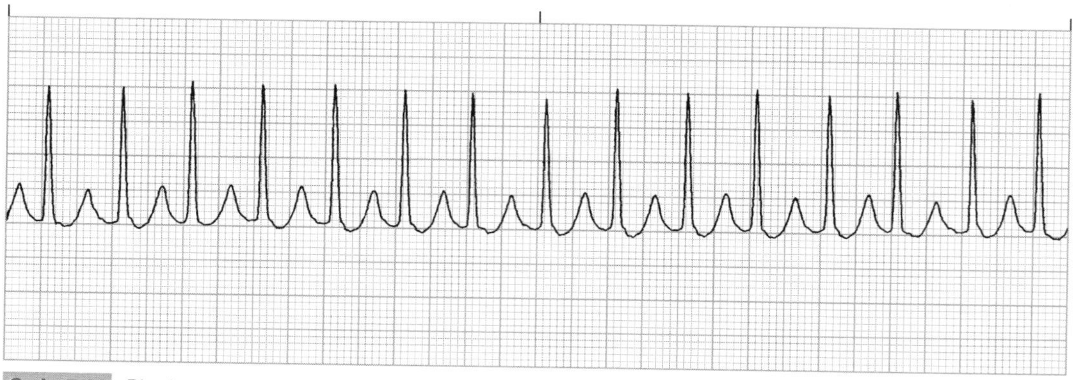

Strip 7.93 Rhythm: _____ Rate: _____ P wave: _____
PR interval: _____ QRS complex: _____
Rhythm interpretation: _____

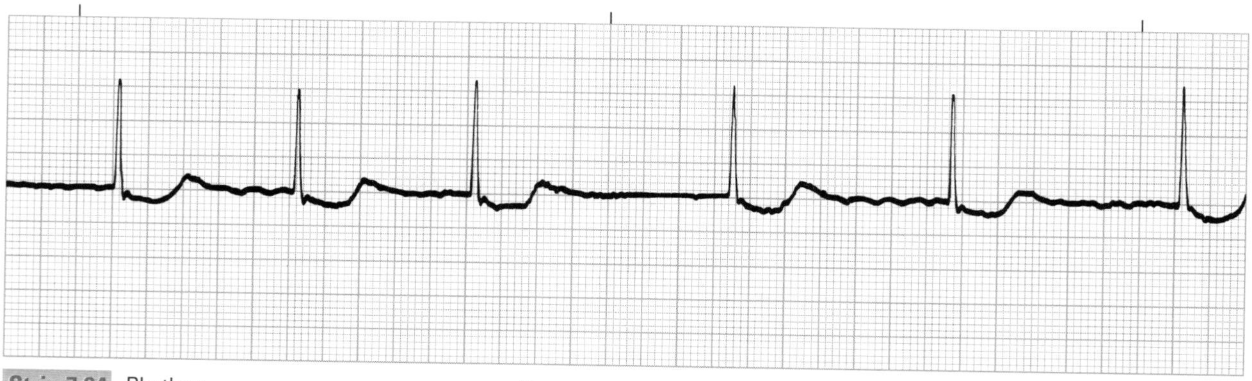

Strip 7.94 Rhythm: _____ Rate: _____ P wave: _____
PR interval: _____ QRS complex: _____
Rhythm interpretation: _____

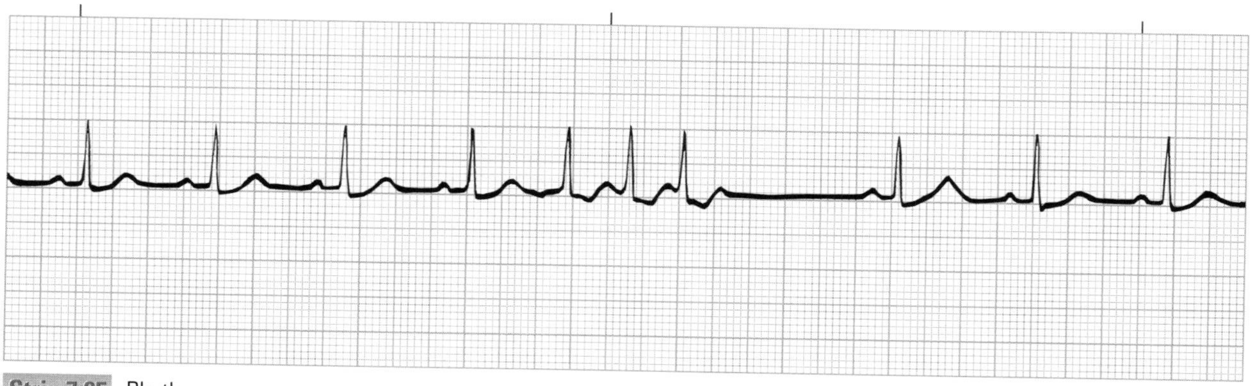

Strip 7.95 Rhythm: _____ Rate: _____ P wave: _____
PR interval: _____ QRS complex: _____
Rhythm interpretation: _____

SKILLBUILDER PRACTICE

This section contains mixed *sinus* and *atrial* rhythm strips, allowing the student to practice differentiating between two rhythm groups before progressing to a new group. As before, analyze the rhythm strips using the five-step process. Interpret the rhythm by comparing the data collected with the ECG characteristics for each rhythm. All strips are lead II, a positive lead, unless otherwise noted. Check your answers with the answer key in the appendix.

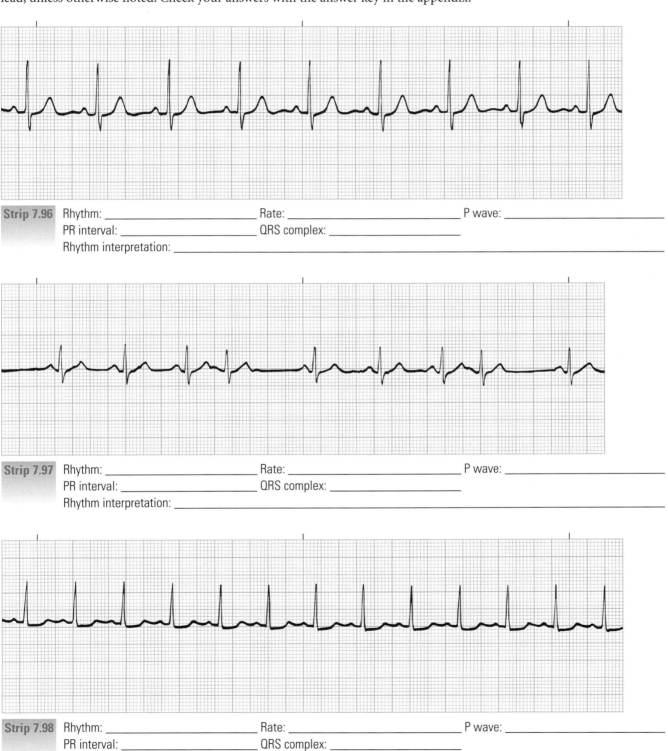

Strip 7.96   Rhythm: _____ Rate: _____ P wave: _____
PR interval: _____ QRS complex: _____
Rhythm interpretation: _____

Strip 7.97   Rhythm: _____ Rate: _____ P wave: _____
PR interval: _____ QRS complex: _____
Rhythm interpretation: _____

Strip 7.98   Rhythm: _____ Rate: _____ P wave: _____
PR interval: _____ QRS complex: _____
Rhythm interpretation: _____

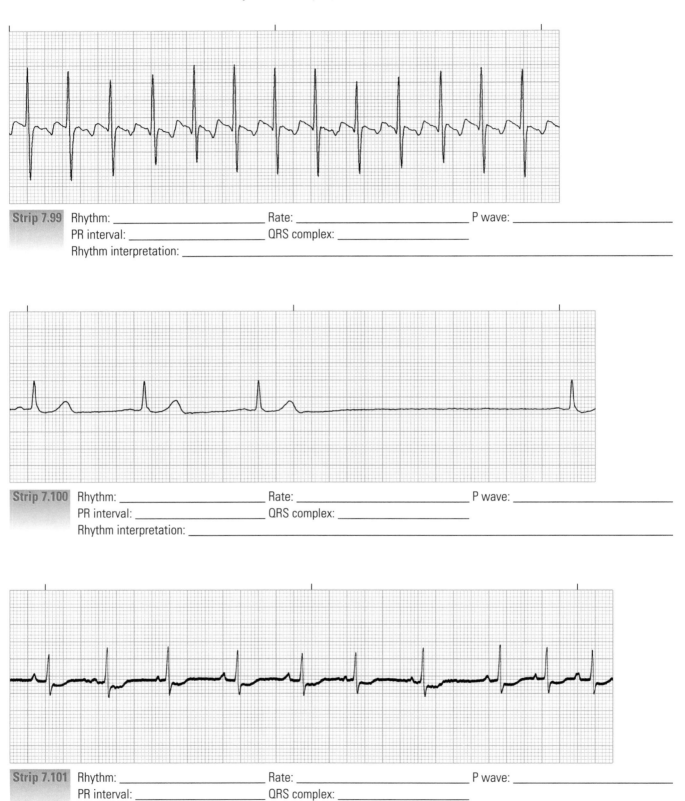

Strip 7.99 Rhythm: _____ Rate: _____ P wave: _____

PR interval: _____ QRS complex: _____

Rhythm interpretation: _____

Strip 7.100 Rhythm: _____ Rate: _____ P wave: _____

PR interval: _____ QRS complex: _____

Rhythm interpretation: _____

Strip 7.101 Rhythm: _____ Rate: _____ P wave: _____

PR interval: _____ QRS complex: _____

Rhythm interpretation: _____

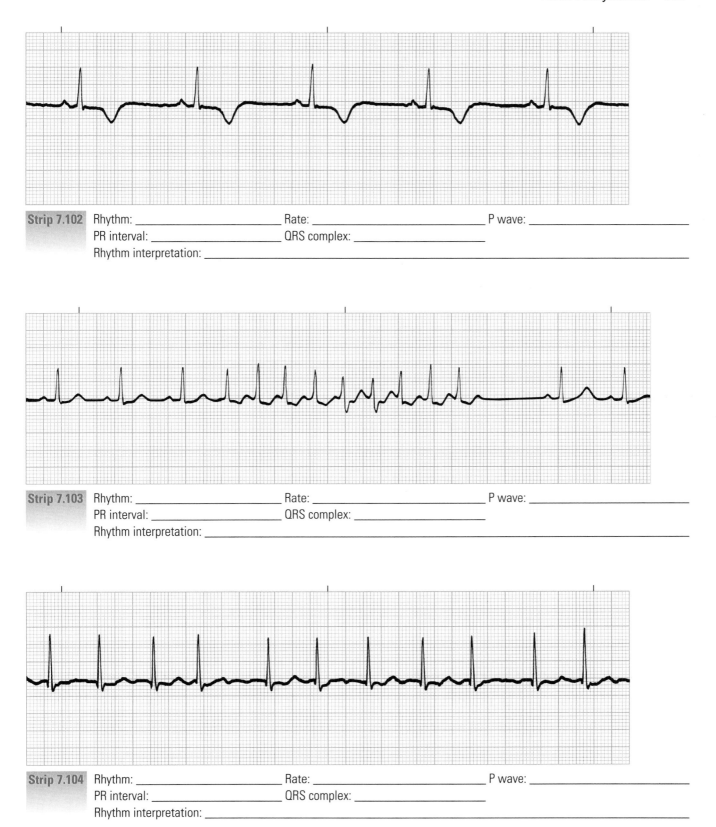

Strip 7.102 Rhythm: _____ Rate: _____ P wave: _____
PR interval: _____ QRS complex: _____
Rhythm interpretation: _____

Strip 7.103 Rhythm: _____ Rate: _____ P wave: _____
PR interval: _____ QRS complex: _____
Rhythm interpretation: _____

Strip 7.104 Rhythm: _____ Rate: _____ P wave: _____
PR interval: _____ QRS complex: _____
Rhythm interpretation: _____

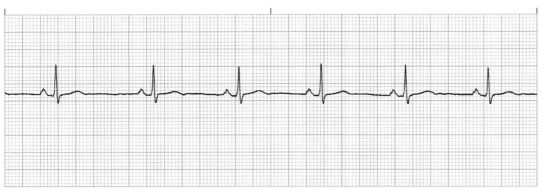

Strip 7.105 Rhythm: _____ Rate: _____ P wave: _____
PR interval: _____ QRS complex: _____
Rhythm interpretation: _____

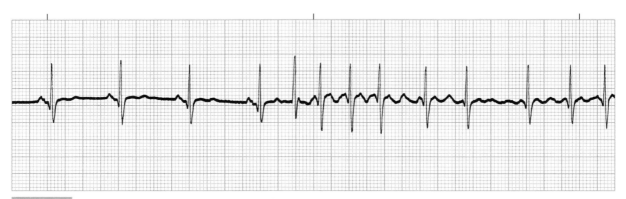

Strip 7.106 Rhythm: _____ Rate: _____ P wave: _____
PR interval: _____ QRS complex: _____
Rhythm interpretation: _____

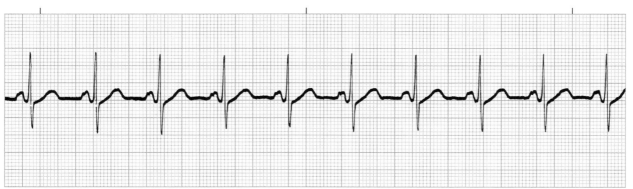

Strip 7.107 Rhythm: _____ Rate: _____ P wave: _____
PR interval: _____ QRS complex: _____
Rhythm interpretation: _____

eight

Junctional Arrhythmias and AV Blocks

Junctional Rhythms—Overview

The atrioventricular (AV) node is located in the lower portion of the right atrium. The bundle of His connects the AV node to the two bundle branches. Together, the AV node and the bundle of His are called the AV junction. The AV node doesn't contain pacemaker cells—the main function of the AV node is to slow conduction of the electrical impulse through the AV node to allow the atria to contract and complete filling of the ventricles prior to ventricular contraction. The bundle of His has pacemaker cells that are responsible for pacing function. Arrhythmias originating in the AV junction are called junctional rhythms (Figure 8.1).

The inherent firing rate of the junctional pacemaker cells is 40 to 60 beats per minute. A rhythm occurring at this rate is called a *junctional rhythm*. Other rhythms originating in the AV junctional area include *premature junctional contraction*, *accelerated junctional rhythm*, and *junctional tachycardia*.

When the AV junction is functioning as the pacemaker of the heart, the electrical impulse produces a wave of depolarization that spreads backward (*retrograde*) into the atria as well as forward (*antegrade*) into the ventricles. The location of the P wave in relation to the QRS complex depends on the speed of antegrade and retrograde conduction:

- If the electrical impulse from the AV junction depolarizes the atria first and then depolarizes the ventricles, the P wave will be in front of the QRS complex.
- If the electrical impulse from the AV junction depolarizes the ventricles first and then depolarizes the atria, the P wave will be after the QRS complex.
- If the electrical impulse from the AV junction depolarizes both the atria and the ventricles simultaneously, the P wave will be hidden in the QRS complex.

Retrograde stimulation of the atria is just opposite the direction of atrial depolarization when normal sinus rhythm is present and produces negative P waves (instead of upright) in lead II (a positive lead). The PR interval is short (0.10 second or less). The ventricles are depolarized normally, resulting in a normal duration QRS complex. Identifying features of junctional rhythms are summarized in Figure 8.2.

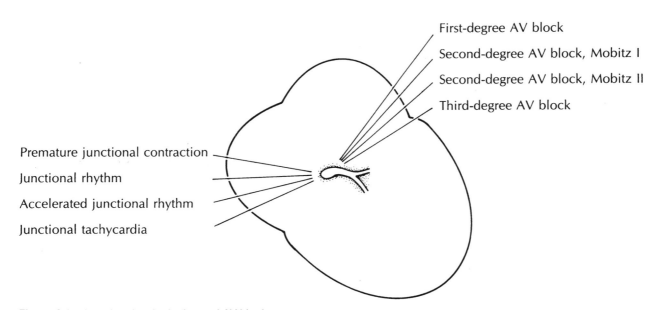

First-degree AV block
Second-degree AV block, Mobitz I
Second-degree AV block, Mobitz II
Third-degree AV block

Premature junctional contraction
Junctional rhythm
Accelerated junctional rhythm
Junctional tachycardia

Figure 8.1 Junctional arrhythmias and AV blocks.

Lead II   Lead II   Lead II

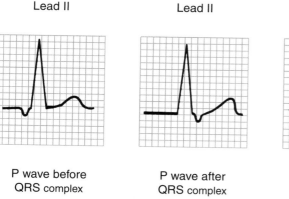

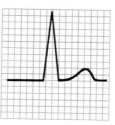

P wave before   P wave after   P wave hidden in
QRS complex   QRS complex   QRS complex

Figure 8.2   Identifying features of junctional rhythms.
- P waves inverted in lead II.
- P waves will occur in one of three patterns:
  – Immediately before the QRS complex
  – Immediately after the QRS complex
  – Hidden within the QRS complex
- PR interval will be short (0.10 second or less).
- QRS complex will be normal (0.10 second or less).

Lead II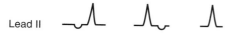

Figure 8.3   Premature junctional contractions will appear as a single beat in any of the above three patterns.

Premature Junctional Contraction

A premature junctional contraction (PJC) (Figures 8.3 through 8.6 and Box 8.1) is an early beat that originates in an ectopic pacemaker site in the AV junction, interrupting the regularity of the basic rhythm, which is usually a sinus rhythm. Like the premature atrial contraction (PAC), the PJC is characterized by a premature, abnormal P wave followed by a normal duration QRS complex and a pause that is usually noncompensatory. The premature beat occurs in addition to an underlying rhythm. Therefore, both the underlying rhythm and the premature beat must

box 8.1	Premature Junctional Contraction (PJC): Identifying ECG Features
Rhythm:	Underlying rhythm usually regular; irregular with PJC.
Rate:	That of the underlying rhythm.
P waves:	P waves associated with the PJC will be premature, will be inverted in lead II, and will occur immediately before the QRS complex, will occur immediately after the QRS complex, or are hidden within the QRS complex.
PR interval:	Short (0.10 second or less).
QRS complex:	Premature; normal duration (0.10 second or less).

be identified (for example, normal sinus rhythm with a PJC). Some differences exist, however, between the two premature beats. Because atrial depolarization occurs in a retrograde fashion with the PJC, the P wave associated with

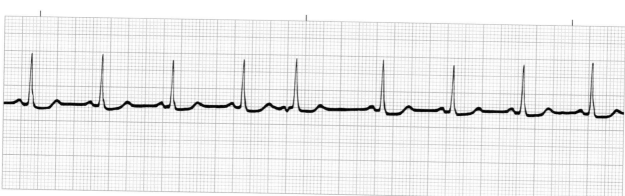

Figure 8.4   Normal sinus rhythm with one premature junctional contraction (PJC).

Rhythm: Basic rhythm regular; irregular with PJC
Rate: Basic rhythm rate 75 beats/minute
P waves: Sinus P waves with basic rhythm; inverted P wave before PJC
PR interval: 0.16 second (basic rhythm); 0.08 to 0.10 second (PJC)
QRS complex: 0.06 to 0.08 second (basic rhythm and PJC)
Comment: ST segment depression is present.

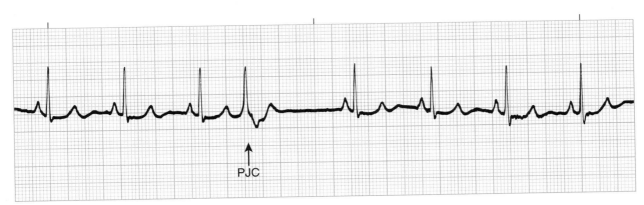

Figure 8.5	**Normal sinus rhythm with one PJC.**
Rhythm:	Basic rhythm regular; irregular with PJC
Rate:	Basic rhythm rate 72
P waves:	Sinus P waves with basic rhythm; inverted P wave after PJC (4th QRS complex)
PR interval:	0.14 to 0.16 second (basic rhythm); 0.06 to 0.08 second PJC
QRS complex:	0.06 to 0.08 second (basic rhythm); 0.08 second PJC
Comment:	A U wave is present.

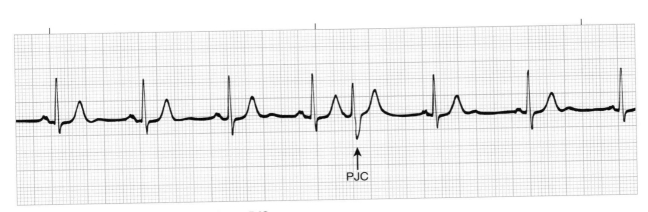

Figure 8.6	**Normal sinus rhythm with one PJC.**
Rhythm:	Basic rhythm regular; irregular with PJC
Rate:	Basic rhythm rate 63; rate slows to 56 following PJC owing to rate suppression (common following a pause in the basic rhythm)
P waves:	Sinus P waves with basic rhythm; P wave associated with PJC is hidden in the QRS complex
PR interval:	0.12 to 0.18 second (basic rhythm)
QRS complex:	0.08 second (basic rhythm); 0.10 second PJC
Comment:	A U wave is present.

the premature beat will be negative in lead II (a positive lead). The inverted P waves will occur immediately before the QRS complex, will occur immediately after the QRS complex, or will be hidden within the QRS complex. The PR interval will be short (0.10 second or less). Figure 8.4 shows a PJC with the P wave before the QRS complex; Figure 8.5 shows a PJC with the P wave after the QRS complex; and in Figure 8.6 the P wave is hidden within the QRS. PJCs are less common than PACs or premature ventricular contractions (PVCs) (discussed in Chapter 9).

Inverted P waves in lead II may also occur with PACs if the pacemaker site is located in the lower atria near the AV junction, but the associated PR interval will be normal duration (not short like the PJC).

If difficulty is encountered in differentiating PJCs from PACs, keep the following in mind: PACs are much more common than PJCs. As a result, narrow complex premature beats are more likely to be PACs. A comparison of ectopic atrial beats and ectopic junctional beats is shown in Figure 8.7. PJCs occur in the same pattern as PACs: as a single beat; in bigeminal, trigeminal, or quadrigeminal patterns; or in pairs (see Figure 8.8). A series of three or more consecutive junctional beats is considered a rhythm (junctional rhythm, accelerated junctional

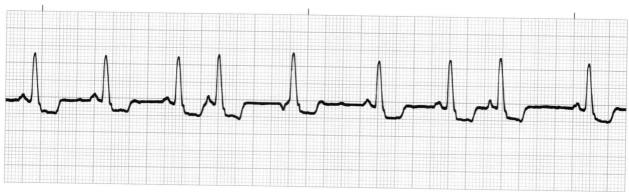

Figure 8.7 **Normal sinus rhythm with two premature atrial contractions (PACs) (4th and 8th complexes) and one junctional escape beat (5th complex).**

Rhythm:	Regular (basic rhythm); irregular with PACs and junctional escape beat
Rate:	75 beats/minute (basic rhythm)
P waves:	Sinus (basic rhythm); pointed P waves with PACs; inverted P waves with junctional escape beat
PR interval:	0.14 second (basic rhythm); 0.12 second (PACs); 0.10 second (junctional escape beat)
QRS complex:	0.08 to 0.10 second (basic rhythm); 0.08 second (PACs and junctional escape beat).

rhythm, or junctional tachycardia). Differentiation of the rhythm depends on the heart rate.

Like PACs, the premature junctional impulse may be conducted to the ventricles abnormally (aberrantly). This results in a wide QRS complex. A PJC associated with a wide QRS complex is called a PJC with aberrancy, indicating that conduction through the ventricles is abnormal. Because of the wide QRS complex, PJCs with aberrancy must be differentiated from PVCs.

Conditions associated with PJCs include ingestion of substances such as caffeine, alcohol, or tobacco; electrolyte imbalances; hypoxia; congestive heart failure; coronary artery disease; and enhanced automaticity of the AV junction caused by digitalis toxicity (the most

common cause). PJCs may also occur without apparent cause.

Frequent PJCs are best treated by correcting the underlying cause: decreasing or eliminating the consumption of caffeine, alcohol, or tobacco; correcting electrolyte imbalances; administering oxygen; treating congestive heart failure; and assessing digitalis levels. Frequent PJCs (more than 6 per minute) may precede the development of a more serious junctional arrhythmia, such as junctional tachycardia.

Occasionally, an ectopic beat will occur late instead of early. This beat is called a junctional escape beat (see Figures 8.7 and 8.9). Junctional escape beats usually occur during a pause in the underlying rhythm (following sinus

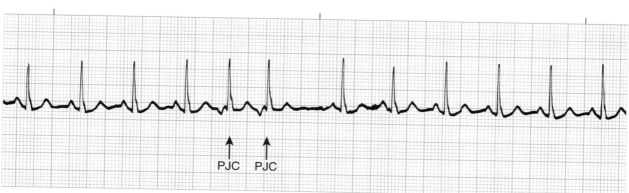

Figure 8.8 **Normal sinus rhythm with paired PJCs.**

Rhythm:	Basic rhythm regular; irregular following paired PJCs
Rate:	Basic rhythm rate 100
P waves:	Sinus P waves with basic rhythm; inverted P waves with PJCs
PR interval:	0.12 to 0.14 second basic rhythm; 0.08 second with PJCs
QRS complex:	0.06 to 0.08 second (basic rhythm and PJCs).

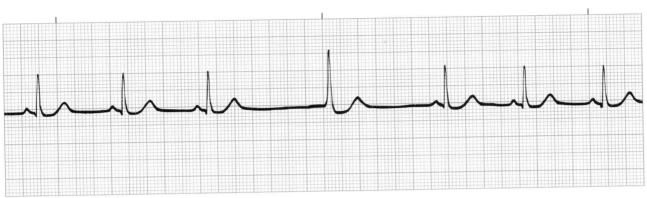

Figure 8.9   Normal sinus rhythm with a pause followed by a junctional escape beat.

Rhythm: Regular with basic rhythm; irregular with escape beat
Rate: 63 beats/minute (basic rhythm)
P waves: Sinus P waves with basic rhythm; P waves hidden in QRS with junctional escape beat
PR interval: 0.12 to 0.14 second (basic rhythm)
QRS complex: 0.06 to 0.10 second (basic rhythm); 0.08 second (junctional escape beat).

arrest or block, after premature beats or nonconducted PACs, or during the pause associated with Mobitz I heart block). The pause in the rhythm allows a focus in the AV junction to "escape" and pace the heart. The morphologic features of the late beat will be the same as the PJC. Escape beats act as an electrical backup to maintain the heart rate and require no treatment.

Junctional Rhythm

Junctional rhythm (Figures 8.10 through 8.13 and Box 8.2) is an arrhythmia originating in the AV junction with a rate between 40 and 60 beats per minute. Junctional rhythm is the normal rhythm of the AV junction. Junctional rhythm most often occurs when the heart rate of the dominant pacemaker (usually the sinus node) becomes less than the heart rate of the AV junction. When this occurs, a focus in the AV junction can "escape" and pace the heart at the inherent firing rate of the AV junction. For this reason, junctional rhythm is sometimes referred to as junctional escape rhythm. Junctional rhythm can also occur following a pause in the underlying rhythm (following sinus arrest or block, after premature beats or nonconducted

box 8.2	Junctional Rhythm: Identifying ECG Features
Rhythm:	Regular
Rate:	40 to 60 beats/minute
P waves:	Inverted in lead II and occurs immediately before the QRS complex, occurs immediately after the QRS complex, or is hidden within the QRS complex
PR interval:	Short (0.10 second or less)
QRS complex:	Normal (0.10 second or less)

PACs, or during the pause associated with Mobitz I heart block).

Junctional rhythm is regular with a heart rate between 40 and 60 beats per minute. The P waves are inverted in lead II (a positive lead) and will occur immediately before the QRS complex, will occur immediately after the QRS complex, or will be hidden within the QRS complex. The PR interval is short (0.10 second or less). The QRS duration is normal. Junctional rhythm has the same ECG features as accelerated junctional rhythm and junctional tachycardia. The rhythm is differentiated from the other junctional rhythms by the heart rate. Junctional rhythm is not a common rhythm.

Junctional rhythm may be seen in acute myocardial infarction (particularly inferior wall MI), increased parasympathetic tone, disease of the sinoatrial (SA) node, and hypoxia. It can also occur in patients taking digitalis, calcium channel blockers, or beta-blockers.

The slow rate and loss of normal atrial contraction (atrial kick) secondary to retrograde atrial depolarization may cause a decrease in cardiac output. Treatment

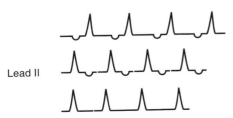

Lead II

Figure 8.10 Junctional rhythm will appear as a continuous rhythm at a rate of 40 to 60 beats/minute in either of the above three patterns.

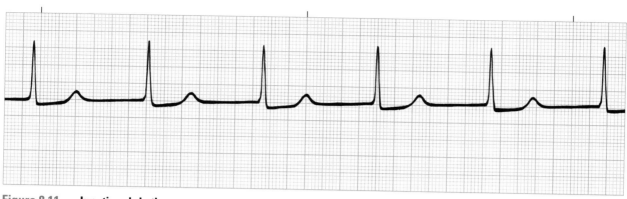

Figure 8.11   Junctional rhythm.

Rhythm:	Regular
Rate:	47 beats/minute
P waves:	Hidden in QRS complex
PR interval:	Not measurable
QRS complex:	0.06 to 0.08 second
Comment:	ST segment depression is present.

for symptomatic junctional rhythm includes following the protocols for significant bradycardia (atropine, pacing, and vasopressors to increase blood pressure). Treatment should also be directed at identifying and correcting the underlying cause of the rhythm if possible. All medications should be reviewed and discontinued if indicated.

Accelerated Junctional Rhythm

Accelerated junctional rhythm (Figures 8.14 through 8.16 and Box 8.3) is an arrhythmia originating in the AV junction with a rate between 60 and 100 beats per minute. The term "accelerated" denotes a rhythm that occurs at a rate that exceeds the junctional escape rate of 40 to 60 but isn't fast enough to be junctional tachycardia.

Accelerated junctional rhythm is regular with a heart rate between 60 and 100 beats per minute.

The P waves are inverted in lead II (a positive lead) and will occur immediately before the QRS complex, will occur immediately after the QRS complex, or will be hidden within the QRS complex. The PR interval is short (0.10 second or less). The QRS duration is normal. Accelerated junctional rhythm has the same ECG features as junctional rhythm and junctional tachycardia. This rhythm is differentiated from the other junctional rhythms by the heart rate. Accelerated junctional rhythm is not a common rhythm.

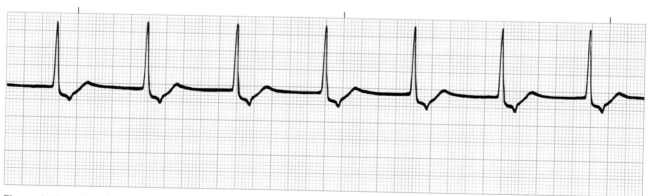

Figure 8.12   Junctional rhythm.

Rhythm:	Regular
Rate:	60 beats/minute
P waves:	Inverted after QRS complex
PR interval:	0.10 second
QRS complex:	0.06 to 0.08 second.

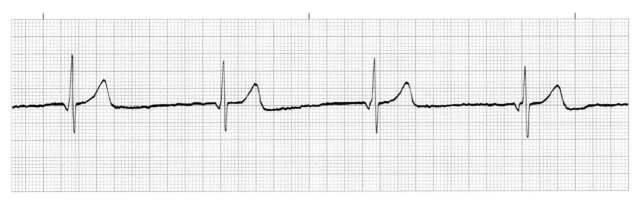

Figure 8.13   Junctional rhythm.

Rhythm:	Regular
Rate:	35 beats/minute
P waves:	Inverted before the QRS
PR interval:	0.06 to 0.08 second
QRS complex:	0.06 to 0.08 second.

Lead II

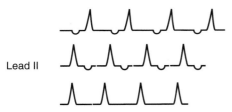

Figure 8.14   Accelerated junctional rhythm will appear as a continuous rhythm at a rate of 60 to 100 beats/minute in any of the above three patterns.

box 8.3   Accelerated Junctional Rhythm: Identifying ECG Features

Rhythm:	Regular
Rate:	60 to 100 beats/minute
P waves:	Inverted in lead II and occurs immediately before the QRS complex, occurs immediately after the QRS complex, or is hidden within the QRS complex
PR interval:	Short (0.10 second or less)
QRS complex:	Normal (0.10 second or less)

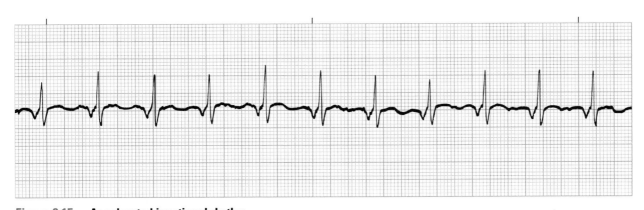

Figure 8.15   Accelerated junctional rhythm.

Rhythm:	Regular
Rate:	94 beats/minute
P waves:	Inverted before QRS complex
PR interval:	0.08 second
QRS complex:	0.08 to 0.10 second.

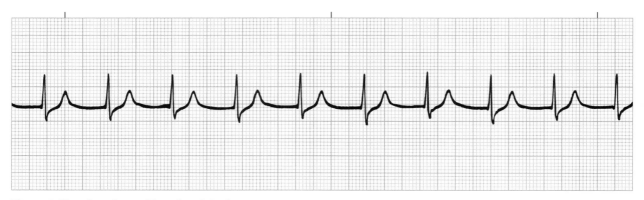

Figure 8.16   Accelerated junctional rhythm.

Rhythm: Regular
Rate: 84 beats/minute
P waves: Hidden in QRS complex
PR interval: Not measurable
QRS complex: 0.06 to 0.08 second.

Accelerated junctional rhythm may result from enhanced automaticity of the AV junction caused by digitalis toxicity (the most common cause). The rhythm may also be caused by damage to the AV junction from myocardial infarction, especially inferior wall MI.

Usually, the heart rate associated with accelerated junctional rhythm isn't a problem because it corresponds to that of the sinus node (60 to 100 beats per minute). Problems are more likely to occur from the loss of the atrial kick secondary to retrograde depolarization of the atria, resulting in a reduction in cardiac output. Treatment is directed at reversing the consequences of reduced cardiac output, if present, as well as identifying and correcting the underlying cause of the rhythm. All medications should be reviewed and discontinued if indicated.

Paroxysmal Junctional Tachycardia

Paroxysmal junctional tachycardia (PJT) (Figures 8.17 and 8.18 and Box 8.4) is an arrhythmia originating in the AV junction with a heart rate exceeding 100 beats per minute. Junctional tachycardia commonly starts and stops abruptly (like PAT) and is often precipitated by a premature junctional complex. Three or more PJCs in a row at a rate exceeding 100 per minute constitute a run of junctional tachycardia.

Junctional tachycardia is regular with a heart rate exceeding 100 beats per minute. The P waves are inverted in lead II (a positive lead) and will occur immediately before the QRS complex, will occur immediately after the QRS complex, or will be hidden within the QRS complex. The PR interval will be short (0.10 second or less). The QRS duration is normal. Junctional tachycardia has the same ECG features as junctional rhythm and accelerated junctional rhythm. This rhythm is differentiated from the other junctional

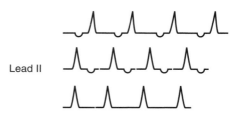

Lead II

Figure 8.17   Paroxysmal junctional tachycardia will appear as a continuous rhythm at a rate exceeding 100 beats/minute in any of the above three patterns.

rhythms by the heart rate. Junctional tachycardia is not a common rhythm.

Junctional tachycardia may result from enhanced automaticity of the AV junction caused by digitalis toxicity (the most common cause). The rhythm may also be caused by damage to the AV junction from myocardial infarction, especially inferior wall MI.

Junctional tachycardia may lead to a decrease in cardiac output related to the faster heart rate as well as the loss

box 8.4	Paroxysmal Junctional Tachycardia: Identifying ECG Features
Rhythm:	Regular
Rate:	Greater than 100 beats/minute
P waves:	Inverted in lead II and occurs immediately before the QRS complex, occurs immediately after the QRS complex, or is hidden within the QRS complex
PR interval:	Short (0.10 second or less)
QRS complex:	Normal (0.10 second or less)

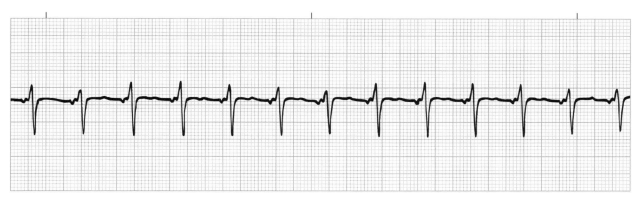

Figure 8.18   **Paroxysmal junctional tachycardia.**

Rhythm: Regular
Rate: 107 beats/minute
P waves: Inverted before QRS complex
PR interval: 0.08 second
QRS complex: 0.08 to 0.10 second.

of the atrial kick secondary to retrograde depolarization of the atria. Treatment is directed at reversing the consequences of reduced cardiac output, as well as identifying and correcting the underlying cause of the rhythm. All medications should be reviewed and discontinued if indicated.

AV Heart Blocks—Overview

The term heart block is used to describe arrhythmias in which there is delayed conduction or failed conduction of impulses through the AV node into the ventricles. Normally, the AV node acts as a bridge between the atria and ventricles. The PR interval is primarily a measure of conduction between the initial stimulation of the atria and the initial stimulation of the ventricles. This measurement is normally 0.12 to 0.20 second.

The site of pathology of the AV blocks may be at the level of the AV node, the bundle of His, or the bundle branches. When located at the level of the AV node or bundle of His, the QRS complexes will be normal duration. The QRS complex will be wide if the site of pathology is located in the bundle branches.

AV blocks are classified into first-degree, second-degree (types I and II), and third-degree AV block. This classification system is based on the degree (type) of block and the location of the block. It is important to remember that the PR interval is the key to identifying the type of block present. The width of the QRS complex and the ventricular rate are keys to differentiating the location of the block (the lower the location of the block in the conduction system, the wider the QRS complexes and the slower the ventricular rate).

In first-degree AV block (the mildest form), the electrical impulses are delayed in the AV node longer than normal, but all impulses are conducted to the ventricles. In second-degree AV block (types I and II), some impulses are conducted to the ventricles and some are blocked. The most extreme form of heart block is third-degree AV block, in which no impulses are conducted from the atria to the ventricles. The clinical significance of an AV block depends on the degree of block, the ventricular rate, and the patient response.

The ability to accurately diagnose AV blocks depends on a systematic approach. The following steps are suggested:

- Look for the P wave. Is there one P wave before each QRS or more than one?
- Measure the regularity of the atrial rhythm (the P-P interval) and the ventricular rhythm (the R-R interval).
- Measure the PR interval. Is the PR interval consistent or does it vary? *Remember, the PR interval is the key to identifying the type of AV block present.*
- Look at the QRS complex. Is it narrow or wide? *Remember, the width of the QRS complex and the ventricular rate are keys to identifying the location of the block.*

First-Degree AV Block

In first-degree heart block (Figure 8.19 and Box 8.5), all components of the ECG tracing are usually normal except the PR interval. The sinus impulse is normally conducted to the AV node, where it's delayed longer than usual before being conducted to the ventricles. This delay in the AV node results in a prolonged PR interval (greater than 0.20 second). This rhythm is reflected on the ECG by a

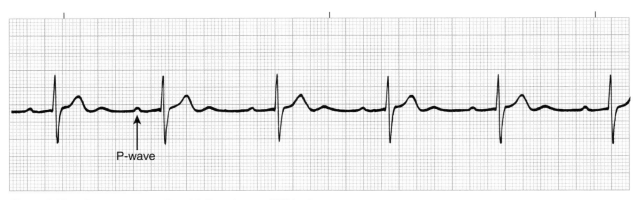

Figure 8.19 **Sinus bradycardia with first-degree AV block.**

Rhythm: Regular
Rate: 48 beats/minute
P waves: Sinus P waves present; one P wave to each QRS complex
PR interval: 0.28 to 0.32 second (remains constant)
QRS complex: 0.08 to 0.10 second
Comment: A U wave is present.

regular rhythm (both atrial and ventricular), one P wave preceding each QRS complex, a consistent but prolonged PR interval, and a narrow QRS complex. This conduction disorder is located at the level of the AV node (thus the narrow QRS complex) and isn't a serious form of heart block. The underlying sinus rhythm is usually identified along with the AV block when interpreting the rhythm (for example, normal sinus rhythm with first-degree AV block).

First-degree AV block may occur from ischemia or injury to the AV node secondary to acute myocardial infarction (usually inferior wall MI), increased parasympathetic tone, drug effects (beta-blockers, calcium channel blockers, digitalis, amiodarone), hyperkalemia, degeneration of the conduction pathways associated with aging, and unknown causes.

First-degree AV block produces no symptoms and requires no treatment. Because first-degree heart block can progress to a higher degree of AV block under certain conditions, the rhythm should continue to be monitored until the block resolves or stabilizes. Drugs causing AV block should be reviewed and discontinued if indicated.

Second-Degree AV Block, Type I (Mobitz I or Wenckebach)

Second-degree AV block, type I, is commonly known as Mobitz I or Wenckebach (for the early 20th century physician who discovered it). In Mobitz I (Figures 8.20 through 8.23 and Box 8.6), most of the impulses are conducted to the ventricles, but some are blocked. In this rhythm, the sinus impulse is normally conducted to the AV node, but each successive impulse has increasing difficulty passing through the AV node, until finally an impulse does not pass through (isn't conducted). This rhythm is reflected on the ECG by P waves that occur at regular intervals across the rhythm strip (regular P-P interval) and PR intervals that progressively lengthen from beat to beat until a P wave appears that is not followed by a QRS complex but instead by a pause. The missing QRS complex (dropped

---

box 8.5 First-Degree AV Block: Identifying ECG Features

Rhythm: Regular
Rate: That of the underlying sinus rhythm; both atrial and ventricular rates will be the same.
P waves: Sinus, one P wave to each QRS complex
PR interval: Consistent; prolonged (greater than 0.20 second)
QRS complex: Normal (0.10 second or less)

---

box 8.6 Second-Degree AV Block (Mobitz I): Identifying ECG Features

Rhythm: Regular atrial rhythm; irregular ventricular rhythm
Rate: Atrial: That of the underlying sinus rhythm
Ventricular: Varies depending on number of impulses conducted through AV node (will be less than the atrial rate)
P waves: Sinus
PR interval: Not consistent (varies); progressively lengthens until a P wave isn't conducted (P wave occurs without the QRS complex); a pause follows the dropped QRS complex.
QRS complex: Normal (0.10 second or less)

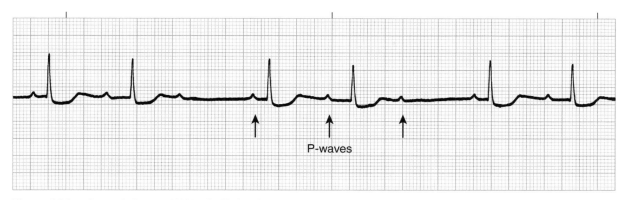

P-waves

Figure 8.20   **Second-degree AV block; Mobitz I.**

Rhythm:	Regular atrial rhythm; irregular ventricular rhythm
Rate:	Atrial: 72 beats/minute
	Ventricular: 50 beats/minute
P waves:	Sinus P waves present
PR interval:	Progressively lengthens from 0.20 to 0.32 second
QRS complex:	0.06 to 0.08 second
Comment:	ST segment depression is present.

beat) causes the ventricular rhythm (the R-R interval) to be irregular. After each dropped beat, the cycle repeats itself. The overall appearance of the rhythm demonstrates group beating (groups of beats separated by pauses) and is a distinguishing characteristic of Mobitz I. Escape beats (atrial, junctional, or ventricular) may occasionally occur during the pause in the ventricular rhythm and may obscure the diagnosis because they interrupt the group beating pattern (see Figure 8.22). The location of the conduction disturbance is at the level of the AV node, and therefore, the QRS complex will be narrow.

Mobitz I can be confused with the nonconducted PAC (see Figure 8.23). Both rhythms have episodes where P waves are not followed by a QRS complex, but instead

by a pause. To differentiate between the two rhythms, one must examine the configuration of the P waves and measure the P-P regularity. The nonconducted PAC will have an abnormal P wave and will occur prematurely. In Mobitz I, the P wave is normal and occurs on schedule, not prematurely.

Mobitz I is common following acute inferior wall myocardial infarction owing to AV node ischemia. Other causes include increased parasympathetic (vagal) tone, effects of medications (digitalis, beta-blockers, calcium channel blockers), and hyperkalemia. Mobitz I may also occur as a normal variant in athletes because of a physiologic increase in vagal tone. Mobitz I, under certain conditions, may progress to a higher degree of AV block, but generally, this

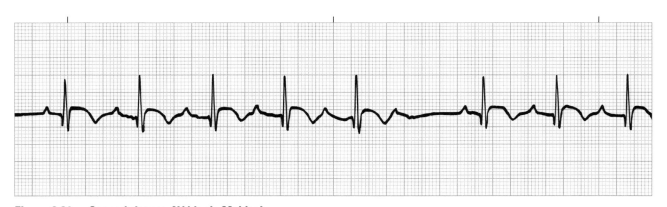

Figure 8.21   **Second-degree AV block, Mobitz I.**

Rhythm:	Regular atrial rhythm; irregular ventricular rhythm
Rate:	Atrial: 75 beats/minute
	Ventricular: 60 beats/minute
P waves:	Sinus P waves
PR interval:	Progressively lengthens from 0.20 to 0.32 second
QRS complex:	0.08 to 0.10 second.

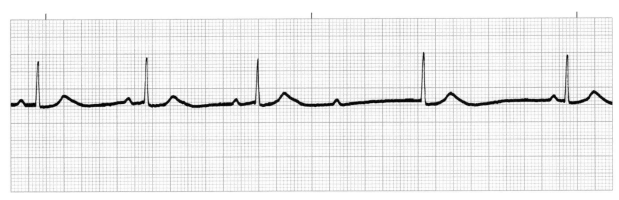

Figure 8.22 **Mobitz I with junctional escape beat (during pause).**

Rhythm:	Regular (atrial rhythm, except during pause); Irregular: ventricular rhythm
Rate:	Atrial (50 beats/minute); ventricular (48 beats/minute)
P waves:	Sinus (basic rhythm); hidden P wave with junctional escape beat
PR interval:	Progressively lengthens from 0.20 to 0.24 second
QRS complex:	0.04 to 0.06 second (basic rhythm); 0.04 second (junctional escape beat).

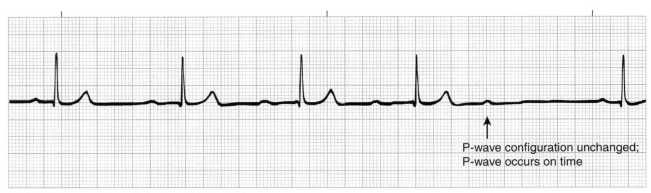

P-wave configuration unchanged;
P-wave occurs on time

MOBITZ I
- Pause in basic ventricular rhythm
- P-P regularity unchanged (P wave occurs on time)
- P wave configuration same as sinus beats
- PR interval of basic rhythm varies

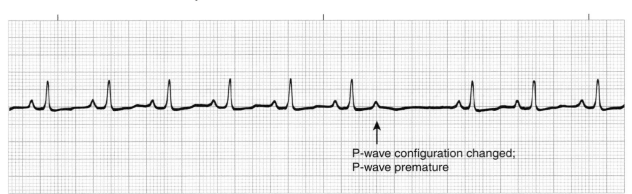

P-wave configuration changed;
P-wave premature

Nonconducted PAC
- Pause in basic ventricular rhythm
- P-P regularity interrupted (P wave occurs prematurely)
- P wave configuration different from sinus beats
- PR interval of basic rhythm remains consistent

Figure 8.23 **Differentiation of the nonconducted premature atrial contraction from Mobitz I.**

is not the case. This type of AV block is usually temporary and resolves spontaneously.

Mobitz I is usually asymptomatic because the ventricular rate is often normal and cardiac output is usually not affected. If the ventricular rate is slow and the patient develops symptoms, protocols for symptomatic bradycardia (atropine, external or transvenous pacing, and vasopressors to increase blood pressure) should be followed. Conduction usually improves in response to the administration of atropine. Drugs causing AV block should be discontinued if indicated.

Second-Degree AV Block, Type II (Mobitz II)

In Mobitz II (Figures 8.24 and 8.25 and Box 8.7), some of the impulses are conducted to the ventricles, but most are blocked. In this rhythm, there is no progressive increase in the PR interval (the PR interval remains consistent). In Mobitz II, there is more than one P wave before each QRS complex (usually two or three, but sometimes more) with only one of the impulses being conducted to the ventricles. The rhythm would be described as Mobitz II with 2:1 or 3:1 AV conduction (see Figures 8.24 and 8.25). The P waves occur at regular intervals across the rhythm strip (regular P-P interval). In Mobitz II with higher conduction ratios (3:1 or more), the P waves may be hidden in the ST segment or T wave (Figure 8.25). The PR interval of the conducted beat may be normal or prolonged but remains consistent. The ventricular rhythm (the R-R interval) is usually regular unless the AV conduction ratio varies (alternating between 2:1, 3:1, 4:1, etc.). The location of the conduction disturbance is below the AV node in the bundle of His or bundle branches. As a result, the QRS complex may be narrow (if located in the bundle of His) or wide (if located in the bundle branches). The most common location is the bundle branches.

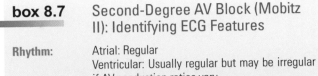

box 8.7	Second-Degree AV Block (Mobitz II): Identifying ECG Features
Rhythm:	Atrial: Regular Ventricular: Usually regular but may be irregular if AV conduction ratios vary
Rate:	Atrial: That of the underlying sinus rhythm Ventricular: Varies depending on number of impulses conducted through AV node (will be less than the atrial rate)
P waves:	Sinus; two or three P waves (sometimes more) before each QRS complex
PR interval:	Consistent; may be normal or prolonged
QRS complex:	Normal if block is located at the level of bundle of His; wide if block is located in bundle branches

Mobitz II is usually associated with an anterior wall myocardial infarction and, unlike Mobitz I, is not the result of increased vagal tone or drug toxicity. Other causes include acute myocarditis and degeneration of the electrical conduction system seen in the elderly.

The patient's response to Mobitz II is usually related to the ventricular rate. If the ventricular rate is within normal limits (rare), the patient may be asymptomatic. More commonly, the ventricular rate is extremely slow, cardiac output is decreased, and symptoms are present (hypotension, shortness of breath, heart failure, chest pain, or syncope). The syncopal episodes, called ***Stokes-Adams syncope***, are caused by a sudden slowing or stopping of the heartbeat.

Mobitz II is less common but more serious than Mobitz I. Mobitz II has the potential to progress suddenly to third-degree AV block or ventricular standstill (asystole) with little or no warning. Treatment usually includes pacemaker therapy. External pacing can be used for treatment of symptomatic Mobitz II until transvenous pacing can be initiated. Atropine is not recommended for Mobitz II

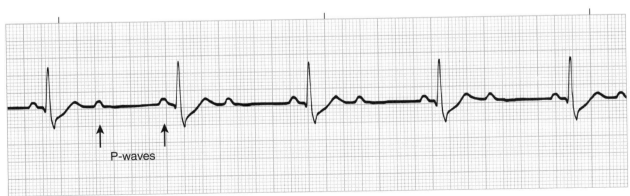

Figure 8.24   Second-degree AV block, Mobitz II with 2:1 AV conduction.

Rhythm:	Regular atrial and ventricular rhythm
Rate:	Atrial, 82 beats/minute; ventricular, 41 beats/minute
P waves:	Two sinus P waves to each QRS
PR interval:	0.16 second (remains consistent)
QRS complex:	0.12 to 0.14 second.

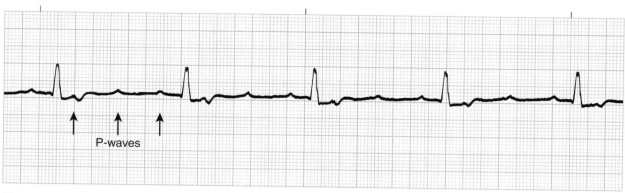

Figure 8.25   Second-degree AV block, Mobitz II with 3:1 AV conduction.

Rhythm:	Regular atrial and ventricular rhythm
Rate:	Atrial, 123 beats/minute; ventricular, 41 beats/minute
P waves:	Three sinus P waves to each QRS
PR interval:	0.24 to 0.26 second (remains consistent)
QRS complex:	0.12 second.

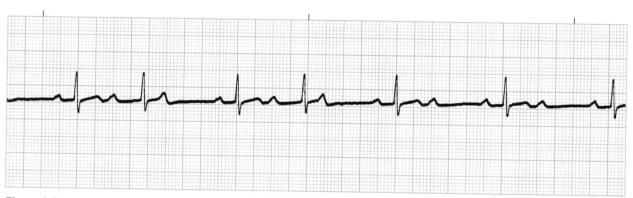

Figure 8.26   Mobitz I. This strip shows a typical Wenckebach pattern during the first part of the strip changing to a 2:1 conduction ratio at the end of the strip. Even though 2:1 conduction is seen (common with Mobitz II), the presence of a Wenckebach pattern confirms the diagnosis of Mobitz I.

Rhythm:	Atrial (regular); ventricular (irregular)
Rate:	Atrial (100 beats/minute); ventricular (60 beats/minute)
P waves:	Sinus
PR interval:	Progressively lengthens from 0.24 to 0.36 second
QRS complex:	0.06 to 0.08 second.

with wide QRS complexes because it may result in further slowing of the ventricular rate by increasing the number of impulses conducted through the AV node (more P waves) and delivering more impulses than the diseased bundles can handle (less QRS complexes). Vasopressors may be used to increase blood pressure. Unresolved Mobitz II will require a permanent pacemaker.

A 2:1 conduction ratio is common with Mobitz II (two P waves to each QRS complex). A 2:1 conduction ratio may also occasionally occur with Mobitz I. In Mobitz I with 2:1 conduction, every other impulse is not conducted and the ECG shows two P waves to one QRS complex. The only difference on the ECG would be a narrow QRS (seen in Mobitz I) and a wide QRS (seen more commonly, but not exclusively, with Mobitz II). Typically, if Mobitz I with 2:1 conduction is present, an occasional Wenckebach pattern

will usually assert itself when a longer rhythm strip is viewed, thus confirming the diagnosis of Mobitz I. Figure 8.26 shows such an example.

The AV block strips with consistent 2:1 AV conduction and a narrow QRS complex have been interpreted in the answer keys as Mobitz II with a notation that clinical correlation may be necessary to determine a definite diagnosis.

Third-Degree AV Block (Complete Heart Block)

Second-degree AV blocks (both Mobitz I and Mobitz II) are types of incomplete blocks because the AV junction conducts at least some of the impulses to the ventricles.

Third-degree AV block (Figures 8.27 and 8.28 and Box 8.8) represents complete absence of conduction between the atria and the ventricles. Thus, this rhythm is often called complete heart block.

With third-degree heart block, the atria and ventricles beat independently of each other, and there's no relationship between atrial activity and ventricular activity (AV dissociation). The atria are usually paced by the sinus node at its inherent rate of 60 to 100 beats per minute, and the ventricles are either paced by a pacemaker in the AV junction at a rate of 40 to 60 beats per minute or in the ventricles at a rate of 30 to 40 beats per minute. The P waves occur at regular intervals across the rhythm strip (regular P-P interval), but have no relationship to the QRS complexes, and therefore will be seen marching across the rhythm strip hiding inside QRS complexes or in the ST segment or T wave. The "hidden" P waves can be found by measuring the regularity of the atrial rhythm (the P-P interval). The PR intervals vary greatly. Both the atrial rhythm and the ventricular rhythm are usually regular. The width of the QRS complex and the ventricular rate reflect the location of the blockage. If the block is at the level of the AV node or bundle of His, the QRS complex will be narrow and the ventricular rate will be between 40 and 60 beats per minute. If the blockage is in the bundle branches, the QRS complex will be wide and the ventricular rate much slower (40 beats per minute or less). Generally, complete heart block with wide QRS complexes tends to be less stable than complete heart block with narrow QRS complexes.

Complete heart block associated with inferior wall MI is usually a result of a block at the level of the AV node or bundle of His. The rhythm is usually stable, and the ventricles are paced by a junctional pacemaker with narrow QRS complexes and a ventricular rate of 40 to 60 beats per minute. Third-degree AV block associated with an inferior wall MI often resolves on its own. Complete heart block associated with an anterior wall MI is usually a result of a block within the bundle branches.

box 8.8	Third-Degree AV Block (Complete Heart Block): Identifying ECG Features
Rhythm:	Atrial: Regular Ventricular: Regular
Rate:	Atrial: That of the underlying sinus rhythm Ventricular: 40 to 60 beats/minutes if paced by AV junction; 30 to 40 beats/minute (or less) if paced by the ventricles; will be less than the atrial rate
P waves:	Sinus P waves with no constant relationship to the QRS complex; P waves can be found hidden in QRS complexes, ST segments, and T waves
PR interval:	Not consistent (varies)
QRS complex:	Normal if block is located at the level of AV node or bundle of His; wide if block is located at the level of bundle branches

The rhythm is usually unstable and the ventricles are paced by a ventricular pacemaker with wide QRS complexes and a ventricular rate of 40 beats per minute or less. Third-degree AV block associated with an anterior MI often does not resolve on its own and may require permanent pacing.

Causes of third-degree heart block include coronary heart disease, myocardial infarction, congenital heart disease, cardiac surgery, and digitalis toxicity, and in older individuals who have chronic degenerative changes in their conduction system. It has also been reported with Lyme disease.

The patient's response to complete heart block is usually related to the ventricular rate and individual tolerance. If the rhythm is of gradual onset and the heart has time to compensate for the slow ventricular rate, the patient may be relatively asymptomatic with minor symptoms such as weakness, fatigue, dizziness, or exercise intolerance. This is often seen in individuals who have developed degenerative changes in their conduction system over a period of time. If the rhythm occurs suddenly with an abrupt decrease in

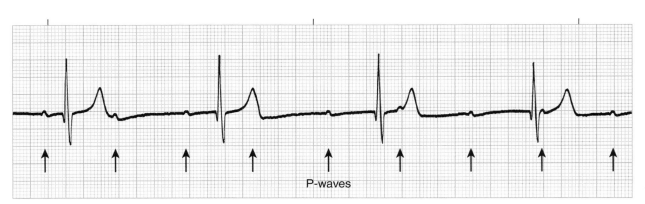

P-waves

Figure 8.27   **Third-degree AV block.**

Rhythm:	Regular (atrial); regular (ventricular) off by 2 squares
Rate:	Atrial (75 beats/minute); ventricular (33 to 34 beats/minute)
P waves:	Sinus P waves (have no relationship to QRS complexes; found hidden in QRS complexes, ST segments, and T waves)
PR interval:	Varies greatly (not consistent)
QRS complex:	0.12 second
Comment:	The ventricles are being paced by a ventricular focus since the QRS duration is wide.

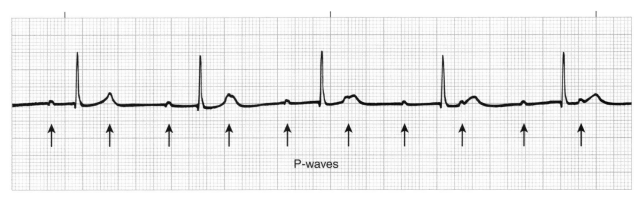

P-waves

Figure 8.28 **Third-degree AV block.**

Rhythm:	Regular atrial and ventricular rhythm
Rate:	Atrial: 88 beats/minute
	Ventricular: 43 beats/minute
P waves:	Sinus P waves
PR interval:	Varies greatly (is not consistent)
QRS complex:	0.06 to 0.08 second
Comment:	The ventricles are being paced by the AV node since the QRS duration is within normal limits.

ventricular rate, the patient is usually symptomatic (hypotension, dyspnea, heart failure, chest pain, or Stokes-Adams syncope). This often occurs following acute MI.

Regardless of its cause, compete heart block is a serious and potentially life-threatening arrhythmia. Third-degree AV block, like Mobitz II, can quickly progress to ventricular standstill with little or no warning. Treatment usually involves pacemaker therapy. External pacing can be used for treatment of symptomatic third-degree AV block until transvenous pacing can be initiated. Third-degree heart block with narrow QRS complexes may occasionally respond to atropine. Atropine is not recommended for third-degree AV block with wide QRS complexes because it may result in further slowing of the ventricular rate. Vasopressors may be used to treat hypotension. Unresolved compete heart block will require a permanent pacemaker.

Tips on Heart Blocks

To distinguish one heart block from another, remember these important tips:
- Measure the P-P interval. The P-P interval is regular in *all* the blocks. If you measure the P-P interval, you will be able to track the P waves. This is very important in finding hidden P waves seen in third-degree AV block or Mobitz II with higher conduction ratios (3:1 or more).
- Measure the R-R interval. First-degree and third-degree heart blocks have a regular ventricular rhythm. Mobitz I has an irregular ventricular rhythm. The ventricular rhythm in Mobitz II may be regular or irregular, depending on conduction ratios.
- Measure the PR interval. If the PR interval is consistent, choose between first-degree and Mobitz II heart block. First-degree heart block has one P wave to each QRS, whereas Mobitz II heart block has two or more P waves

to each QRS. If the PR interval is not consistent, choose between Mobitz I and third-degree heart block. In Mobitz I, the PR interval is not consistent and the ventricular rhythm is irregular. In third-degree heart block, the PR interval is not consistent and the ventricular rhythm is regular.

Table 8.1 compares the ECG features of each type of heart block. A **pull-out arrhythmia summary** of the junctional rhythms and heart blocks can be found in Table 8.2 at the back of the book. This may be used as a *quick guide to assist with rhythm interpretation.*

table 8.1 AV Block Comparisons

PR constant	PR varies
First-degree	***Second-degree, Mobitz I***
PR constant	PR varies
PR prolonged; one P wave to each QRS	PR progressively gets longer until a QRS is dropped
Regular atrial rhythm; regular ventricular rhythm	Regular atrial rhythm; irregular ventricular rhythm
Second-degree, Mobitz II	***Third-degree***
PR constant`	PR varies
PR normal or prolonged; two or three P waves (possibly more) to each QRS	P waves have no constant relationship to QRS (found hidden in QRS complexes, ST segments, and T waves)
Regular atrial rhythm; regular ventricular rhythm (unless conduction ratios vary)	Regular atrial rhythm; regular ventricular rhythm

RHYTHM STRIP PRACTICE: JUNCTIONAL ARRHYTHMIAS AND AV BLOCKS

Analyze the following rhythm strips by following the five basic steps:

- Determine *rhythm regularity.*
- Calculate *heart rate* (this usually refers to the ventricular rate, but if atrial rate differs, you need to calculate both).
- Identify and examine *P waves.*
- Measure *PR interval.*
- Measure *QRS complex.*

Interpret the rhythm by comparing this data with the ECG characteristics for each rhythm. All rhythm strips are lead II, a positive lead, unless otherwise noted. Check your answers with the answer key in the appendix.

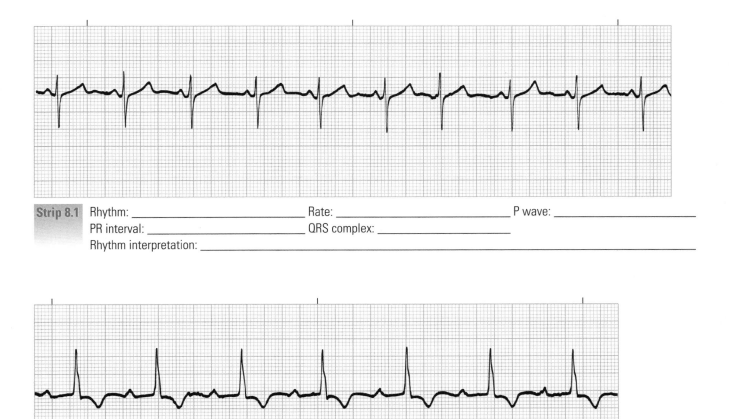

Strip 8.1 Rhythm: _____ Rate: _____ P wave: _____
PR interval: _____ QRS complex: _____
Rhythm interpretation: _____

Strip 8.2 Rhythm: _____ Rate: _____ P wave: _____
PR interval: _____ QRS complex: _____
Rhythm interpretation: _____

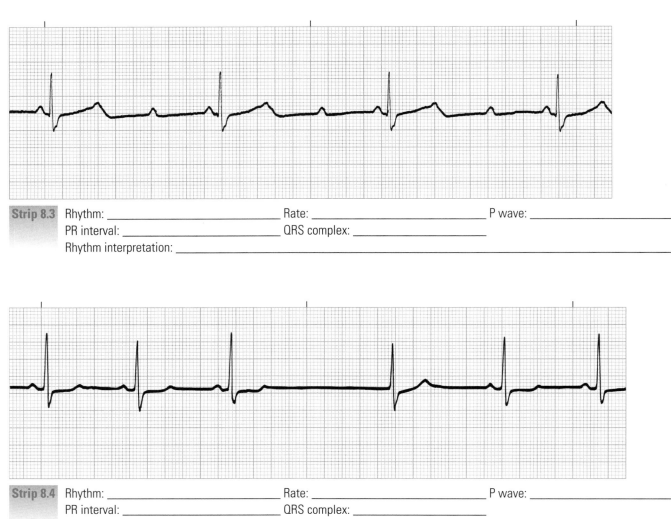

Strip 8.3 Rhythm: _____   Rate: _____   P wave: _____
PR interval: _____   QRS complex: _____
Rhythm interpretation: _____

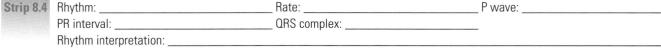

Strip 8.4 Rhythm: _____   Rate: _____   P wave: _____
PR interval: _____   QRS complex: _____
Rhythm interpretation: _____

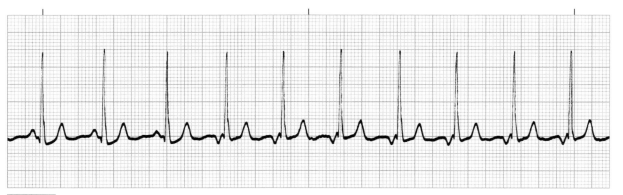

Strip 8.5 Rhythm: _____   Rate: _____   P wave: _____
PR interval: _____   QRS complex: _____
Rhythm interpretation: _____

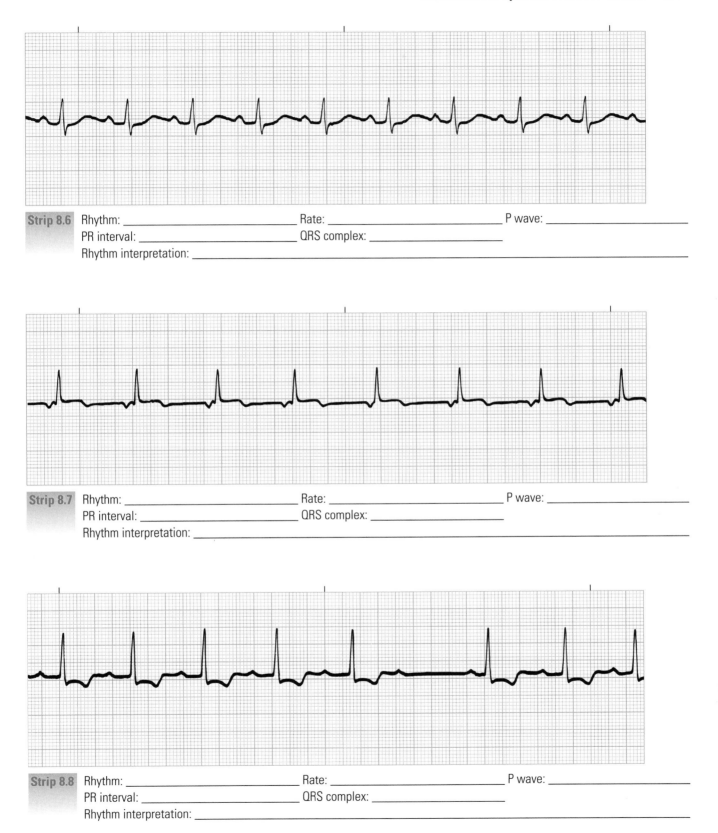

Strip 8.6   Rhythm: _____   Rate: _____   P wave: _____
PR interval: _____   QRS complex: _____
Rhythm interpretation: _____

Strip 8.7   Rhythm: _____   Rate: _____   P wave: _____
PR interval: _____   QRS complex: _____
Rhythm interpretation: _____

Strip 8.8   Rhythm: _____   Rate: _____   P wave: _____
PR interval: _____   QRS complex: _____
Rhythm interpretation: _____

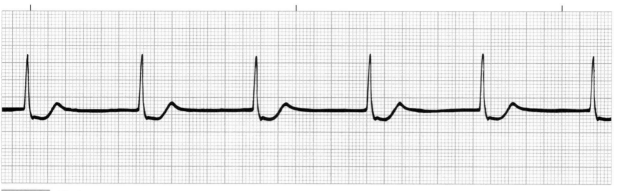

Strip 8.9   Rhythm: _____ Rate: _____ P wave: _____
PR interval: _____ QRS complex: _____
Rhythm interpretation: _____

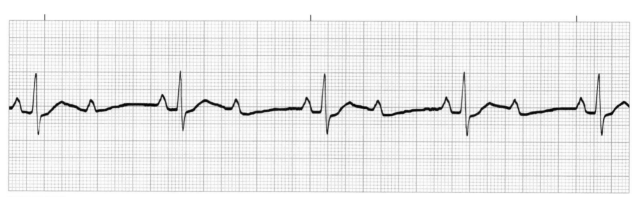

Strip 8.10   Rhythm: _____ Rate: _____ P wave: _____
PR interval: _____ QRS complex: _____
Rhythm interpretation: _____

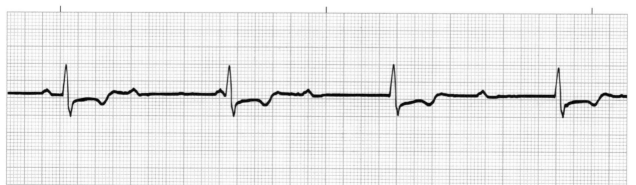

Strip 8.11   Rhythm: _____ Rate: _____ P wave: _____
PR interval: _____ QRS complex: _____
Rhythm interpretation: _____

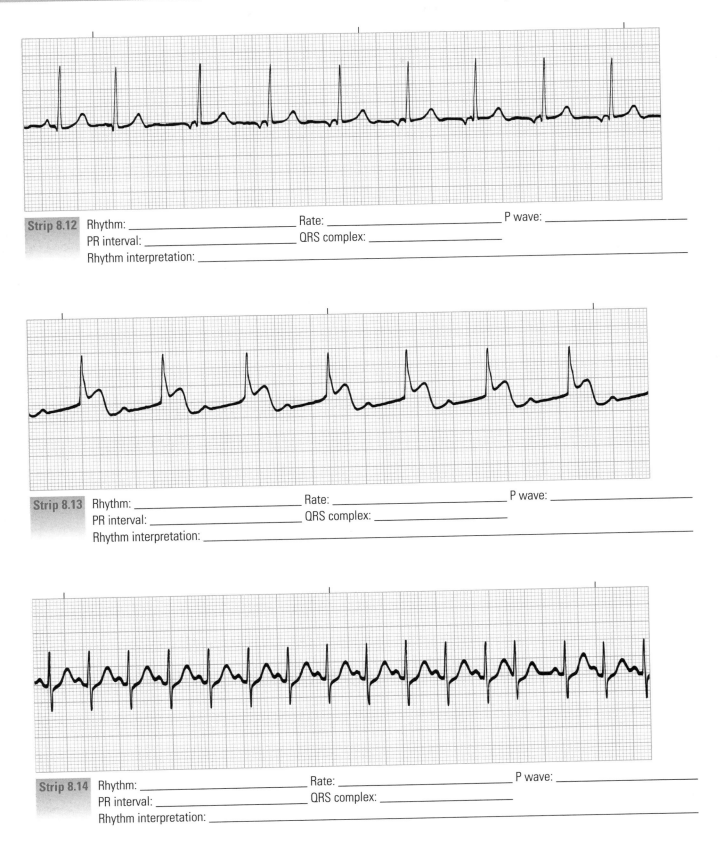

Strip 8.12 Rhythm: _____ Rate: _____ P wave: _____

PR interval: _____ QRS complex: _____

Rhythm interpretation: _____

Strip 8.13 Rhythm: _____ Rate: _____ P wave: _____

PR interval: _____ QRS complex: _____

Rhythm interpretation: _____

Strip 8.14 Rhythm: _____ Rate: _____ P wave: _____

PR interval: _____ QRS complex: _____

Rhythm interpretation: _____

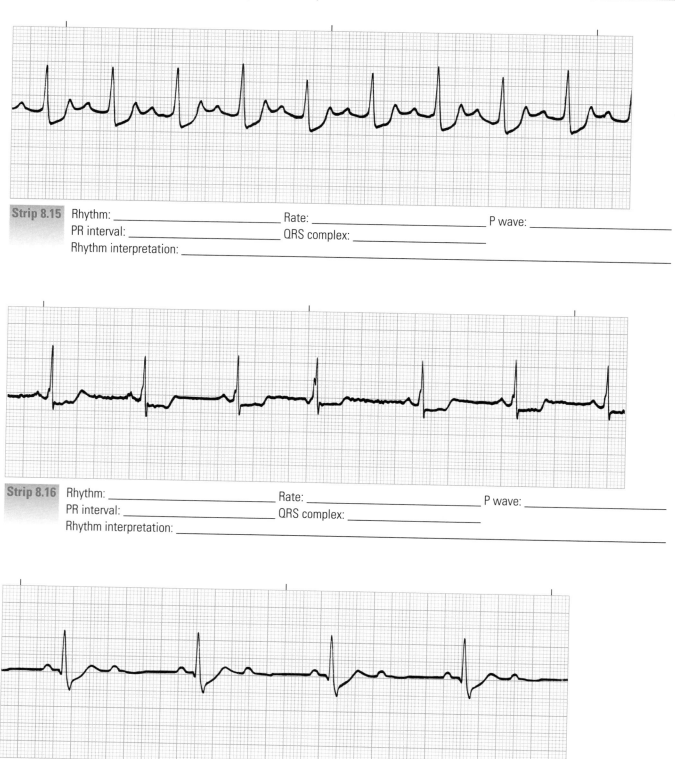

Strip 8.15 Rhythm: _____ Rate: _____ P wave: _____
PR interval: _____ QRS complex: _____
Rhythm interpretation: _____

Strip 8.16 Rhythm: _____ Rate: _____ P wave: _____
PR interval: _____ QRS complex: _____
Rhythm interpretation: _____

Strip 8.17 Rhythm: _____ Rate: _____ P wave: _____
PR interval: _____ QRS complex: _____
Rhythm interpretation: _____

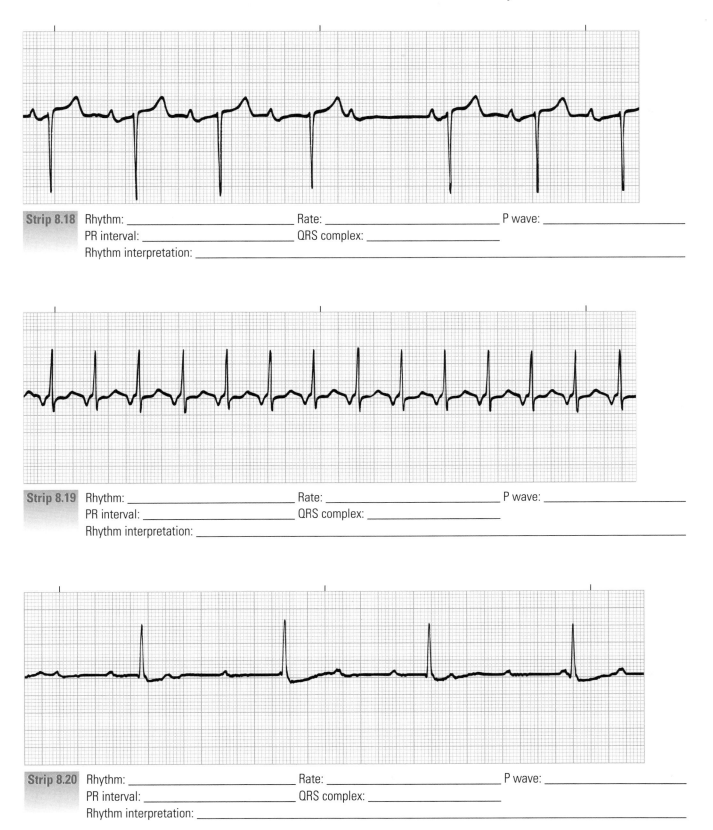

Strip 8.18 Rhythm: _____ Rate: _____ P wave: _____
PR interval: _____ QRS complex: _____
Rhythm interpretation: _____

Strip 8.19 Rhythm: _____ Rate: _____ P wave: _____
PR interval: _____ QRS complex: _____
Rhythm interpretation: _____

Strip 8.20 Rhythm: _____ Rate: _____ P wave: _____
PR interval: _____ QRS complex: _____
Rhythm interpretation: _____

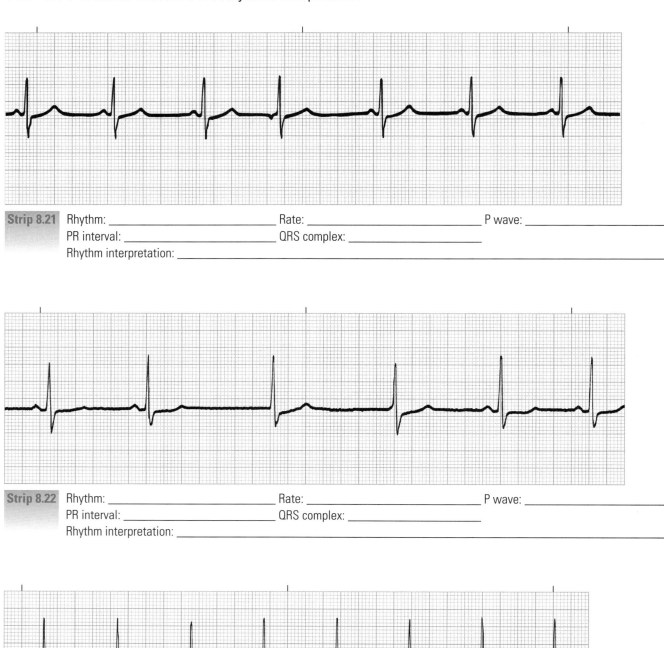

Strip 8.21 Rhythm: _____ Rate: _____ P wave: _____
PR interval: _____ QRS complex: _____
Rhythm interpretation: _____

Strip 8.22 Rhythm: _____ Rate: _____ P wave: _____
PR interval: _____ QRS complex: _____
Rhythm interpretation: _____

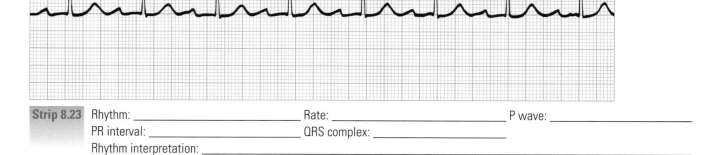

Strip 8.23 Rhythm: _____ Rate: _____ P wave: _____
PR interval: _____ QRS complex: _____
Rhythm interpretation: _____

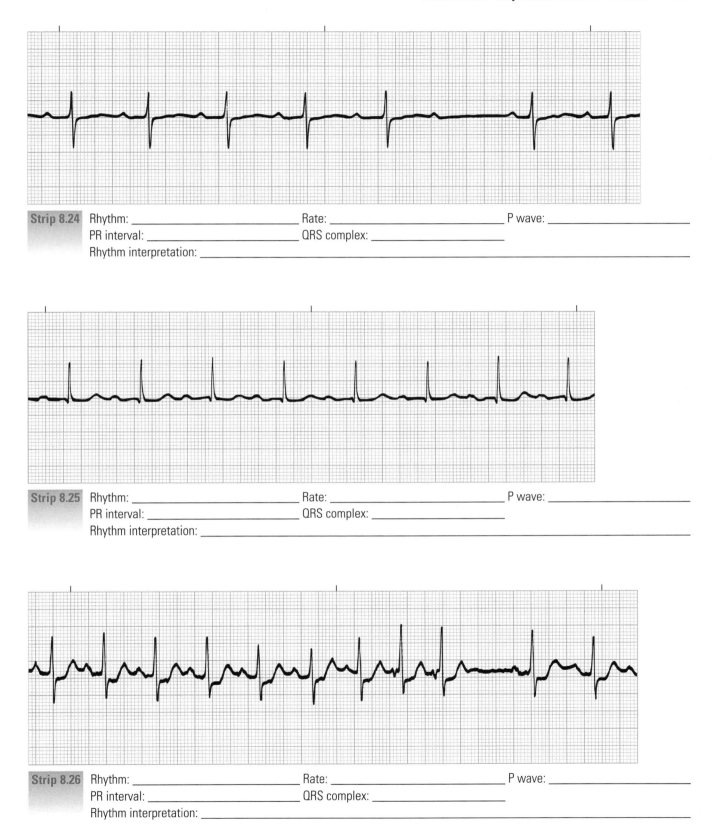

Rhythm: _____ Rate: _____ P wave: _____
PR interval: _____ QRS complex: _____
Rhythm interpretation: _____

Rhythm: _____ Rate: _____ P wave: _____
PR interval: _____ QRS complex: _____
Rhythm interpretation: _____

Rhythm: _____ Rate: _____ P wave: _____
PR interval: _____ QRS complex: _____
Rhythm interpretation: _____

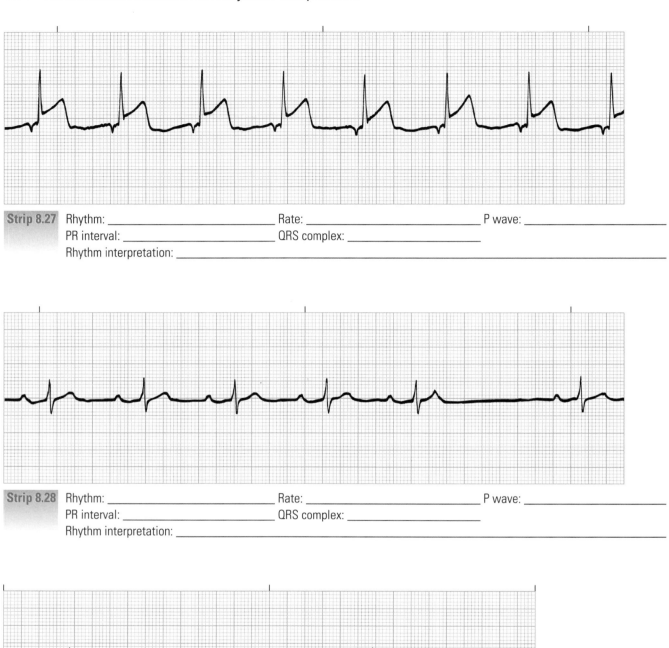

Strip 8.27 Rhythm: _____ Rate: _____ P wave: _____

PR interval: _____ QRS complex: _____

Rhythm interpretation: _____

Strip 8.28 Rhythm: _____ Rate: _____ P wave: _____

PR interval: _____ QRS complex: _____

Rhythm interpretation: _____

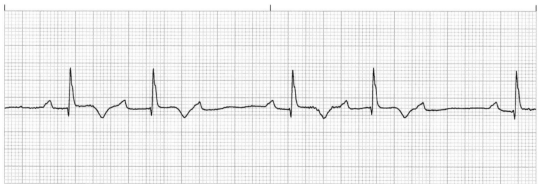

Strip 8.29 Rhythm: _____ Rate: _____ P wave: _____

PR interval: _____ QRS complex: _____

Rhythm interpretation: _____

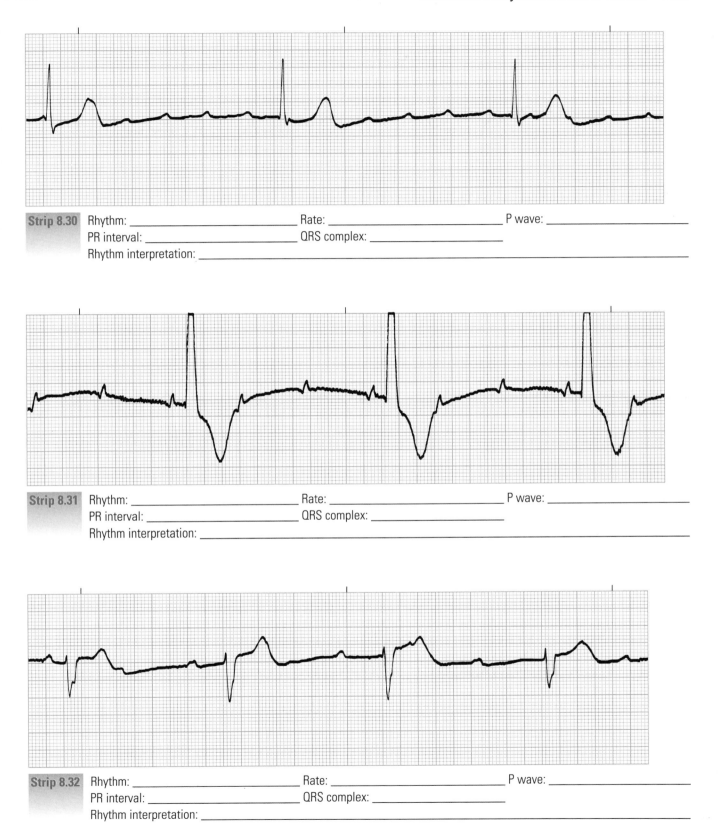

Strip 8.30 Rhythm: _____ Rate: _____ P wave: _____
PR interval: _____ QRS complex: _____
Rhythm interpretation: _____

Strip 8.31 Rhythm: _____ Rate: _____ P wave: _____
PR interval: _____ QRS complex: _____
Rhythm interpretation: _____

Strip 8.32 Rhythm: _____ Rate: _____ P wave: _____
PR interval: _____ QRS complex: _____
Rhythm interpretation: _____

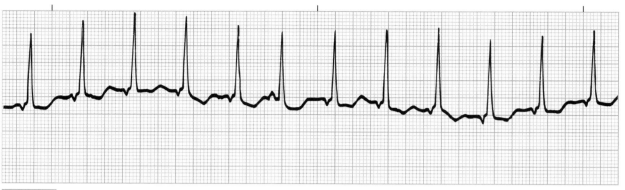

Strip 8.33 Rhythm: _____ Rate: _____ P wave: _____

PR interval: _____ QRS complex: _____

Rhythm interpretation: _____

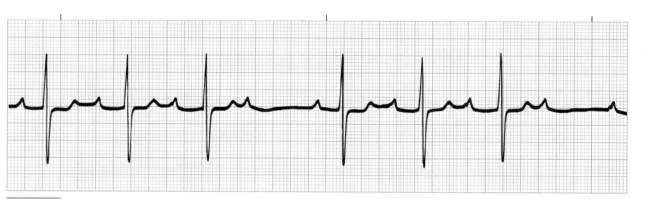

Strip 8.34 Rhythm: _____ Rate: _____ P wave: _____

PR interval: _____ QRS complex: _____

Rhythm interpretation: _____

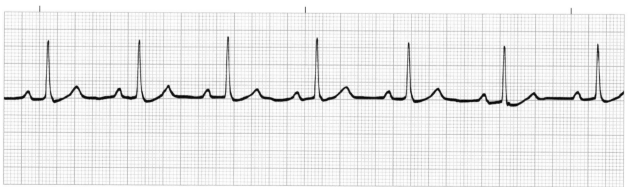

Strip 8.35 Rhythm: _____ Rate: _____ P wave: _____

PR interval: _____ QRS complex: _____

Rhythm interpretation: _____

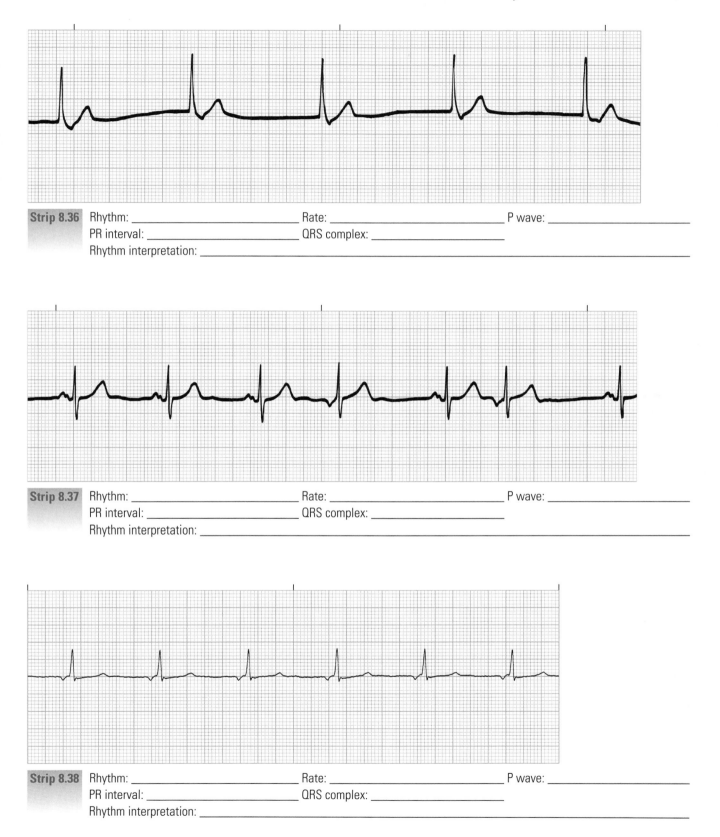

Strip 8.36   Rhythm: _____   Rate: _____   P wave: _____
PR interval: _____   QRS complex: _____
Rhythm interpretation: _____

Strip 8.37   Rhythm: _____   Rate: _____   P wave: _____
PR interval: _____   QRS complex: _____
Rhythm interpretation: _____

Strip 8.38   Rhythm: _____   Rate: _____   P wave: _____
PR interval: _____   QRS complex: _____
Rhythm interpretation: _____

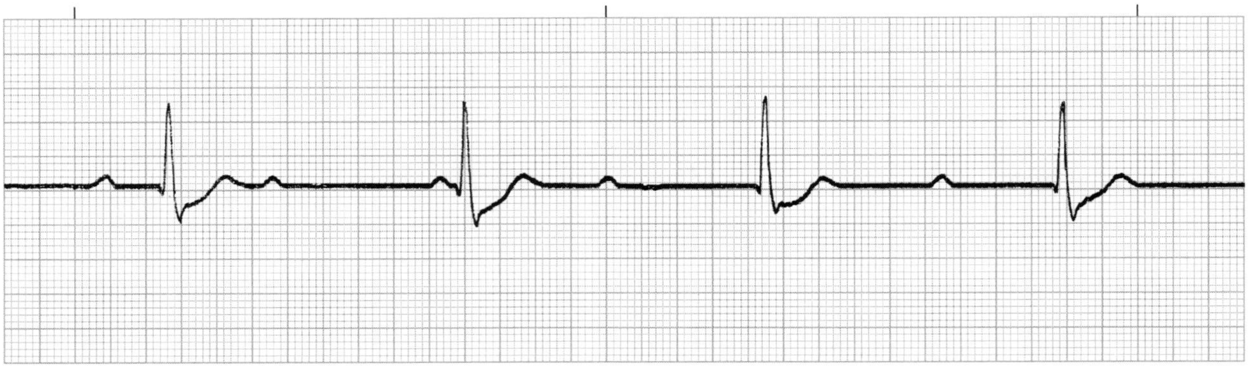

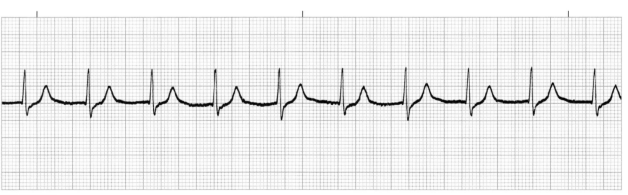

Strip 8.39   Rhythm: _____   Rate: _____   P wave: _____
PR interval: _____   QRS complex: _____
Rhythm interpretation: _____

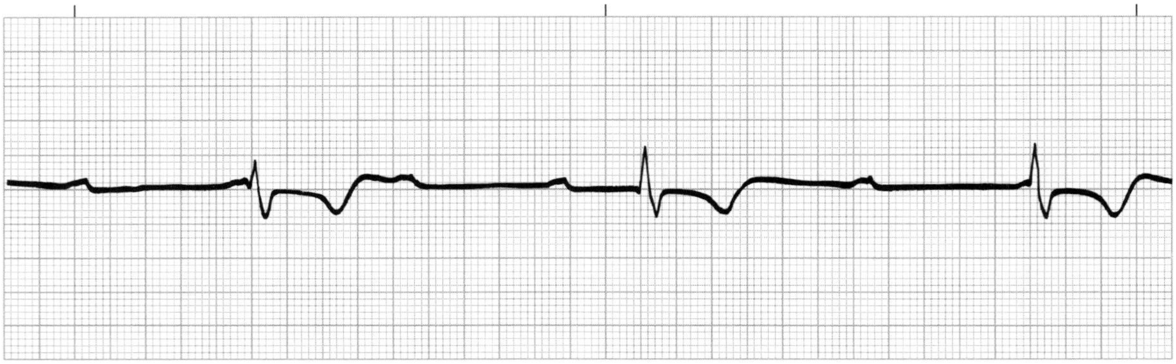

Strip 8.40   Rhythm: _____   Rate: _____   P wave: _____
PR interval: _____   QRS complex: _____
Rhythm interpretation: _____

Strip 8.41   Rhythm: _____   Rate: _____   P wave: _____
PR interval: _____   QRS complex: _____
Rhythm interpretation: _____

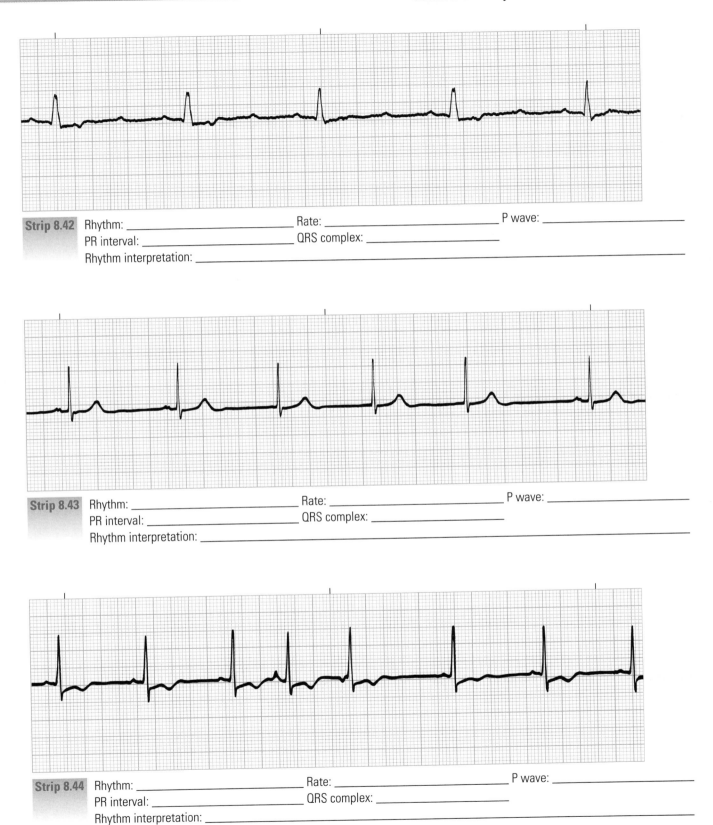

Strip 8.42 Rhythm: _____ Rate: _____ P wave: _____

PR interval: _____ QRS complex: _____

Rhythm interpretation: _____

Strip 8.43 Rhythm: _____ Rate: _____ P wave: _____

PR interval: _____ QRS complex: _____

Rhythm interpretation: _____

Strip 8.44 Rhythm: _____ Rate: _____ P wave: _____

PR interval: _____ QRS complex: _____

Rhythm interpretation: _____

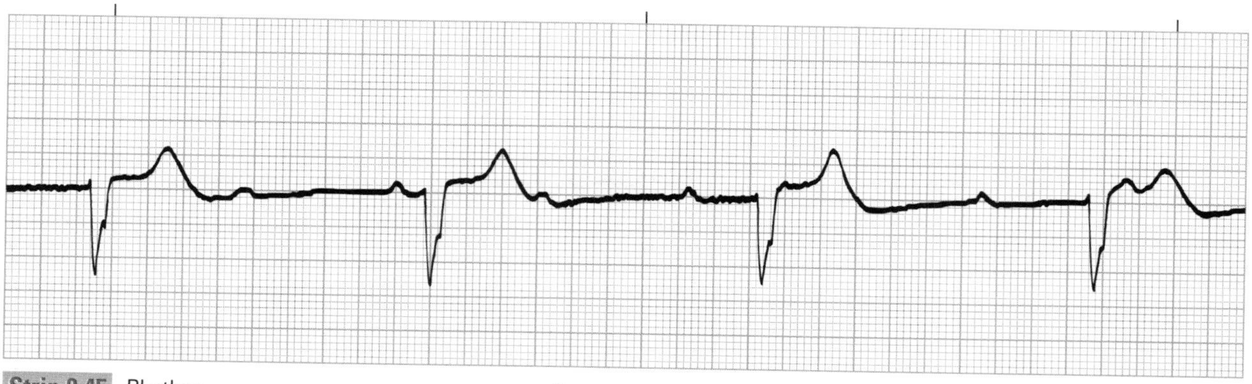

Strip 8.45 Rhythm: _____ Rate: _____ P wave: _____
PR interval: _____ QRS complex: _____
Rhythm interpretation: _____

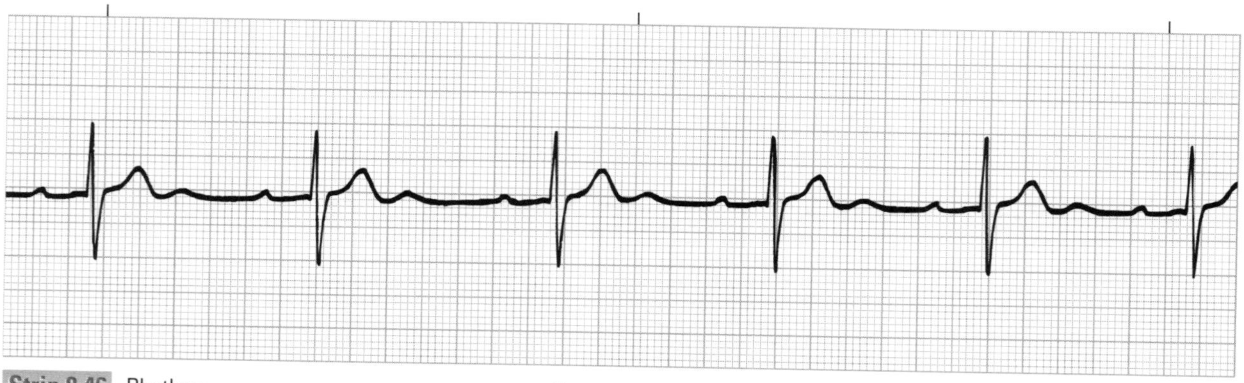

Strip 8.46 Rhythm: _____ Rate: _____ P wave: _____
PR interval: _____ QRS complex: _____
Rhythm interpretation: _____

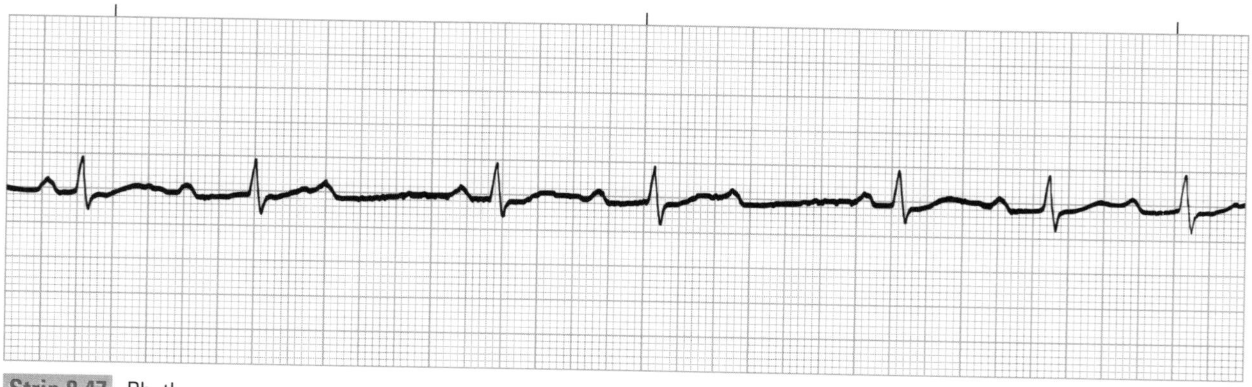

Strip 8.47 Rhythm: _____ Rate: _____ P wave: _____
PR interval: _____ QRS complex: _____
Rhythm interpretation: _____

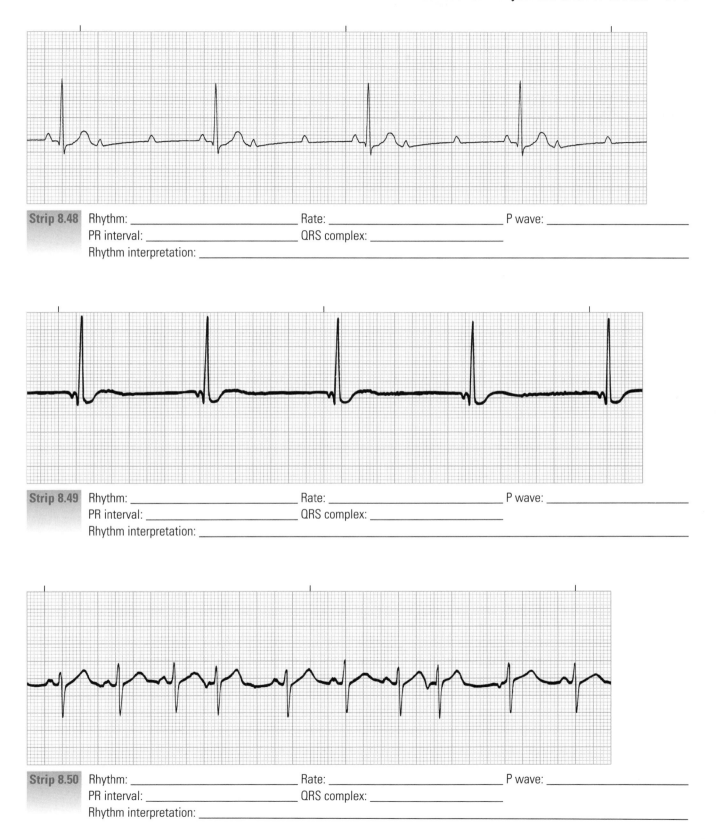

Strip 8.48 Rhythm: _____ Rate: _____ P wave: _____

PR interval: _____ QRS complex: _____

Rhythm interpretation: _____

Strip 8.49 Rhythm: _____ Rate: _____ P wave: _____

PR interval: _____ QRS complex: _____

Rhythm interpretation: _____

Strip 8.50 Rhythm: _____ Rate: _____ P wave: _____

PR interval: _____ QRS complex: _____

Rhythm interpretation: _____

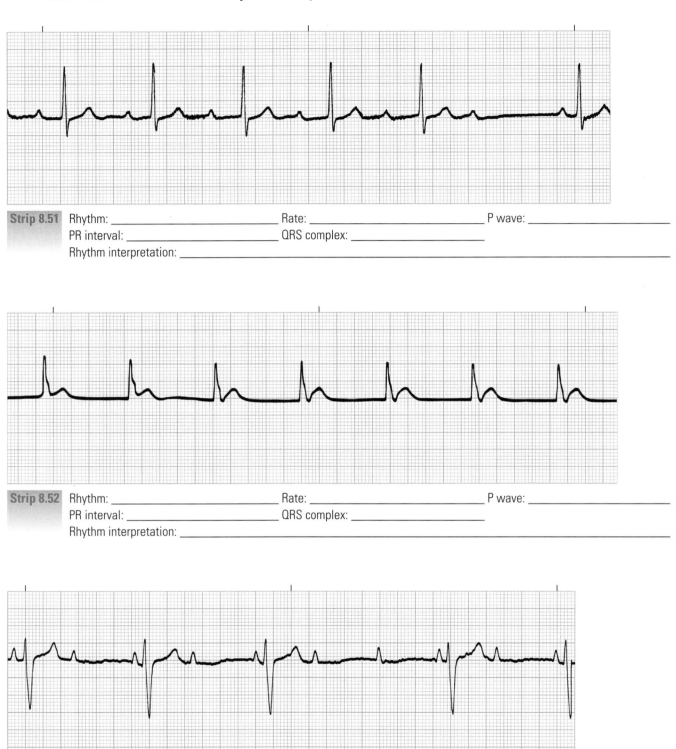

Strip 8.51 Rhythm: _____ Rate: _____ P wave: _____
PR interval: _____ QRS complex: _____
Rhythm interpretation: _____

Strip 8.52 Rhythm: _____ Rate: _____ P wave: _____
PR interval: _____ QRS complex: _____
Rhythm interpretation: _____

Strip 8.53 Rhythm: _____ Rate: _____ P wave: _____
PR interval: _____ QRS complex: _____
Rhythm interpretation: _____

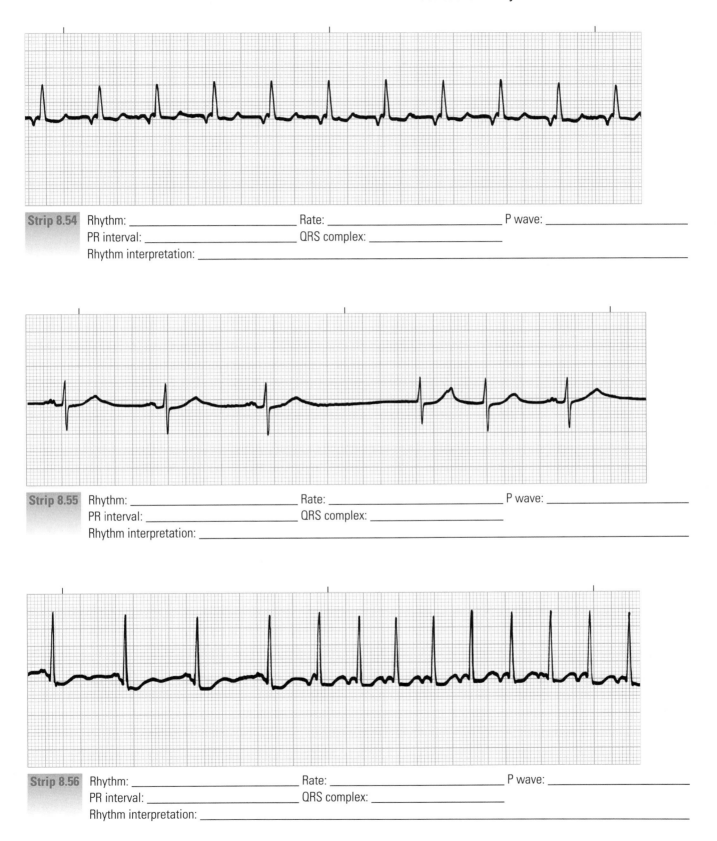

Strip 8.54 Rhythm: _____ Rate: _____ P wave: _____
PR interval: _____ QRS complex: _____
Rhythm interpretation: _____

Strip 8.55 Rhythm: _____ Rate: _____ P wave: _____
PR interval: _____ QRS complex: _____
Rhythm interpretation: _____

Strip 8.56 Rhythm: _____ Rate: _____ P wave: _____
PR interval: _____ QRS complex: _____
Rhythm interpretation: _____

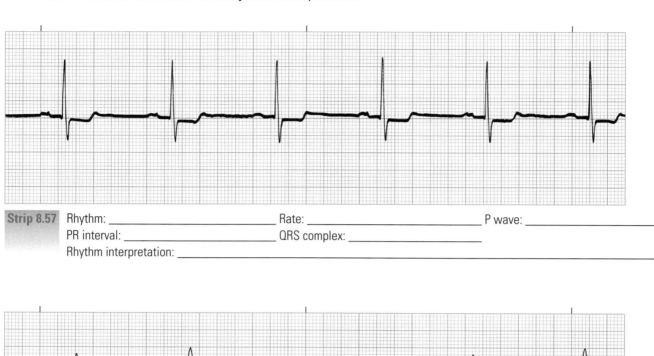

Strip 8.57   Rhythm: _____   Rate: _____   P wave: _____
PR interval: _____   QRS complex: _____
Rhythm interpretation: _____

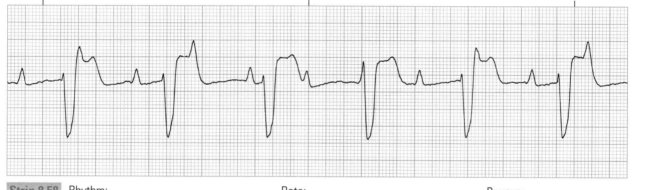

Strip 8.58   Rhythm: _____   Rate: _____   P wave: _____
PR interval: _____   QRS complex: _____
Rhythm interpretation: _____

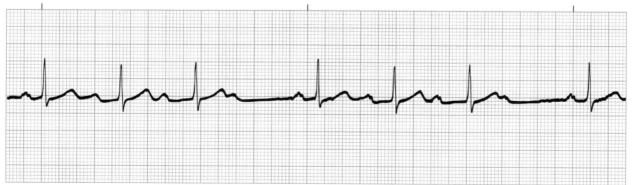

Strip 8.59   Rhythm: _____   Rate: _____   P wave: _____
PR interval: _____   QRS complex: _____
Rhythm interpretation: _____

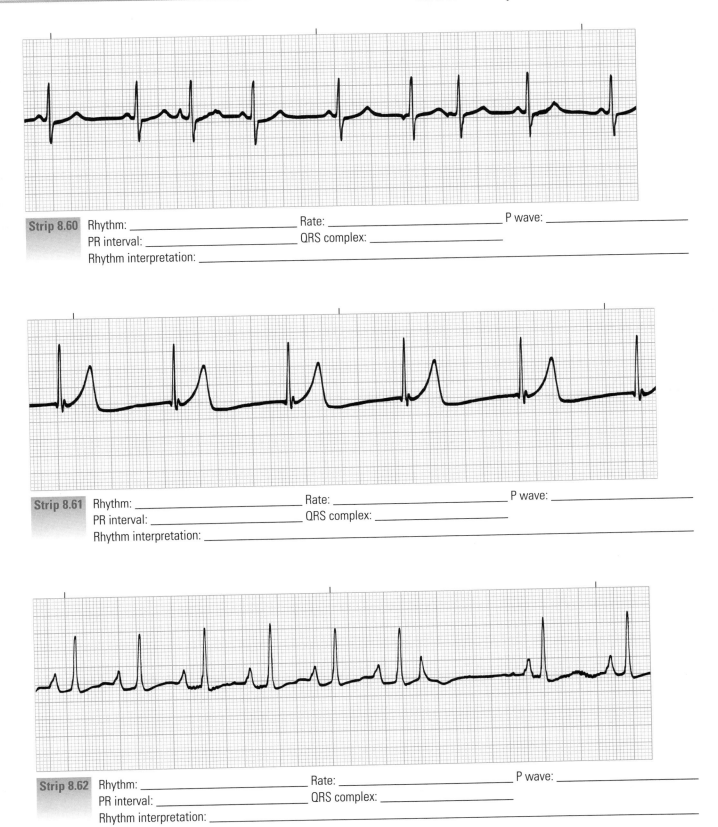

Strip 8.60 Rhythm: _____ Rate: _____ P wave: _____
PR interval: _____ QRS complex: _____
Rhythm interpretation: _____

Strip 8.61 Rhythm: _____ Rate: _____ P wave: _____
PR interval: _____ QRS complex: _____
Rhythm interpretation: _____

Strip 8.62 Rhythm: _____ Rate: _____ P wave: _____
PR interval: _____ QRS complex: _____
Rhythm interpretation: _____

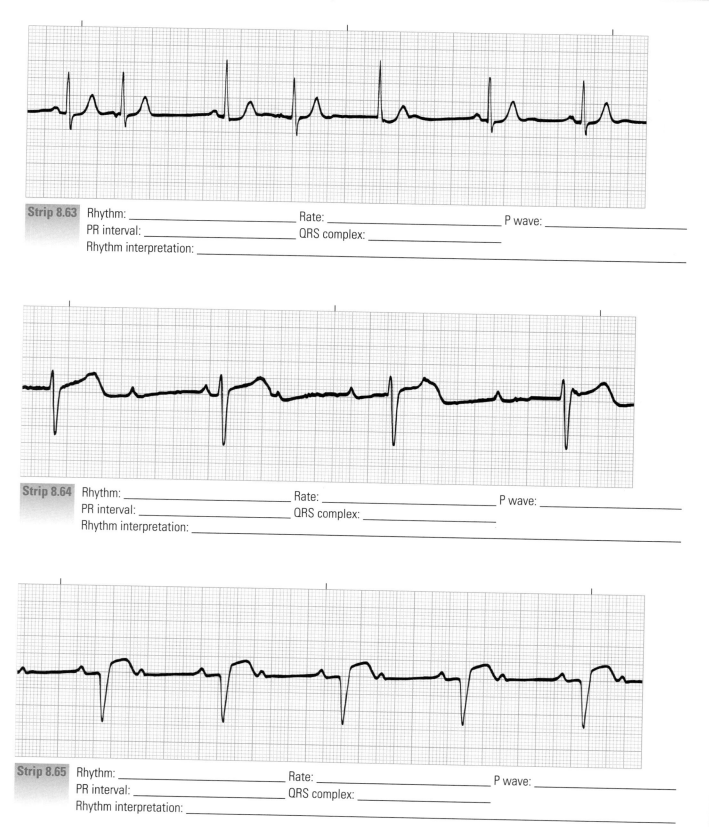

Strip 8.63 Rhythm: _____ Rate: _____ P wave: _____
PR interval: _____ QRS complex: _____
Rhythm interpretation: _____

Strip 8.64 Rhythm: _____ Rate: _____ P wave: _____
PR interval: _____ QRS complex: _____
Rhythm interpretation: _____

Strip 8.65 Rhythm: _____ Rate: _____ P wave: _____
PR interval: _____ QRS complex: _____
Rhythm interpretation: _____

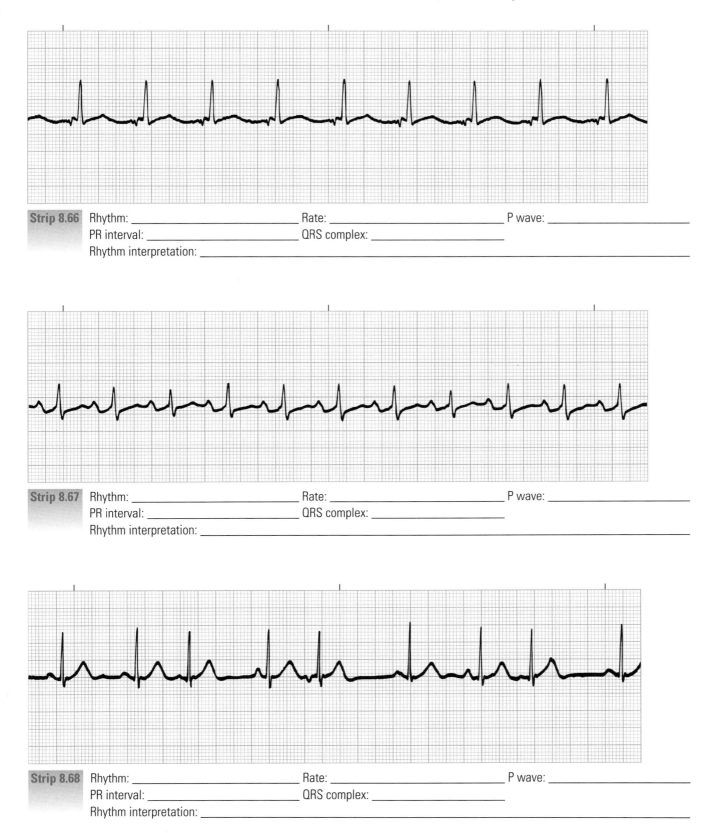

Strip 8.66 Rhythm: _____ Rate: _____ P wave: _____

PR interval: _____ QRS complex: _____

Rhythm interpretation: _____

Strip 8.67 Rhythm: _____ Rate: _____ P wave: _____

PR interval: _____ QRS complex: _____

Rhythm interpretation: _____

Strip 8.68 Rhythm: _____ Rate: _____ P wave: _____

PR interval: _____ QRS complex: _____

Rhythm interpretation: _____

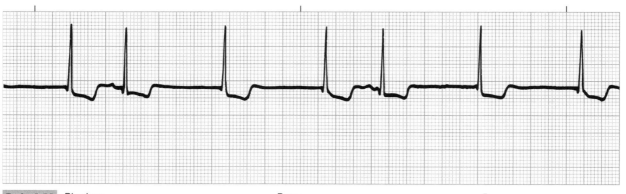

Strip 8.69 Rhythm: _____ Rate: _____ P wave: _____
PR interval: _____ QRS complex: _____
Rhythm interpretation: _____

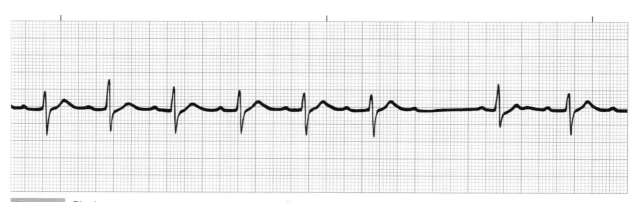

Strip 8.70 Rhythm: _____ Rate: _____ P wave: _____
PR interval: _____ QRS complex: _____
Rhythm interpretation: _____

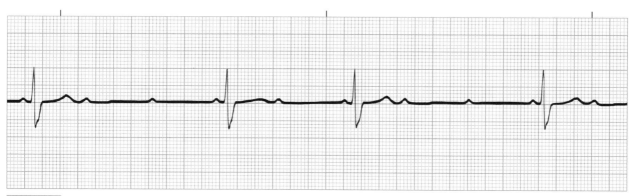

Strip 8.71 Rhythm: _____ Rate: _____ P wave: _____
PR interval: _____ QRS complex: _____
Rhythm interpretation: _____

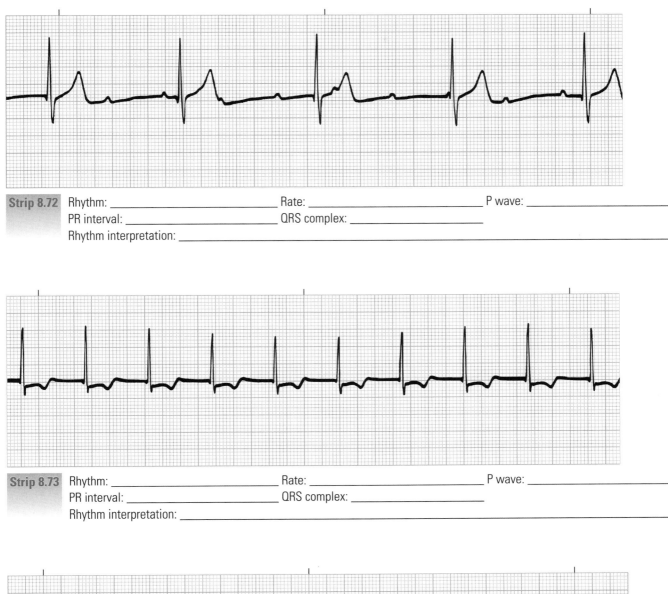

Strip 8.72 Rhythm: _____ Rate: _____ P wave: _____
PR interval: _____ QRS complex: _____
Rhythm interpretation: _____

Strip 8.73 Rhythm: _____ Rate: _____ P wave: _____
PR interval: _____ QRS complex: _____
Rhythm interpretation: _____

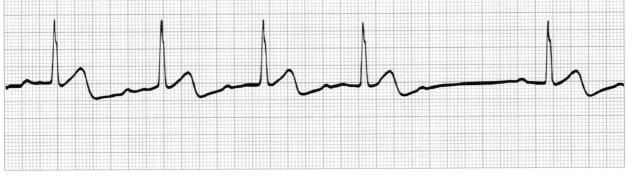

Strip 8.74 Rhythm: _____ Rate: _____ P wave: _____
PR interval: _____ QRS complex: _____
Rhythm interpretation: _____

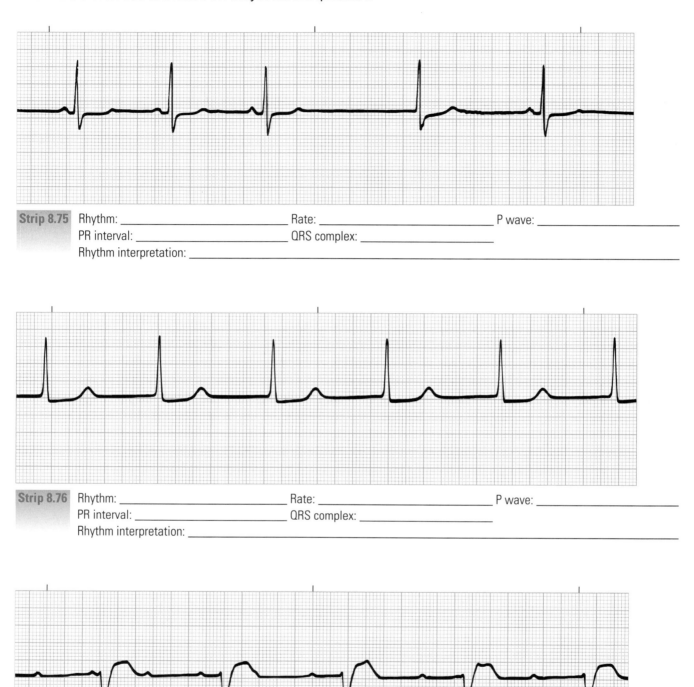

Strip 8.75   Rhythm: _____   Rate: _____   P wave: _____
PR interval: _____   QRS complex: _____
Rhythm interpretation: _____

Strip 8.76   Rhythm: _____   Rate: _____   P wave: _____
PR interval: _____   QRS complex: _____
Rhythm interpretation: _____

Strip 8.77   Rhythm: _____   Rate: _____   P wave: _____
PR interval: _____   QRS complex: _____
Rhythm interpretation: _____

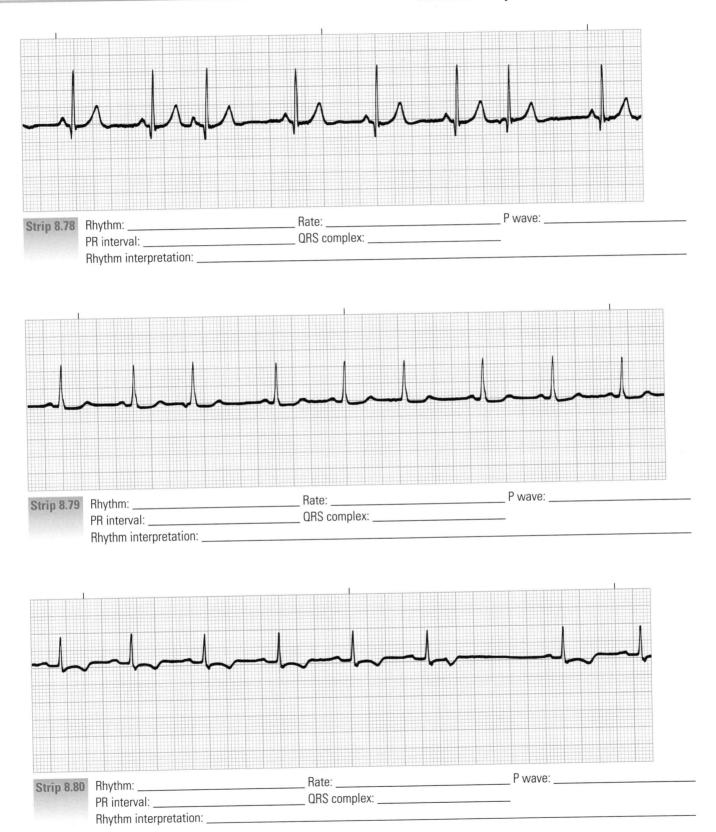

Strip 8.78 Rhythm: _____ Rate: _____ P wave: _____
PR interval: _____ QRS complex: _____
Rhythm interpretation: _____

Strip 8.79 Rhythm: _____ Rate: _____ P wave: _____
PR interval: _____ QRS complex: _____
Rhythm interpretation: _____

Strip 8.80 Rhythm: _____ Rate: _____ P wave: _____
PR interval: _____ QRS complex: _____
Rhythm interpretation: _____

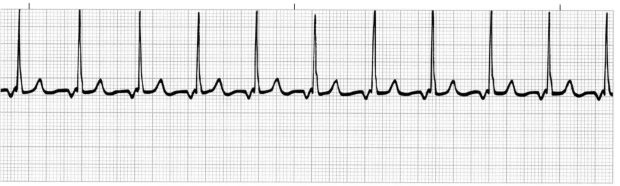

Strip 8.81 Rhythm: _____ Rate: _____ P wave: _____
PR interval: _____ QRS complex: _____
Rhythm interpretation: _____

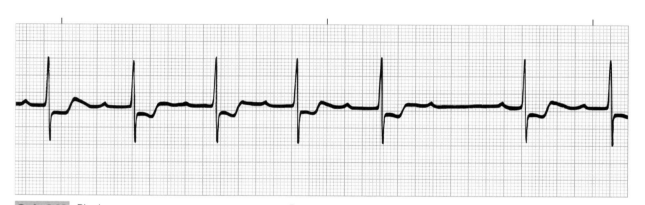

Strip 8.82 Rhythm: _____ Rate: _____ P wave: _____
PR interval: _____ QRS complex: _____
Rhythm interpretation: _____

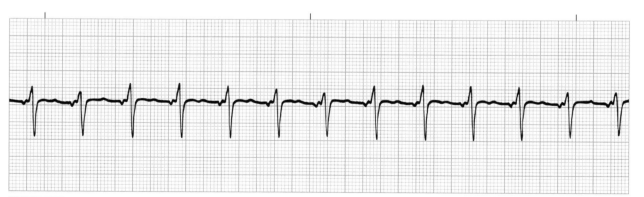

Strip 8.83 Rhythm: _____ Rate: _____ P wave: _____
PR interval: _____ QRS complex: _____
Rhythm interpretation: _____

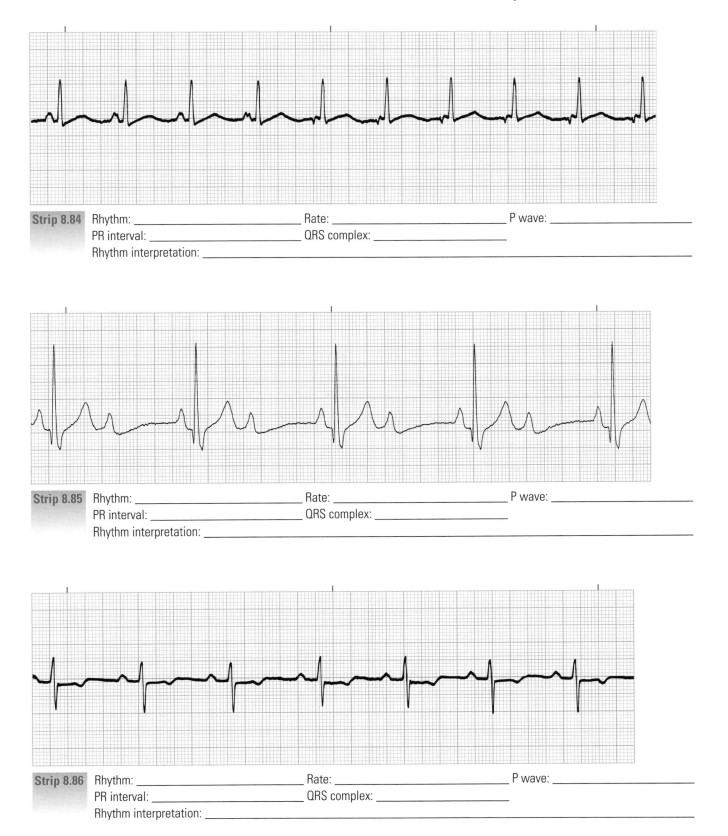

Strip 8.84 Rhythm: _____ Rate: _____ P wave: _____

PR interval: _____ QRS complex: _____

Rhythm interpretation: _____

Strip 8.85 Rhythm: _____ Rate: _____ P wave: _____

PR interval: _____ QRS complex: _____

Rhythm interpretation: _____

Strip 8.86 Rhythm: _____ Rate: _____ P wave: _____

PR interval: _____ QRS complex: _____

Rhythm interpretation: _____

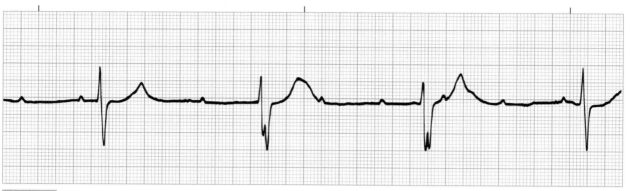

Strip 8.87 Rhythm: _____ Rate: _____ P wave: _____
PR interval: _____ QRS complex: _____
Rhythm interpretation: _____

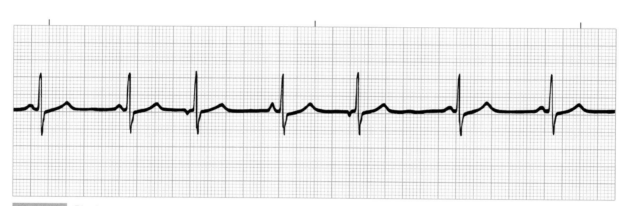

Strip 8.88 Rhythm: _____ Rate: _____ P wave: _____
PR interval: _____ QRS complex: _____
Rhythm interpretation: _____

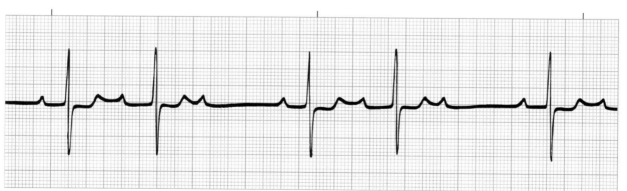

Strip 8.89 Rhythm: _____ Rate: _____ P wave: _____
PR interval: _____ QRS complex: _____
Rhythm interpretation: _____

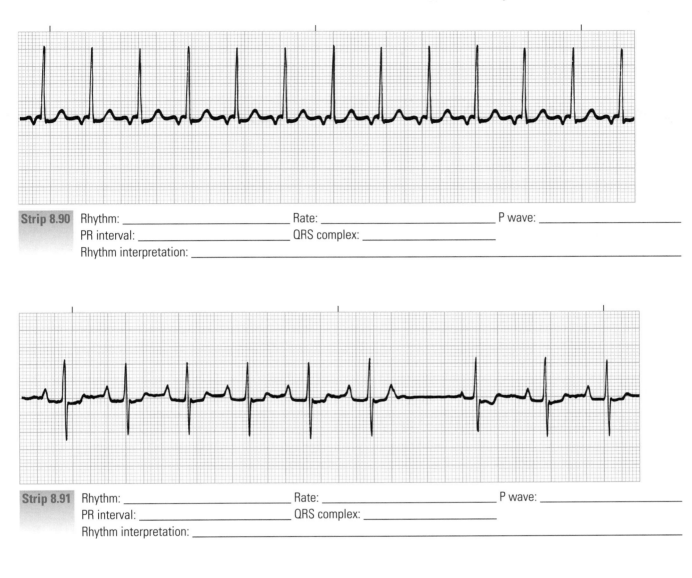

Strip 8.90 Rhythm: _____ Rate: _____ P wave: _____

PR interval: _____ QRS complex: _____

Rhythm interpretation: _____

Strip 8.91 Rhythm: _____ Rate: _____ P wave: _____

PR interval: _____ QRS complex: _____

Rhythm interpretation: _____

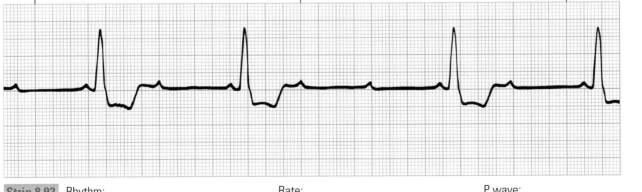

Strip 8.92 Rhythm: _____ Rate: _____ P wave: _____

PR interval: _____ QRS complex: _____

Rhythm interpretation: _____

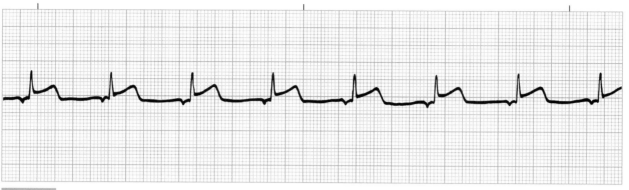

Strip 8.93 Rhythm: _____ Rate: _____ P wave: _____
PR interval: _____ QRS complex: _____
Rhythm interpretation: _____

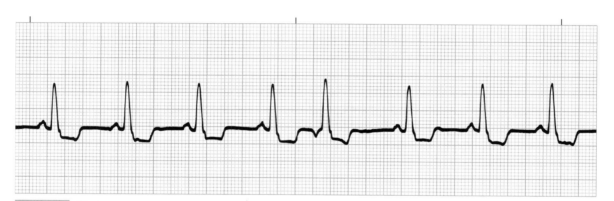

Strip 8.94 Rhythm: _____ Rate: _____ P wave: _____
PR interval: _____ QRS complex: _____
Rhythm interpretation: _____

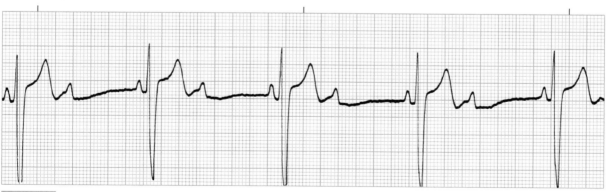

Strip 8.95 Rhythm: _____ Rate: _____ P wave: _____
PR interval: _____ QRS complex: _____
Rhythm interpretation: _____

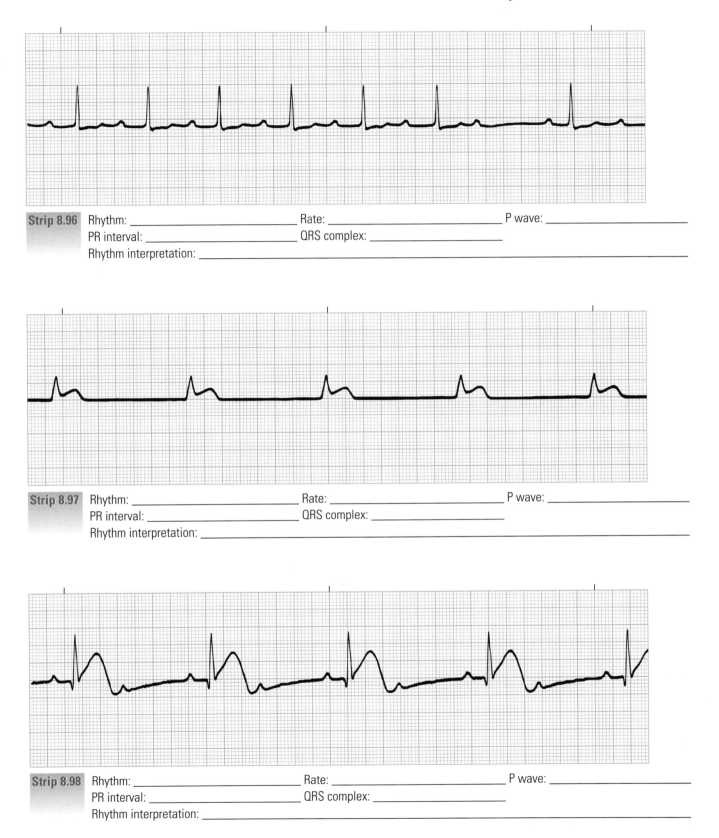

Strip 8.96 Rhythm: _____ Rate: _____ P wave: _____
PR interval: _____ QRS complex: _____
Rhythm interpretation: _____

Strip 8.97 Rhythm: _____ Rate: _____ P wave: _____
PR interval: _____ QRS complex: _____
Rhythm interpretation: _____

Strip 8.98 Rhythm: _____ Rate: _____ P wave: _____
PR interval: _____ QRS complex: _____
Rhythm interpretation: _____

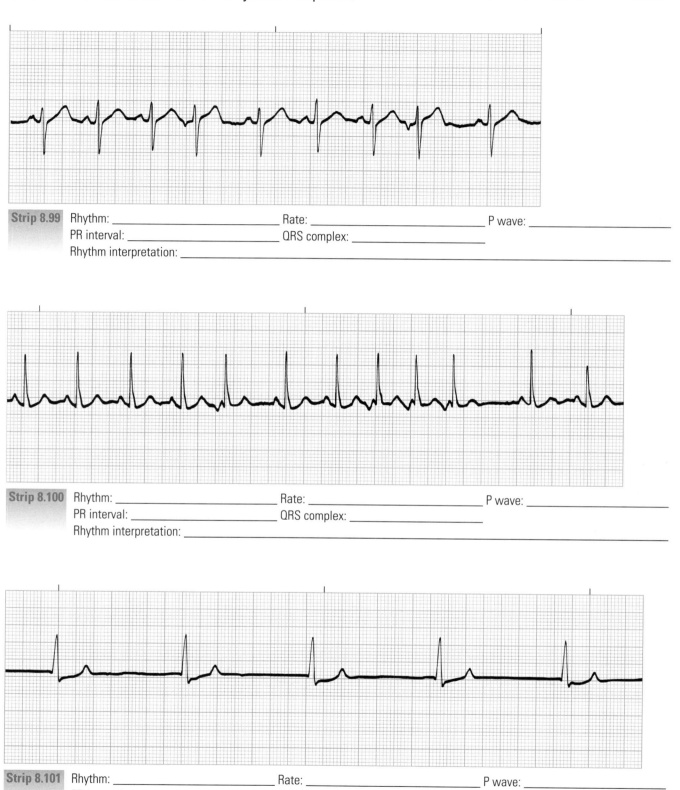

Strip 8.99 Rhythm: _____ Rate: _____ P wave: _____

PR interval: _____ QRS complex: _____

Rhythm interpretation: _____

Strip 8.100 Rhythm: _____ Rate: _____ P wave: _____

PR interval: _____ QRS complex: _____

Rhythm interpretation: _____

Strip 8.101 Rhythm: _____ Rate: _____ P wave: _____

PR interval: _____ QRS complex: _____

Rhythm interpretation: _____

SKILLBUILDER PRACTICE

This section contains mixed *sinus, atrial,* and *junctional* and *AV block* rhythm strips, allowing the student to practice differentiating between three rhythm groups before progressing to a new group. As before, analyze the rhythm strips using the five-step process. Interpret the rhythm by comparing the data collected with the ECG characteristics for each rhythm. All strips are lead II, a positive lead, unless otherwise noted. Check your answers with the answer key in the appendix.

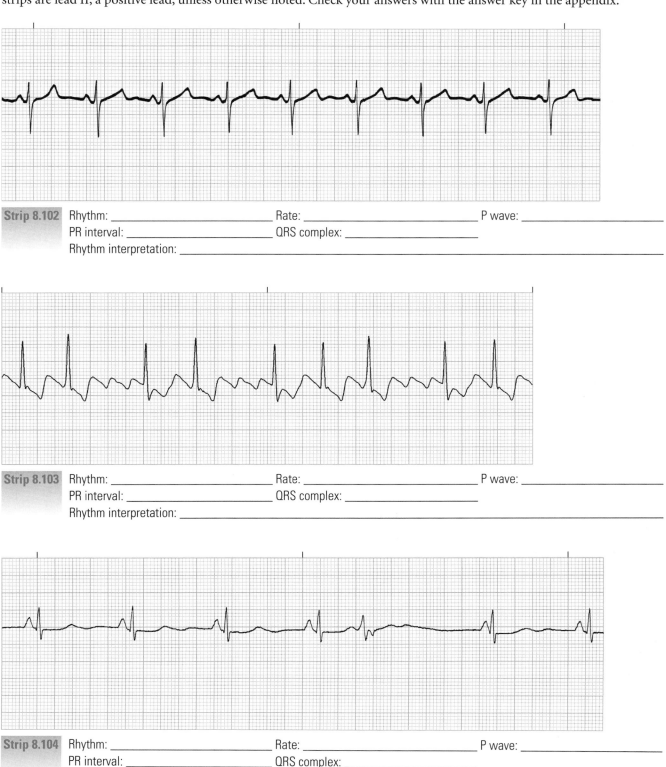

Strip 8.102   Rhythm: _____   Rate: _____   P wave: _____
PR interval: _____   QRS complex: _____
Rhythm interpretation: _____

Strip 8.103   Rhythm: _____   Rate: _____   P wave: _____
PR interval: _____   QRS complex: _____
Rhythm interpretation: _____

Strip 8.104   Rhythm: _____   Rate: _____   P wave: _____
PR interval: _____   QRS complex: _____
Rhythm interpretation: _____

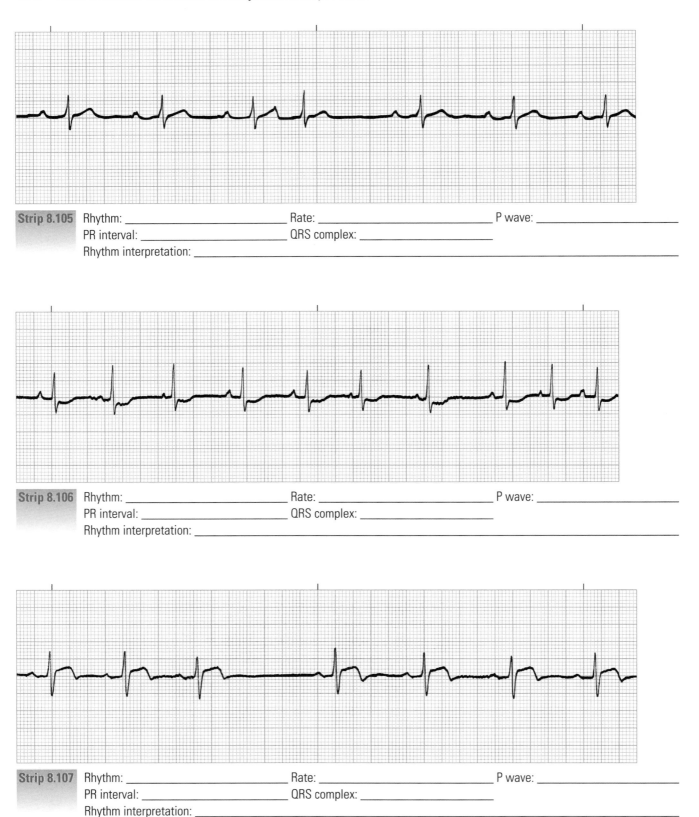

Strip 8.105 Rhythm: _____ Rate: _____ P wave: _____

PR interval: _____ QRS complex: _____

Rhythm interpretation: _____

Strip 8.106 Rhythm: _____ Rate: _____ P wave: _____

PR interval: _____ QRS complex: _____

Rhythm interpretation: _____

Strip 8.107 Rhythm: _____ Rate: _____ P wave: _____

PR interval: _____ QRS complex: _____

Rhythm interpretation: _____

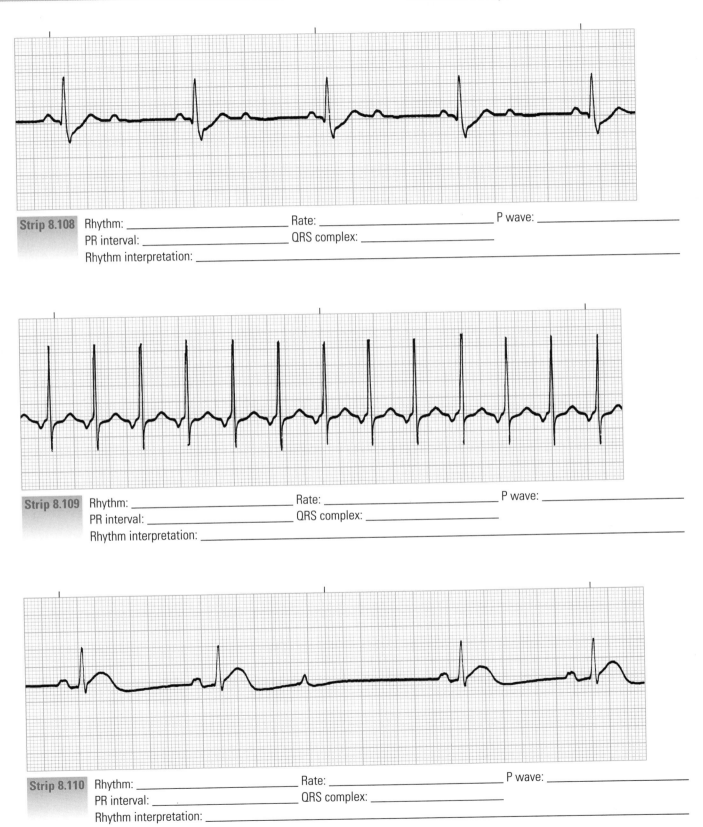

Strip 8.108   Rhythm: _____   Rate: _____   P wave: _____
PR interval: _____   QRS complex: _____
Rhythm interpretation: _____

Strip 8.109   Rhythm: _____   Rate: _____   P wave: _____
PR interval: _____   QRS complex: _____
Rhythm interpretation: _____

Strip 8.110   Rhythm: _____   Rate: _____   P wave: _____
PR interval: _____   QRS complex: _____
Rhythm interpretation: _____

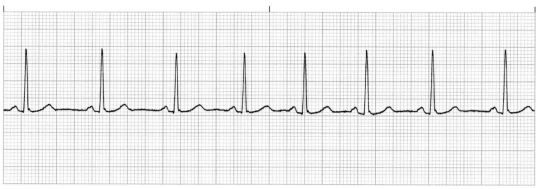

Strip 8.111 Rhythm: _____ Rate: _____ P wave: _____
PR interval: _____ QRS complex: _____
Rhythm interpretation: _____

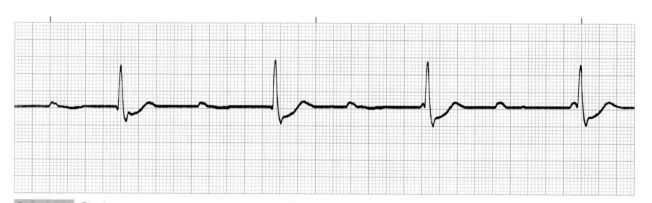

Strip 8.112 Rhythm: _____ Rate: _____ P wave: _____
PR interval: _____ QRS complex: _____
Rhythm interpretation: _____

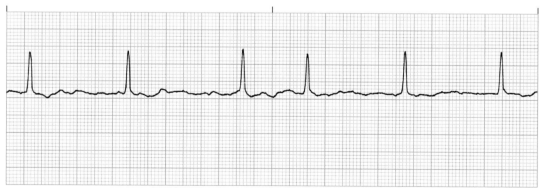

Strip 8.113 Rhythm: _____ Rate: _____ P wave: _____
PR interval: _____ QRS complex: _____
Rhythm interpretation: _____

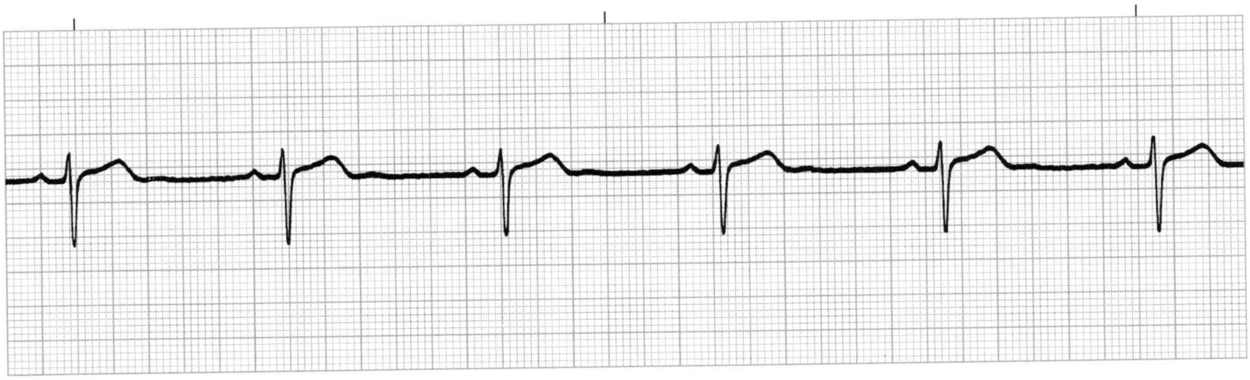

Strip 8.114 Rhythm: _____ Rate: _____ P wave: _____

PR interval: _____ QRS complex: _____

Rhythm interpretation: _____

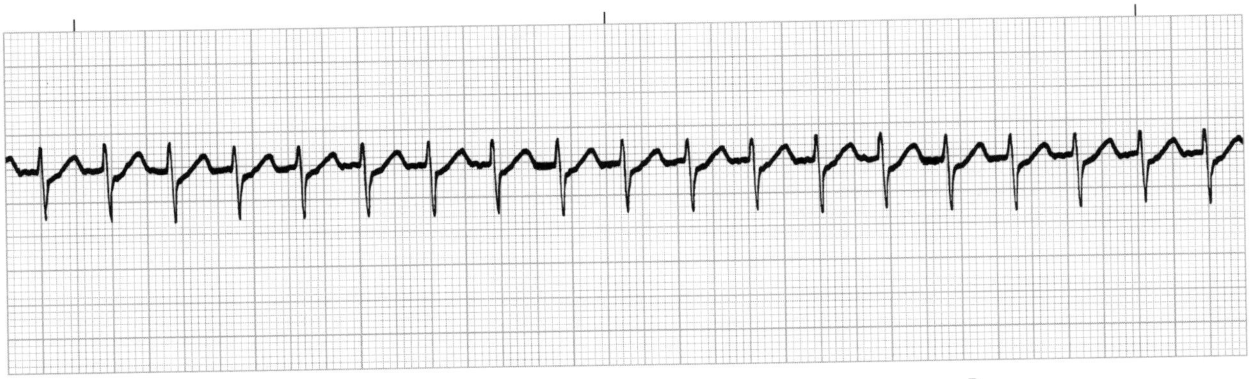

Strip 8.115 Rhythm: _____ Rate: _____ P wave: _____

PR interval: _____ QRS complex: _____

Rhythm interpretation: _____

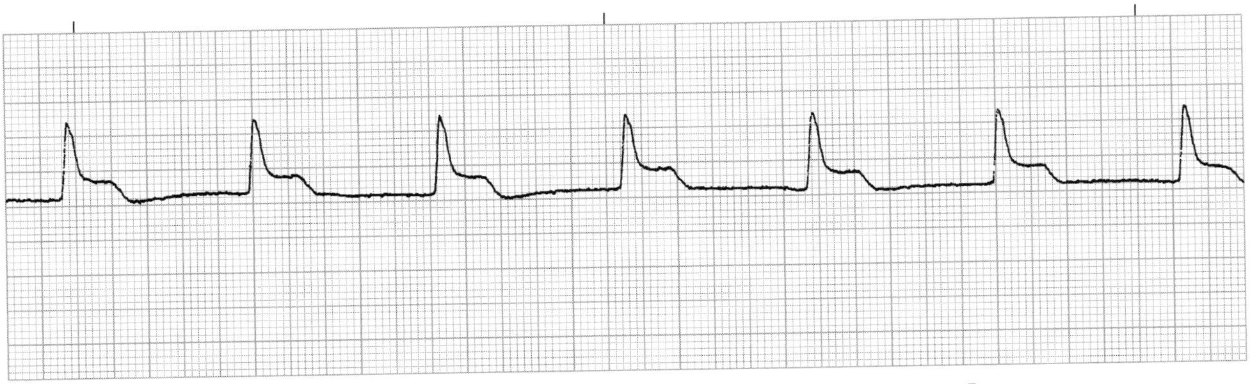

Strip 8.116 Rhythm: _____ Rate: _____ P wave: _____

PR interval: _____ QRS complex: _____

Rhythm interpretation: _____

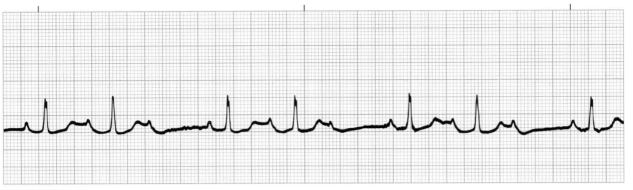

Strip 8.117 Rhythm: _____ Rate: _____ P wave: _____

PR interval: _____ QRS complex: _____

Rhythm interpretation: _____

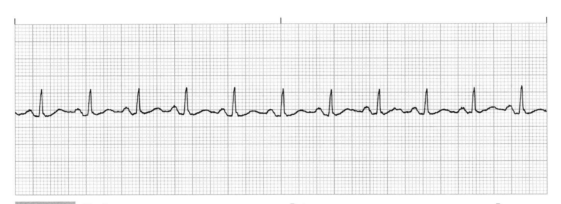

Strip 8.118 Rhythm: _____ Rate: _____ P wave: _____

PR interval: _____ QRS complex: _____

Rhythm interpretation: _____

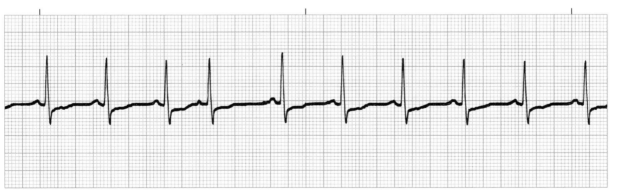

Strip 8.119 Rhythm: _____ Rate: _____ P wave: _____

PR interval: _____ QRS complex: _____

Rhythm interpretation: _____

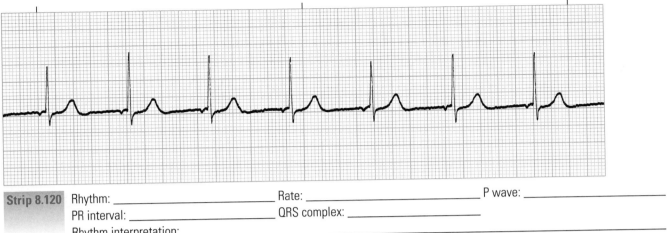

Strip 8.120   Rhythm: _____ Rate: _____ P wave: _____

PR interval: _____ QRS complex: _____

Rhythm interpretation: _____

nine

Ventricular Arrhythmias and Bundle-Branch Block

Overview

The three preceding chapters have focused on **supraventricular** arrhythmias. Supraventricular arrhythmias refer to those rhythms that originate above the bundle branches and include the sinus, atrial, and junctional rhythms. The electrical impulse produced by supraventricular rhythms follows the normal conduction pathway causing simultaneous depolarization of the right and left ventricles, resulting in normal ventricular depolarization and a narrow QRS complex of 0.10 second or less. Ventricular beats and rhythms (Figure 9.1) originate below the bundle of His in a pacemaker site in either the right or left ventricle. When impulses arise in the ventricles, the impulse does not enter the normal conduction pathway but instead travels through muscle fibers in such a way that slows the electrical movement and changes the direction of the impulses. Therefore, ventricular depolarization is abnormal, resulting in QRS complexes that are abnormally shaped and prolonged (0.12 second or greater in duration).

Since ventricular depolarization is abnormal, ventricular repolarization will also be abnormal, resulting in changes in the ST segments and T waves. The ST segments and T waves will slope in the opposite direction from the main QRS deflection (if the ectopic QRS complex is predominantly negative, the ST segment is usually elevated and the T wave positive; if the ectopic QRS complex is predominantly positive, the ST segment is usually depressed and the T wave negative). A P wave is not produced in ventricular rhythms.

Ventricular arrhythmias include premature ventricular contractions (PVCs), idioventricular rhythm (IVR), accelerated idioventricular rhythm (AIVR), ventricular tachycardia (VT), ventricular fibrillation (VF), and ventricular standstill (asystole). All of these rhythms are associated with a wide QRS complex (except ventricular fibrillation and ventricular standstill, which do not have QRS complexes). Because the ventricles are the least efficient of the heart's pacemakers, most of these rhythms are (or have the potential to be) life threatening and demand prompt recognition and treatment.

The electrical impulse in bundle-branch block originates in the sinus node, not in ventricular tissue, but a discussion of bundle-branch block is included in this rhythm group because of the location of the block in the bundle branches (located within the ventricles) and the wide QRS complex.

Bundle-Branch Block (BBB)

The intraventricular conduction system consists of the right bundle branch and the left main bundle branch, which divides into two fascicles: an anterior fascicle and a posterior fascicle. Block may occur in any part of this conduction system. Normally, the electrical impulses travel through the right bundle branch and the left bundle branch

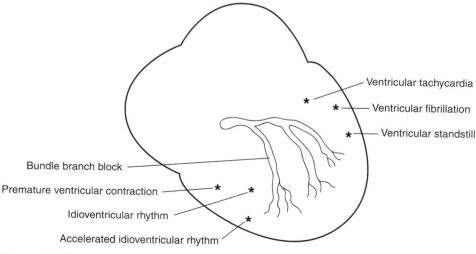

Figure 9.1 Ventricular arrhythmias and bundle-branch block.

and its fascicles at the same time, causing simultaneous depolarization of the right and left ventricles, resulting in normal ventricular depolarization and a narrow QRS duration of 0.10 second or less. When one of the bundle branches is blocked, the electrical impulse travels down the intact bundle, depolarizing that ventricle first, and then the impulse progresses through the interventricular septum to depolarize the other ventricle. Depolarization of one ventricle before the other is called sequential depolarization or asynchronous depolarization. Depolarization of the ventricles is delayed, resulting in a wide QRS complex of 0.12 second or greater.

The typical bundle-branch block appearance on the ECG is that of a normal sinus rhythm with a wide QRS complex (Figures 9.2 and 9.3). However, it may also be present with atrial fibrillation (Figure 9.4) and atrial

box 9.1	Bundle-Branch Block: Identifying ECG Features
Rhythm:	Regular
Rate:	That of the underlying rhythm (usually sinus)
P waves:	Sinus
PR interval:	Normal (0.12 to 0.20 second)
QRS complex:	Wide (0.12 second or greater)

flutter. A notched R wave is a common QRS complex pattern (see Figure 9.3). Identifying ECG features are listed in Box 9.1. Although the presence of a bundle-branch block can be recognized by a monitoring lead, differentiating between right and left bundle-branch block requires a 12-lead electrocardiogram.

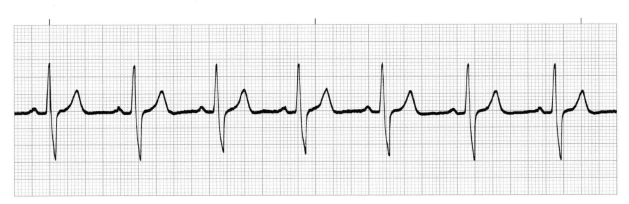

Figure 9.2   Normal sinus rhythm with bundle-branch block.

Rhythm:	Regular (off by 2 squares)
Rate:	60 to 65 beats/minute
P waves:	Sinus
PR interval:	0.16 to 0.20 second
QRS complex:	0.12 to 0.14 second.

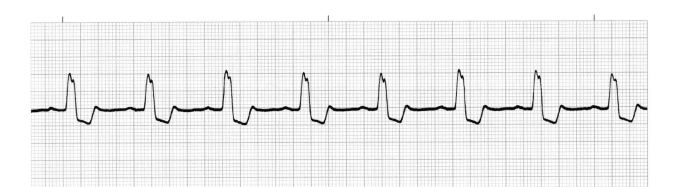

Figure 9.3   Normal sinus rhythm with bundle-branch block.

Rhythm:	Regular
Rate:	68 beats/minute
P waves:	Sinus
PR interval:	0.20 second
QRS complex:	0.12 to 0.14 second
Comment:	A notched R wave is a common pattern with BBB.

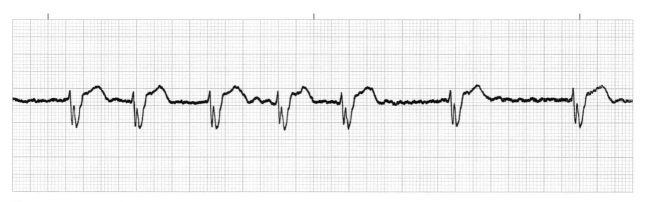

Figure 9.4	**Atrial fibrillation with bundle-branch block.**
Rhythm:	Irregular
Rate:	70 beats/minute
P waves:	Fibrillatory waves present
PR interval:	Not measurable
QRS complex:	0.16 second.

Right bundle-branch block (RBBB) may be present in healthy individuals with no apparent underlying heart disease but more commonly occurs in the presence of coronary artery disease (the most common cause). Other causes of RBBB include hypertensive heart disease, congenital heart disease, myocarditis, following acute MI, heart failure, cardiomyopathy, as a result of scar tissue that develops after heart surgery, and degenerative disease of the electrical conduction system. RBBB may be temporary or chronic.

Left bundle-branch block (LBBB) is rarely seen in individuals with healthy hearts. The most common cause is hypertensive heart disease. Other causes are the same as with RBBB. Left bundle-branch block may be temporary or chronic.

Specific treatment is usually not indicated for a bundle-branch block. Cardiac pacing may be indicated if the bundle-branch block develops as a result of acute MI or in the presence of AV block.

Premature Ventricular Contraction (PVC)

A premature ventricular contraction (Figures 9.5 through 9.14 and Box 9.2) is a premature ectopic impulse that arises below the bundle of His in the ventricles. PVCs occur as a result of enhanced automaticity of a focus in the ventricles, reentry involving the ventricles, or triggered activity occurring during ventricular repolarization. PVCs have the following characteristics:

- The QRS is premature.
- A P wave isn't associated with the PVC. Normally, the P wave of the underlying rhythm (usually sinus) is

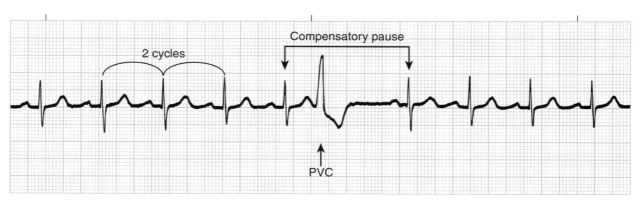

Figure 9.5	**Normal sinus rhythm with one PVC.**
Rhythm:	Basic rhythm regular; irregular with PVC
Rate:	Basic rhythm rate 88 beats/minute
P waves:	Sinus with basic rhythm
PR interval:	0.18 to 0.20 second
QRS complex:	0.06 to 0.08 second (basic rhythm). 0.12 second (PVC)
Comment:	The interval from the beat preceding the PVC to the beat following the PVC is equal to two cardiac cycles and represents a full compensatory pause.

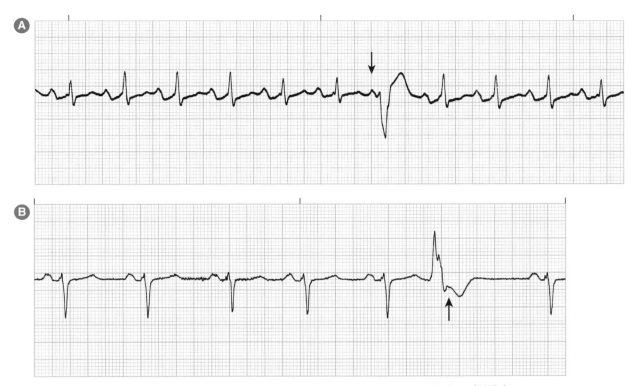

Figure 9.6   Sinus P waves occurring before and after premature ventricular contractions (PVCs).
The sinus P waves of the underlying rhythm can be seen just before the PVC in **(A)** and after the PVC in the ST segment in **(B)**. These P waves are associated with the underlying rhythm (not the PVC) and usually are hidden within the wide QRS of the PVC.

A. Normal sinus rhythm with first-degree AV block and one PVC.

B. Sinus arrhythmia with bundle-branch block and one PVC.

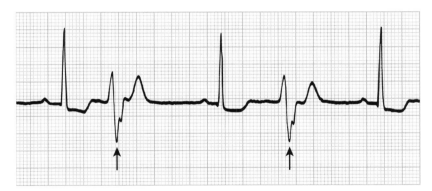

Figure 9.7   Bigeminal PVCs.

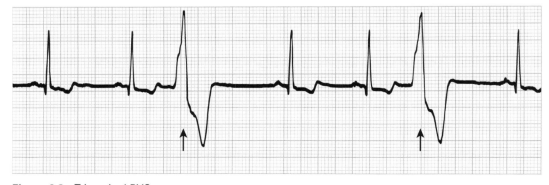

Figure 9.8   Trigeminal PVCs.

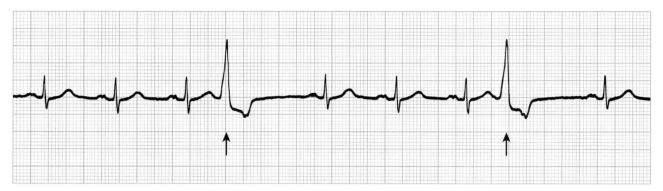

Figure 9.9 Quadrigeminal PVCs.

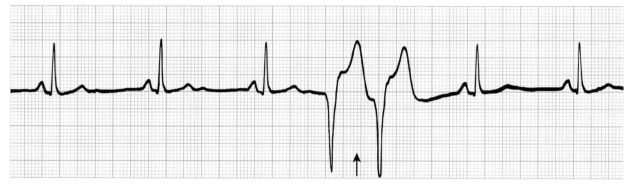

Figure 9.10 Paired PVCs.

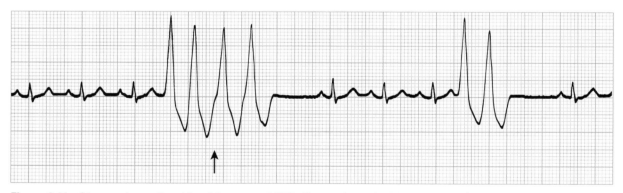

Figure 9.11 Sinus tachycardia with a 4-beat run of PVCs (burst of ventricular tachycardia) and paired PVCs.

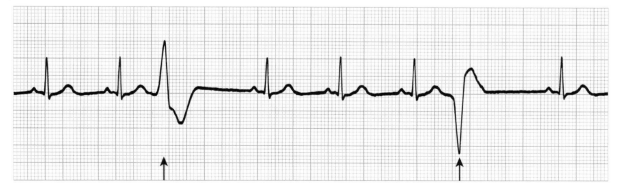

Figure 9.12 Multifocal PVCs.

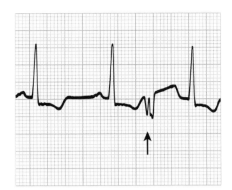

Figure 9.13   Interpolated PVC.

box 9.2	Premature Ventricular Contraction (PVC): Identifying ECG Features
Rhythm:	Underlying rhythm usually regular; irregular with PVC
Rate:	That of the underlying rhythm (usually sinus)
P waves:	None associated with PVC; P waves associated with the underlying sinus rhythm can occasionally be seen just before the PVC or after the PVC in the ST segment or T wave; usually, these P waves are hidden in the QRS complex.
PR interval:	Not measurable
QRS complex:	Premature QRS complex; wide (0.12 second or greater)

obscured within the PVC, but sometimes, it appears just before or after the PVC in the ST segment or T wave (see Figure 9.6).

- The QRS is wide (0.12 second or greater), and the morphology is different from the QRS complexes of the underlying rhythm.
- The ST segment and T-wave slope in the opposite direction from the main QRS deflection (if the ectopic QRS complex is predominantly negative, the ST segment is usually elevated and the T wave positive; if the ectopic QRS complex is predominantly positive, the ST segment is usually depressed and the T wave negative).
- The pause associated with the PVC is usually compensatory (the measurement from the beat before the PVC to the beat after the PVC is equal to two R-R intervals of the underlying rhythm [see Figure 9.5]). The underlying rhythm must be regular to determine a compensatory pause.

PVCs may occur in various patterns. They may appear as a single beat (see Figure 9.5), every other beat (bigeminal pattern, see Figure 9.7), every third beat (trigeminal pattern, see Figure 9.8), every fourth beat (quadrigeminal pattern, see Figure 9.9), in pairs (also called couplets, see Figure 9.10), or in runs (see Figure 9.11). A run of three or more consecutive PVCs constitutes a rhythm. The rate will determine which rhythm is present (idioventricular rhythm, accelerated idioventricular rhythm, or ventricular tachycardia).

PVCs that look the same in the same lead are called *unifocal PVCs*. These PVCs originate from a single ectopic focus in the ventricles. PVCs that appear different from one another in the same lead are called *multifocal PVCs* (see

Figure 9.12). These PVCs usually originate from different ectopic sites but sometimes may fire from a single site and are conducted along different routes in the ventricles, resulting in a QRS that differs in morphology in the same lead.

A PVC sandwiched between two normally conducted sinus beats, without greatly disturbing the regularity of the underlying rhythm, is called an *interpolated PVC* (see Figure 9.13). The compensatory pause, usually associated with the PVC, is absent.

R-on-T PVC (see Figure 9.14) is a term used to describe a PVC that falls on the downslope of the preceding T wave. This period corresponds to the relative refractory period of ventricular repolarization when the myocardium is in its most vulnerable state electrically. During this period, the myocardial cells have repolarized enough to respond to a strong stimulus. Stimulation of the ventricle at this time may precipitate repetitive ventricular contractions, resulting in ventricular tachycardia or ventricular fibrillation.

PVCs are among the most commonly seen arrhythmias. PVCs may occur in individuals with a healthy heart but are more common in older individuals with heart disease. Common causes of PVCs include myocardial ischemia or infarction; hypoxia; hypertension; cardiomyopathy; congestive heart failure; mitral valve prolapse; cardiac contusion; myocarditis; high levels of adrenaline because of stress; ingestion of substances such as alcohol, tobacco, caffeine, cocaine, and amphetamines; drugs such as digoxin, aminophylline, tricyclic antidepressants, and ephedrine-containing decongestants; electrolyte disturbances (especially

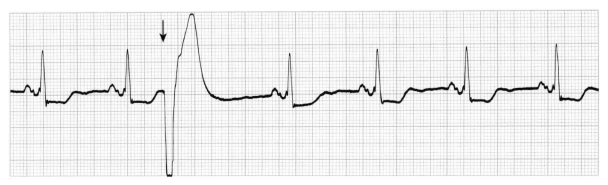

Figure 9.14   R-on-T PVC.

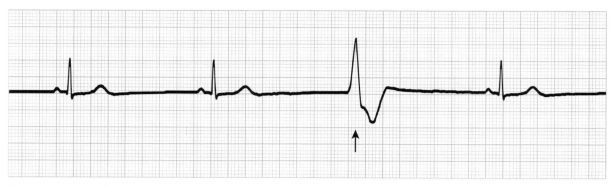

Figure 9.15 Ventricular escape beat.

hypokalemia and hypomagnesemia); a reperfusion arrhythmia after thrombolytic therapy or percutaneous coronary interventions; or following insertion of invasive catheters into the heart, such as pacing leads or a pulmonary artery catheter.

Patients with PVCs may report feeling that the heart has "skipped" or "missed" a beat. This is because there is usually a brief pause in the heartbeat after a PVC when the electrical system of the heart resets. Patients with frequent PVCs may complain of weakness, dizziness, or fainting if their frequency diminishes cardiac output.

Treatment of PVCs depends on the cause, the patient's symptoms, and the clinical setting. Because occasional PVCs are a normal finding in healthy individuals, no treatment may be indicated, especially if the person is asymptomatic. Initially, a search should be made for possible reversible causes (such as oxygen for hypoxia; replacement of electrolytes; diuretics for heart failure; elimination of certain drugs; avoidance of alcohol, caffeine, tobacco, and illegal drugs; and administration of antianxiety medications if indicated). Significant PVCs (more than 6 per minute, multifocal PVCs, paired PVCs, R-on-T PVCs, or PVCs in runs of three or more) should be treated with an antiarrhythmic medication, especially in the setting of acute MI or following heart sugary because of the increased risk of ventricular tachycardia or ventricular fibrillation in this setting.

On some occasions, a ventricular beat may occur late instead of early. A late ectopic ventricular beat usually occurs after a pause in the underlying rhythm in which the dominant pacemaker (usually the sinus node) fails to initiate an impulse. If the ventricles are not activated by an impulse from the higher level pacemakers (SA node or AV node) within a certain period of time, a focus in the ventricles may "escape" and pace the heart. These are called ventricular escape beats (Figure 9.15). The ventricular escape beat is a protective mechanism, protecting the heart from slow rates, and no treatment is required.

Idioventricular Rhythm (IVR)

Normally, the pacemaker of the heart that is responsible for triggering each heart beat is the SA node. If the ventricles do not receive triggering signals at a rate high enough from either the SA node or the AV node, a focus in the ventricles can "escape" and become the pacemaker of the heart. For this reason, ventricular rhythm is commonly referred to as ventricular escape rhythm.

Idioventricular rhythm (Figure 9.16 and Box 9.3) is a very slow rhythm originating in the ventricles at a rate of 30 to 40 beats per minute (sometimes less). Because the impulse originates in the ventricles, there is no P wave and

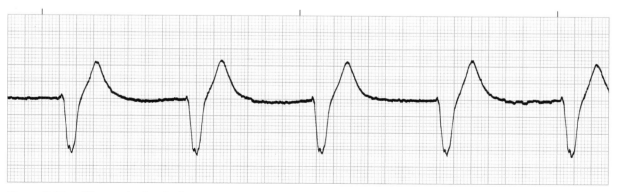

Figure 9.16 Idioventricular rhythm.

Rhythm:	Regular
Rate:	41 beats/minute
P waves:	Absent
PR interval:	Not measurable
QRS complex:	0.22 to 0.24 second.

Idioventricular Rhythm: Identifying ECG Features

Rhythm:	Regular
Rate:	30 to 40 beats/minute (sometimes less)
P waves:	Absent
PR interval:	Not measurable
QRS complex:	Wide (0.12 second or greater)

the QRS is abnormal and wide. The rhythm is usually regular. IVR is the normal rhythm of the ventricles.

IVR may occur intermittently or as a continuous rhythm. Intermittent IVR often occurs in short runs of three or more consecutive ventricular beats and is usually related to increased vagal effect on the SA node, allowing a ventricular focus to take control for a temporary period of time. Treatment is usually unnecessary. Continuous IVR usually occurs in advanced heart disease and is commonly the cardiac rhythm present just before the appearance of the final rhythm, ventricular standstill (asystole). Continuous IVR is generally symptomatic because of the slow rate and the loss of the atrial kick. The rhythm must be treated promptly following the protocols for symptomatic bradycardia (atropine, pacing, and vasopressors

to increase blood pressure). However, treatment is rarely successful.

If the rate of IVR falls below 20 beats per minute and the QRS complexes deteriorate into irregular, wide, indistinguishable waveforms, the rhythm is commonly referred to as an ***agonal rhythm*** or "dying heart" (Figure 9.17). Treatment is usually ineffective at this point.

Accelerated Idioventricular Rhythm (AIVR)

Accelerated idioventricular rhythm (Figures 9.18 and 9.19 and Box 9.4) originates in an ectopic pacemaker site in the ventricles with a rate between 50 and 100 beats per minute. The term accelerated denotes a rhythm that exceeds the inherent idioventricular escape rate of 30 to 40 beats per minute, but isn't fast enough to be ventricular tachycardia. AIVR has the same ECG features as IVR (no P waves; wide, abnormal QRS complex; regular rhythm) but is differentiated by the heart rate. AIVR can occur as a continuous rhythm (see Figure 9.18) or intermittently in short runs of three or more consecutive ventricular beats at a rate of 50 to 100 per minute (see Figure 9.19).

AIVR results when the rate of the ectopic ventricular pacemaker exceeds that of the "higher-order" pacemakers

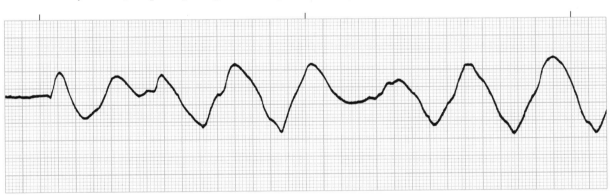

Figure 9.17 Agonal rhythm, sometimes called "dying heart."

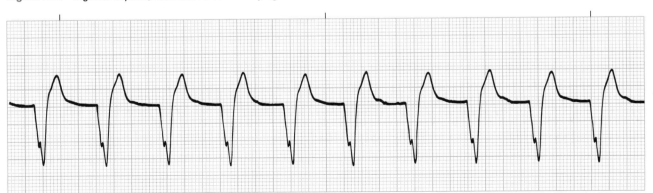

Figure 9.18 **Accelerated idioventricular rhythm.**

Rhythm:	Regular
Rate:	88 beats/minute
P waves:	Absent
PR interval:	Not measurable
QRS complex:	0.14 to 0.16 second.

box 9.4	Accelerated Idioventricular Rhythm: Identifying ECG Features
Rhythm:	Regular
Rate:	50 to 100 beats/minute
P waves:	Absent
PR interval:	Not measurable
QRS complex:	Wide (0.12 second or greater)

(the SA node and AV node). The mechanism is usually enhanced automaticity of the ventricular pacemaker cells, although triggered activity may play a role especially in ischemia and digitalis toxicity.

AIVR is most commonly seen during the reperfusion phase following acute myocardial infarction. It is often associated with increased vagal tone. Other causes include electrolyte abnormalities, cardiomyopathy, congenital heart disease, myocarditis, and digitalis toxicity.

Accelerated idioventricular rhythm is a benign rhythm in most settings, is well tolerated, and is rarely associated with symptoms. If the patient is symptomatic, it is usually related to a decrease in cardiac output from a loss of the atrial kick and not because of the heart rate, which is within a normal range.

Treatment of AIVR with antiarrhythmics is not recommended. Abolishing the ventricular focus may lead to a less desirable rate and rhythm. This rhythm is usually transient, requires no specific therapy, and spontaneously resolves on its own. A "tincture of time" is most often the best remedy.

Ventricular Tachycardia (VT)

Ventricular tachycardia (Figures 9.20 through 9.24 and Box 9.5) is an arrhythmia originating in an ectopic focus in the ventricles discharging impulses at a rate of 140 to 250 beats per minute.

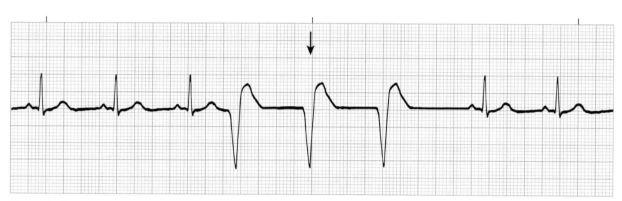

Figure 9.19   **Normal sinus rhythm with 3-beat run of AIVR.**

Rhythm:	Basic rhythm regular; AIVR regular
Rate:	72 beats/minute (basic rhythm). 72 beats/minute (AIVR)
P waves:	Sinus with basic rhythm. None with AIVR
PR interval:	0.14 to 0.16 second (basic rhythm)
QRS complex:	0.08 second (basic rhythm); 0.12 second (AIVR).

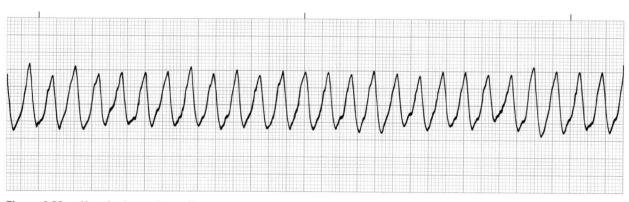

Figure 9.20   **Ventricular tachycardia.**

Rhythm:	Regular
Rate:	250 beats/minute
P waves:	None identified
PR interval:	Not measurable
QRS complex:	0.16 second.

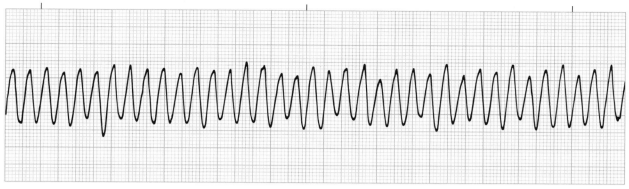

Figure 9.21   **Ventricular flutter.**

Rhythm: Regular
Rate: 300 beats/minute
P waves: None identified
PR interval: Not measurable
QRS complex: 0.12 to 0.16 second.

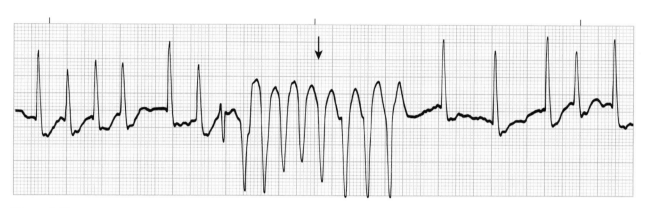

Figure 9.22   **Atrial fibrillation with an 8-beat run of ventricular tachycardia.**

Rhythm: Basic rhythm irregular; VT regular
Rate: Approximately 160 beats/minute (basic rhythm). 250 beats/minute (VT)
P waves: Fibrillation waves in basic rhythm; none with VT
PR interval: Not measurable
QRS complex: 0.06 to 0.08 second (basic rhythm). 0.12 second (VT).

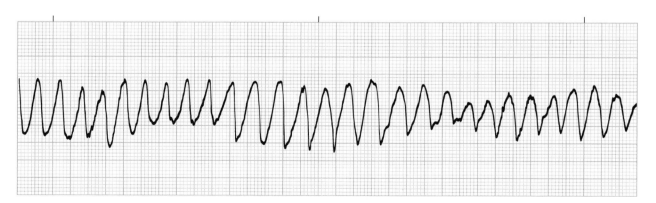

Figure 9.23   **Polymorphic ventricular tachycardia (torsade de pointes).**

Rhythm: Regular
Rate: 250 beats/minute
P waves: None identified
PR interval: Not measurable
QRS complex: 0.12 to 0.16 second or more
Comment: This type of ventricular tachycardia is called *torsade de pointes* (twisting of the points). The QRS changes from negative to positive polarity and appears to twist around the isoelectric line. It is associated with a prolonged QT interval and is refractory to antiarrhythmics. IV magnesium or overdrive pacing has been successful in the treatment of this rhythm.

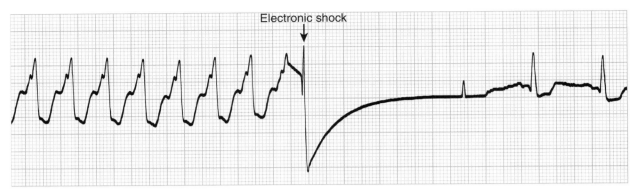

Figure 9.24   Electrical cardioversion of ventricular tachycardia to sinus rhythm.

---

box 9.5   Ventricular Tachycardia (VT): Identifying ECG Features

Rhythm: Regular; can be slightly irregular
Rate: 140 to 250 beats/minute
P waves: No P waves are associated with VT.
PR interval: Not measurable
QRS complex: Wide (0.12 second or greater)

VT occurs as a series of wide, abnormal QRS complexes seen in intermittent runs or as a continuous rhythm. Because of the ventricular origin of the impulse, no P waves are produced. The rhythm is usually regular but may be slightly irregular. The ST segment and T-wave slope in the opposite direction from the main QRS deflection. When the QRS complexes are of the same morphology in the same lead, the rhythm is termed *monomorphic VT* (see Figure 9.20). When the QRS complexes differ in morphology in the same lead, the VT is called *polymorphic VT* (see Figure 9.23).

VT may occasionally occur at rates greater than 250 beats per minute. At such extreme rates, the QRS complexes appear sawtooth in appearance and the rhythm is commonly referred to as ventricular flutter (see Figure 9.21). Ventricular flutter is so rapid that there is virtually no cardiac output. Ventricular flutter is often a precursor to ventricular fibrillation.

The most common cause of monomorphic VT is myocardial scarring from previous myocardial infarction. The scar cannot conduct electrical activity, so there is a reentry circuit around the scar that results in the tachycardia. Ventricular tachycardia can also be caused by enhanced automaticity of a focus in the ventricles or to triggered activity occurring during ventricular repolarization. Other causes include coronary heart disease, occurrence of significant PVCs (more than 6 per minute, paired PVCs, R-on-T PVCs, multifocal PVCs), hypertension, cardiomyopathy, heart failure, electrolyte imbalances, hypoxia, myocarditis, excessive caffeine and alcohol consumption, recreational drugs, stimulation of the endocardium during insertion of a pacing lead or pulmonary artery catheter, and as an effect of myocardial reperfusion following percutaneous coronary interventions or the administration of thrombolytic drugs. Certain medications or conditions may prolong the QT interval, causing the ventricles to be particularly vulnerable to a type of polymorphic VT called torsade de pointes (TdP) (see Figure 9.23).

When VT lasts for less than 30 seconds, it is called nonsustained VT. Ventricular tachycardia occurring in short runs of three or more consecutive PVCs at a rate of 140 to 250 beats per minute is considered a "run" or "burst" of nonsustained VT (see Figures 9.11 and 9.22). Nonsustained VT, unless frequent, usually doesn't cause symptoms, but it can progress into sustained VT. When VT lasts longer than 30 seconds, it is considered sustained VT. Sustained ventricular tachycardia is a life-threatening arrhythmia for two major reasons:

- The rapid ventricular rate and loss of the atrial kick reduce cardiac output. This reduction in cardiac output often compounds the already low cardiac output frequently seen in the diseased hearts in which VT tends to occur.
- The rhythm may degenerate into ventricular fibrillation or asystole.

Treatment is based on the patient's presentation. An "unstable" patient refers to an individual who presents with symptoms such as hypotension, chest pain, shortness of breath, signs of decreased perfusion (i.e., cool, clammy skin; peripheral cyanosis; or decreased level of consciousness). A "stable" patient refers to an individual with normal blood pressure, no chest pain, shortness of breath, or signs of decreased perfusion. As part of the initial assessment, you should check for a pulse. If there is not a pulse (pulseless VT), the rhythm must be treated as ventricular fibrillation. If there is a pulse, protocols for *stable VT* and *unstable VT* are followed.

Treatment Protocols: Stable Monomorphic VT with Pulse

- Amiodarone (150 mg in 100 mL D5W) is given as an intravenous piggyback (IVPB) bolus over 10 minutes. An additional 150-mg IVPB bolus can be repeated in 10 minutes for resistant VT. Once the rhythm converts to a stable rhythm, an amiodarone maintenance infusion should be started to prevent reoccurrence of VT. The amiodarone maintenance infusion (900 mg in 500 mL

D5W) is started at 1 mg per minute for 6 hours, then decreased to 0.5 mg per minute for 18 hours. The total dose of amiodarone (IVPB bolus doses plus maintenance infusion) should not exceed 2.2 g in 24 hours. Oral amiodarone can be started once the maintenance infusion is completed. Elimination of the drug from the body is extremely long (half-life lasts up to 40 days).

- If the rhythm is unresponsive to amiodarone, sedate the patient and perform synchronized cardioversion beginning at 100 J biphasic energy dose, increasing in a stepwise fashion with subsequent attempts.

Some physicians prefer to skip drug therapy and go directly to synchronized cardioversion. Figure 9.24 shows cardioversion of VT to sinus rhythm.

Treatment Protocols: Unstable Monomorphic VT with Pulse

- Sedate the patient (if conscious).
- Convert the rhythm using synchronized cardioversion beginning at 100 J biphasic energy dose, increasing in stepwise fashion with subsequent attempts. Once cardioversion has converted the rhythm, a maintenance infusion of amiodarone is usually started at 1 mg per minute for 6 hours, then decreased to 0.5 mg per minute for 18 hours, followed by oral amiodarone once the maintenance infusion is completed.

Treatment of chronic, recurrent VT usually includes therapy with an oral antiarrhythmic. Patients who are refractory to a pharmacologic approach may require further evaluation, which could include specialized electrophysiologic testing and endocardial mapping with long-term options including the use of an implantable cardioverter defibrillator (ICD) or reentry circuit ablation. Most ICDs are set to initially overdrive pace the ventricle. Pacing the ventricle at a rate faster than the underlying tachycardia can sometimes be effective in terminating the rhythm (this is called antitachycardia pacing). If this fails, the ICD will stop pacing and deliver an electric shock.

Ablation of the reentry circuit involves delivering short pulses of radio frequency current through an intracardiac catheter. It produces a small burn that effectively blocks the part of the circuit supporting the reentrant-type wave.

Torsade de Pointes Ventricular Tachycardia

Torsade de pointes (TdP) (see Figure 9.23) is a form of polymorphic VT. This name is derived from a French term meaning "twisting of the points," which describes a QRS complex that changes polarity (from negative to positive and positive to negative) as it twists around the isoelectric line. TdP is an intermediary arrhythmia between VT and VF.

TdP is most commonly caused by abnormalities of ventricular muscle repolarization. The predisposition to this problem usually manifests on the ECG as a prolongation of the QT interval. A prolonged QT interval indicates a lengthened relative refractory period (vulnerable period) that puts the ventricles at risk for TdP and may result in sudden cardiac death.

TdP is often associated with bradycardia. Antiarrhythmic agents such as quinidine, procainamide, disopyramide, sotalol, and amiodarone may cause QT prolongation. Other causes include phenothiazines, tricyclic antidepressants, certain antibiotics and antihistamines, electrolyte imbalances, and congenital long QT syndrome.

The ventricular rate in TdP is extremely rapid, and the patient usually becomes unstable very quickly. Recognition of TdP is critical, not only because of the rapid deterioration of the patient but also because the treatment plan differs greatly from the treatment of monomorphic VT. Amiodarone, a drug used in treating monomorphic VT, can prolong the QT interval and make matters worse in this situation.

Treatment Protocols: Torsade de Pointes VT

- The initial treatment should be immediate unsynchronized shock at 200 J biphasic energy dose (because of the variability in the QRS complexes in TdP, it may be difficult or impossible to reliably synchronize to a QRS complex). Although TdP is responsive to electrical therapy, the rhythm has a tendency to recur unless the precipitating factors are eliminated.
- Magnesium is the pharmacologic treatment of choice for TdP. Magnesium is usually very effective even in patients with normal magnesium levels. Magnesium acts as an antiarrhythmic and may terminate or prevent recurrent episodes of TdP. Give a loading dose of 1 to 2 g IV diluted in 10 mL D5W slowly over 5 minutes. This is followed by a 0.5 to 1 g IV drip. A side effect of magnesium is hypotension, especially if administered rapidly. Magnesium also reduces neuromuscular tone and close monitoring of deep tendon reflexes is suggested.
- Potassium chloride (like magnesium) is a first-line therapy for TdP. Potassium is essential for maintenance of intracellular tonicity; transmission of nerve impulses; contraction of cardiac, skeletal, and smooth muscles; and maintenance of normal renal function. Depletion usually results from diuretic therapy, diabetic ketoacidosis, severe diarrhea, or inadequate replacement during prolonged parenteral nutrition therapy. Dosage of potassium depends on the serum potassium level, hospital protocols, and physician orders.
- Removing or correcting precipitating factors:
  1. Bradycardia induced: Discontinue drugs that decrease heart rate.
  2. Drug induced: Discontinue drugs that prolong QR interval.
  3. Electrolyte induced: Correct electrolyte abnormalities (magnesium and potassium are considered first-line therapy).

In treatment of congenital prolonged QT syndrome or recurrent TdP VT, an ICD can be used as prophylaxis.

Ventricular Fibrillation

In ventricular fibrillation (Figures 9.25 and 9.26 and Box 9.6), rapid, erratic electrical impulses in the ventricles take over control of the heart. There is no organized depolarization of the ventricles (thus no QRS complexes). Instead, the ventricular muscle quivers, and as a result, there is no effective myocardial contraction or pulse. The resulting rhythm shows wavy, irregular deflections, which vary in size, shape, and amplitude, appearing in a chaotic pattern.

Ventricular fibrillation with large waves is called coarse VF (see Figure 9.25). If the waves are small, the rhythm is called fine VF (see Figure 9.26). Coarse VF waves are generally more irregular than fine VF waves. Fine VF may resemble ventricular asystole and should be confirmed by examining the rhythm in different leads. The distinction between fine VF and coarse VF is significant because

box 9.6	Ventricular Fibrillation (VF): Identifying ECG Features
Rhythm:	Irregular and chaotic
Rate:	Not measurable
P waves:	Absent; wavy, irregular deflections seen, varying in size, shape, and height and representative of quivering of the ventricles instead of contraction; deflections may be small (described as *fine VF*) or large (described as *coarse VF*)
PR interval:	Not measurable
QRS complex:	Absent

coarse VF usually indicates a more recent onset and is more likely to be reversed by early defibrillation. Fine VF usually indicates that the rhythm has been present longer and may require drug therapy and cardiopulmonary

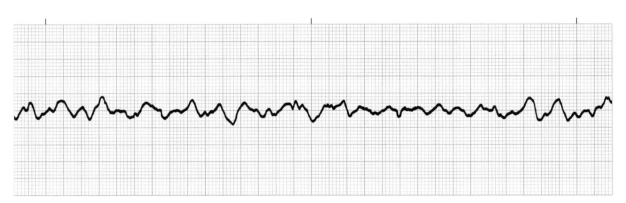

Figure 9.25   Ventricular fibrillation (coarse wave forms).

Rhythm:	Irregular and chaotic
Rate:	Not measurable
P waves:	Recognizable P waves are absent; wavy, irregular deflections are seen, which vary in size, shape, and height representative of quivering of the ventricles instead of contraction
PR interval:	Not measurable
QRS complex:	Absent.

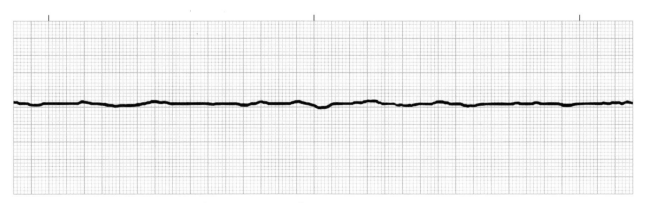

Figure 9.26   Ventricular fibrillation ("fine" wave forms).

Rhythm:	Irregular and chaotic
Rate:	Not measurable
P waves:	Recognizable P waves are absent; wave deflections are chaotic and vary in size, shape, and height
PR interval:	Not measurable
QRS complex:	Absent.

resuscitation (CPR) before defibrillation can be effective. Fine VF will progress to asystole unless the rhythm is treated.

VF is the most common cause of cardiac death in patients with acute MI. Other conditions that may lead to ventricular fibrillation include cardiomyopathy, congenital heart disease, coronary artery disease, hypoxia, myocarditis, electrolyte disturbances, use of illegal drugs such as cocaine and methamphetamine, and electrocution accidents or injury to the heart. VF may be preceded by significant PVCs or VT, but it may also occur spontaneously when there is no discernible heart pathology or other evident cause. VF may also occur during anesthesia, cardiac catheterization procedures, or stimulation of the endocardium during insertion of a pacing lead or a pulmonary artery catheter.

Once ventricular fibrillation occurs, there is no cardiac output, peripheral pulses and blood pressure are absent, and the patient becomes unconscious immediately. Cyanosis and seizure activity may also be present. Death is imminent unless the rhythm is treated immediately.

Treatment Protocols: VF

- Check the pulse and rapidly assess the patient. If there is a pulse and the patient is conscious, VF isn't the problem. ECG artifacts produced by loose or dry electrodes, patient movement, or muscle tremors may resemble VF.
- If there is no pulse and the patient is unconscious, defibrillate at 200 J biphasic energy dose. If the arrest is unwitnessed, perform CPR for five cycles (2 minutes) before the initial shock.
- If unsuccessful, start CPR and establish an IV line. Intubate the patient when possible.
- Administer epinephrine 1 mg IV push and repeat every 3 to 5 minutes.
- Continue CPR for five cycles to circulate drug and then defibrillate at 200 J biphasic energy dose × 1.
- Consider one of the following antiarrhythmics:
  1. Amiodarone 300 mg IV push (dilution in 20 mL D5W is recommended); if VF is refractory or recurs, consider one additional dose of 150 mg IV push in 3 to 5 minutes (dilution in 20 mL D5W is recommended). If drug therapy is successful, a maintenance infusion of amiodarone can be started at 1 mg per minute for 6 hours followed by 0.5 mg per minute for 18 hours (total dose of IV push and maintenance infusion should not exceed 2.2 g in 24 hours). Oral amiodarone can be started following completion of the IV infusion.
  2. Lidocaine 1 to 1.5 mg/kg IV push followed by half the initial dose (0.5 to 0.75 mg/kg IV push) every 5 to 10 minutes to a maximum dose of 3 mg/kg. If drug therapy is successful, a maintenance infusion of lidocaine can be started at 1 to 4 mg per minute. The half-life of lidocaine increases after 24 to 48 hours. Therefore, after 24 hours, the dosage should be reduced or blood levels monitored. Signs of toxicity include

slurred speech, altered consciousness, muscle twitching, seizures, and bradycardia.

Note: All antiarrhythmics have some degree of ***proarrhythmic effects*** (may induce or worsen ventricular arrhythmias). Use of more than one antiarrhythmic compounds the adverse effect, particularly for bradycardia, hypotension, and TdP. Never use more than one agent unless absolutely necessary.

- Continue drug therapy, CPR, and defibrillation attempts (drug-CPR-shock pattern) until rhythm resolves or a decision is made to stop resuscitative efforts.

Ventricular Standstill (Asystole)

Ventricular standstill (Figures 9.27 and 9.28 and Box 9.7) is the absence of all electrical activity in the ventricles. When the ventricles are inactive, there are no QRS complexes. The atria, however, may continue to generate electrical activity, producing P waves. Thus, ventricular standstill has two presentations on the ECG tracing: P waves without QRS complexes (see Figure 9.27) or a straight line (see Figure 9.28). If P waves are present, some form of advanced heart block (Mobitz II second-degree AV block or third-degree AV block) may have preceded the arrhythmia. Ventricular standstill with a straight line usually occurs following such arrhythmias as VT, VF, IVR, and pulseless electrical activity (PEA). Asystole may also occur following termination of a tachyarrhythmia by medication administration, defibrillation, or synchronized cardioversion.

Once ventricular standstill occurs, there is no cardiac output, peripheral pulses and blood pressure are absent, and the patient becomes unconscious immediately. Cyanosis and seizure activity may also be present. Death is imminent unless the arrhythmia is treated immediately. Without cardiac monitoring, ventricular standstill cannot be distinguished from VF at the bedside.

Treatment Protocols: Ventricular Standstill (Asystole)

- Check pulse and rapidly assess the patient. If there is a pulse and the patient is conscious, ventricular standstill is not the problem.

box 9.7	Ventricular Standstill: Identifying ECG Features
Rhythm:	Atrial: If P waves present, will have atrial rhythm Ventricular: None
Rate:	Atrial: If P waves present, will have atrial rate Ventricular: None
P waves:	ECG tracings will show either P waves without a QRS complex or a straight line
PR interval:	Not measurable
QRS complex:	Absent

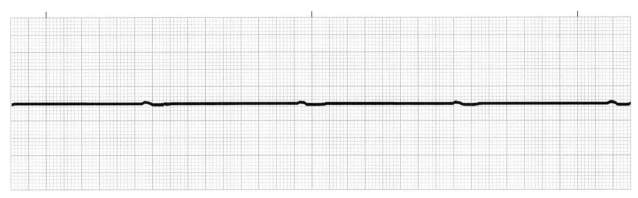

Figure 9.27 **Ventricular standstill (asystole).**

Rhythm: Regular atrial rhythm; no ventricular rhythm
Rate: Atrial: 34 beats/minute; no ventricular rate
P waves: Sinus
PR interval: Not measurable
QRS complex: No QRS present.

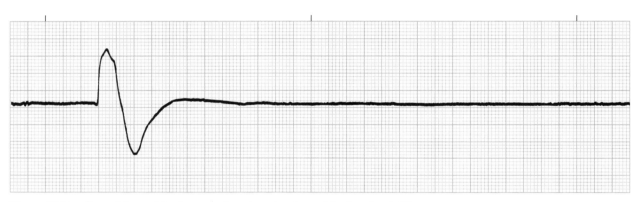

Figure 9.28 **One wide ventricular complex changing to ventricular standstill.**

Rhythm: Not measurable
Rate: Ventricular, 10 beats/minute
P waves: None identified
PR interval: Not measurable
QRS complex: 0.24 or wider.

- Check monitor lead system (a loose electrode pad or lead wire will show a straight line).
- Check rhythm in two leads (low amplitude QRS complexes may look like P waves; fine VF may look like a straight line).
- Start CPR and establish an IV line. Intubate the patient when possible.
- Give epinephrine 1 mg IV push and repeat every 3 to 5 minutes. Continue CPR to circulate the drug.
- Consider the underlying reversible causes of the rhythm (the so-called Hs and Ts):
  ○ Hypovolemia (the most common cause)
  ○ Hypoxia
  ○ Hydrogen ions (acidosis)
  ○ Hypothermia
  ○ Hypo-/hyperkalemia
  ○ Hypoglycemia
  ○ Toxins (drug overdose)
  ○ Tamponade (cardiac)
  ○ Tension pneumothorax
  ○ Thrombosis (coronary or pulmonary)

Pulseless Electrical Activity

Pulseless electrical activity is a clinical situation (not a specific arrhythmia) in which an organized cardiac rhythm (excluding pulseless VT) is observed on the monitor but no pulse is palpated. Causes and treatment of PEA are the same as asystole. PEA has a poor prognosis unless the underlying cause can be quickly identified and managed appropriately.

A **pull-out arrhythmia summary** of the ventricular arrhythmias and bundle-branch block can be found in Table 9.1, at the back of the book. This may be used as a *quick guide to assist with rhythm interpretation.*

RHYTHM STRIP PRACTICE: VENTRICULAR ARRHYTHMIAS AND BUNDLE-BRANCH BLOCKS

Analyze the following rhythm strips by following the five basic steps:

- Determine *rhythm regularity*.
- Calculate *heart rate* (this usually refers to the ventricular rate, but if atrial rate differs, you need to calculate both).
- Identify and examine *P waves*.
- Measure *PR interval*.
- Measure *QRS complex*.

Interpret the rhythm by comparing this data with the ECG characteristics for each rhythm. All rhythm strips are lead II, a positive lead, unless otherwise noted. Check your answers with the answer key in the appendix.

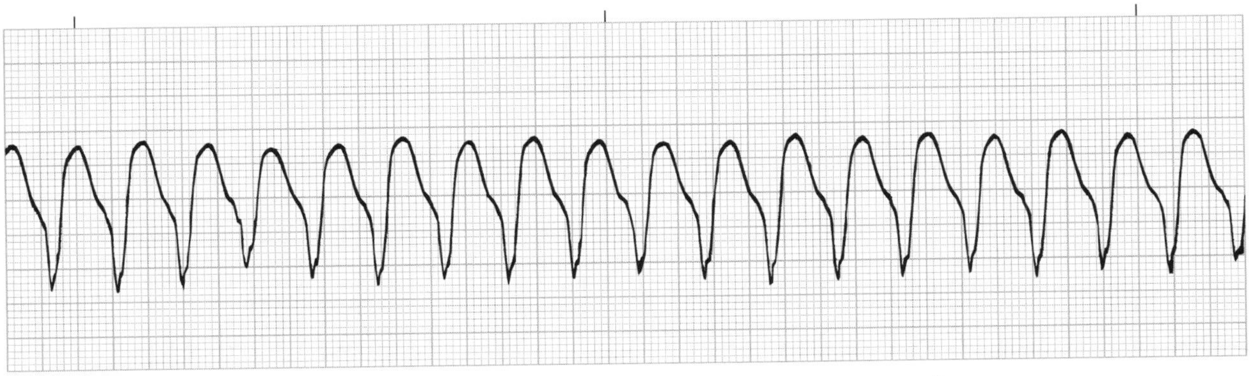

Strip 9.1 Rhythm: _____ Rate: _____ P wave: _____

PR interval: _____ QRS complex: _____

Rhythm interpretation: _____

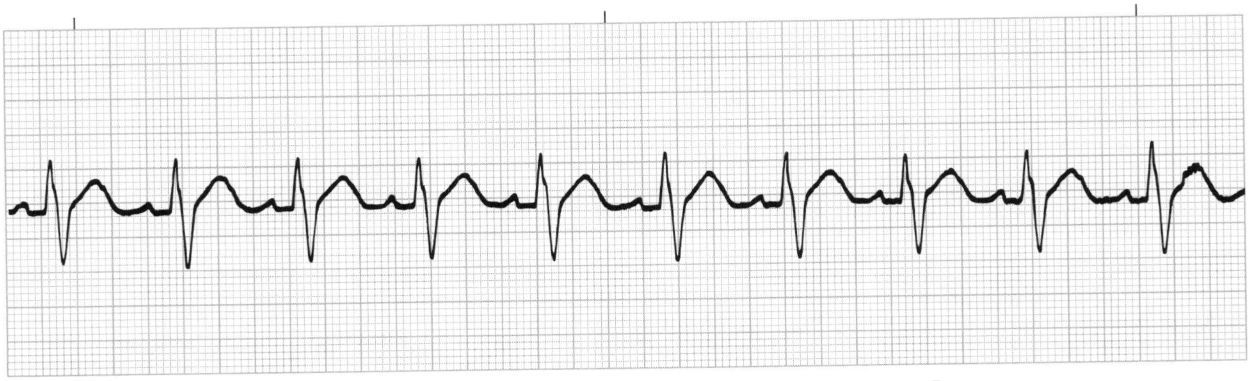

Strip 9.2 Rhythm: _____ Rate: _____ P wave: _____

PR interval: _____ QRS complex: _____

Rhythm interpretation: _____

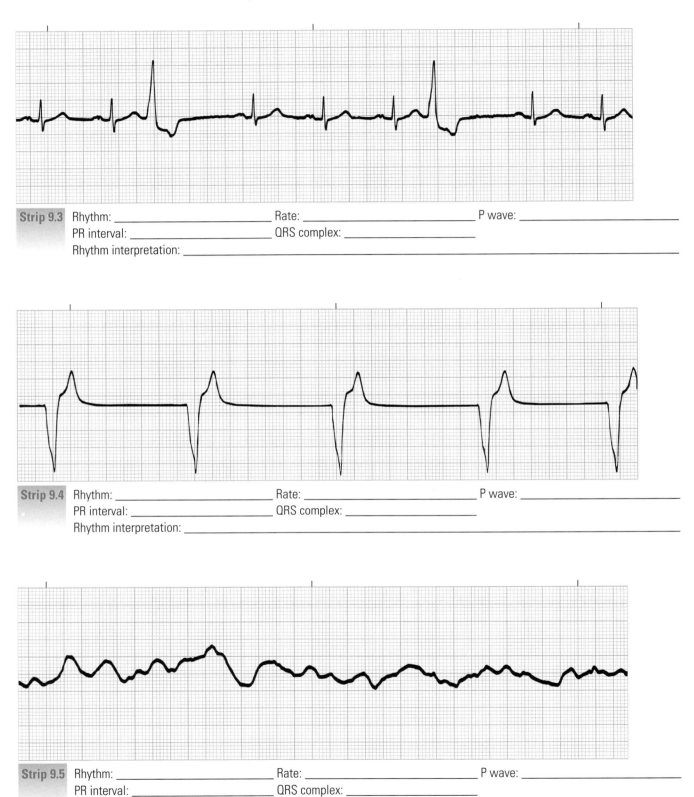

Strip 9.3 Rhythm: _____ Rate: _____ P wave: _____
PR interval: _____ QRS complex: _____
Rhythm interpretation: _____

Strip 9.4 Rhythm: _____ Rate: _____ P wave: _____
PR interval: _____ QRS complex: _____
Rhythm interpretation: _____

Strip 9.5 Rhythm: _____ Rate: _____ P wave: _____
PR interval: _____ QRS complex: _____
Rhythm interpretation: _____

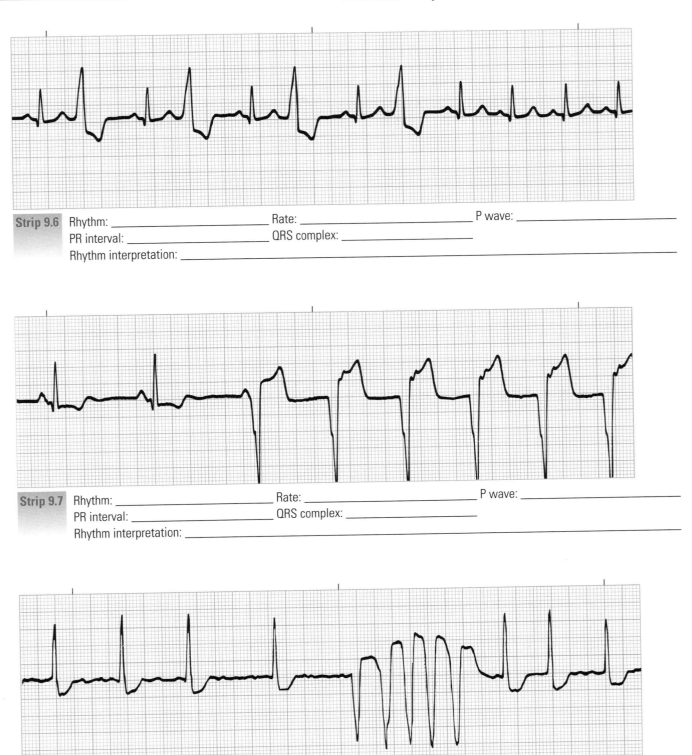

Strip 9.6 Rhythm: _____ Rate: _____ P wave: _____
PR interval: _____ QRS complex: _____
Rhythm interpretation: _____

Strip 9.7 Rhythm: _____ Rate: _____ P wave: _____
PR interval: _____ QRS complex: _____
Rhythm interpretation: _____

Strip 9.8 Rhythm: _____ Rate: _____ P wave: _____
PR interval: _____ QRS complex: _____
Rhythm interpretation: _____

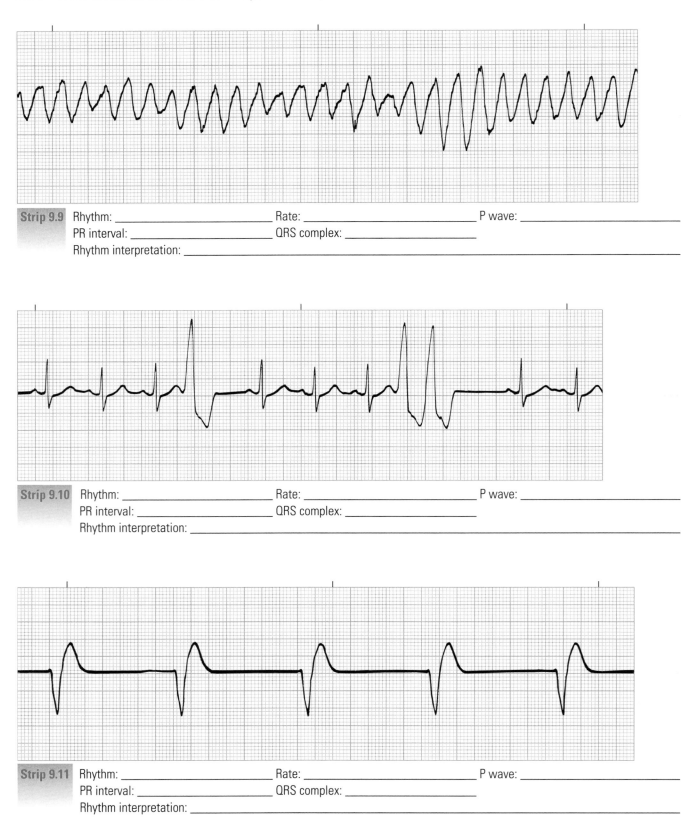

Strip 9.9 Rhythm: _____ Rate: _____ P wave: _____

PR interval: _____ QRS complex: _____

Rhythm interpretation: _____

Strip 9.10 Rhythm: _____ Rate: _____ P wave: _____

PR interval: _____ QRS complex: _____

Rhythm interpretation: _____

Strip 9.11 Rhythm: _____ Rate: _____ P wave: _____

PR interval: _____ QRS complex: _____

Rhythm interpretation: _____

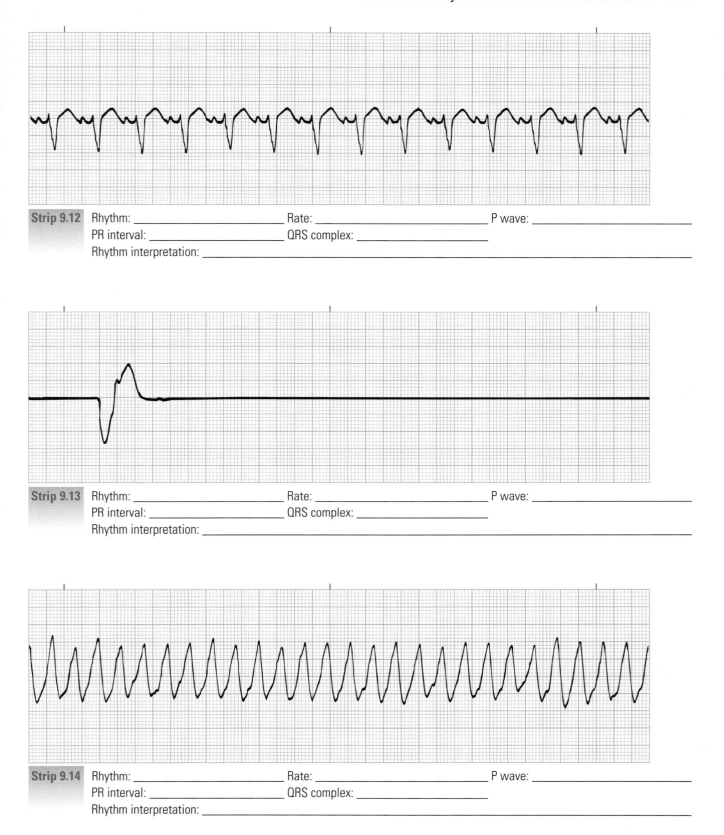

Strip 9.12 Rhythm: _____ Rate: _____ P wave: _____
PR interval: _____ QRS complex: _____
Rhythm interpretation: _____

Strip 9.13 Rhythm: _____ Rate: _____ P wave: _____
PR interval: _____ QRS complex: _____
Rhythm interpretation: _____

Strip 9.14 Rhythm: _____ Rate: _____ P wave: _____
PR interval: _____ QRS complex: _____
Rhythm interpretation: _____

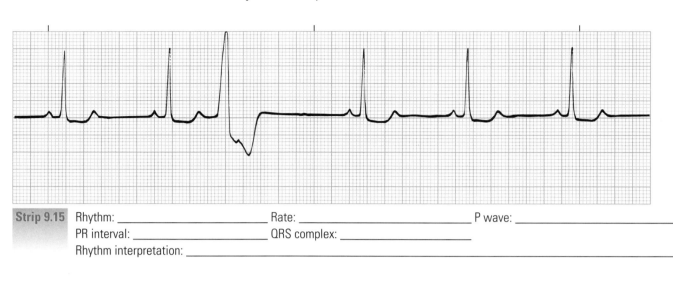

Strip 9.15 Rhythm: _____ Rate: _____ P wave: _____
PR interval: _____ QRS complex: _____
Rhythm interpretation: _____

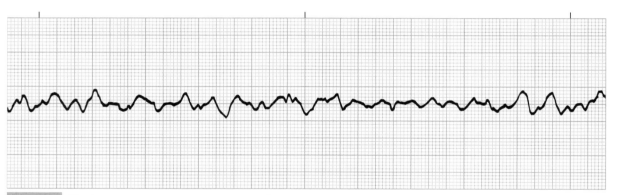

Strip 9.16 Rhythm: _____ Rate: _____ P wave: _____
PR interval: _____ QRS complex: _____
Rhythm interpretation: _____

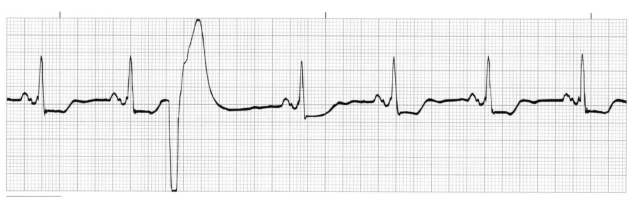

Strip 9.17 Rhythm: _____ Rate: _____ P wave: _____
PR interval: _____ QRS complex: _____
Rhythm interpretation: _____

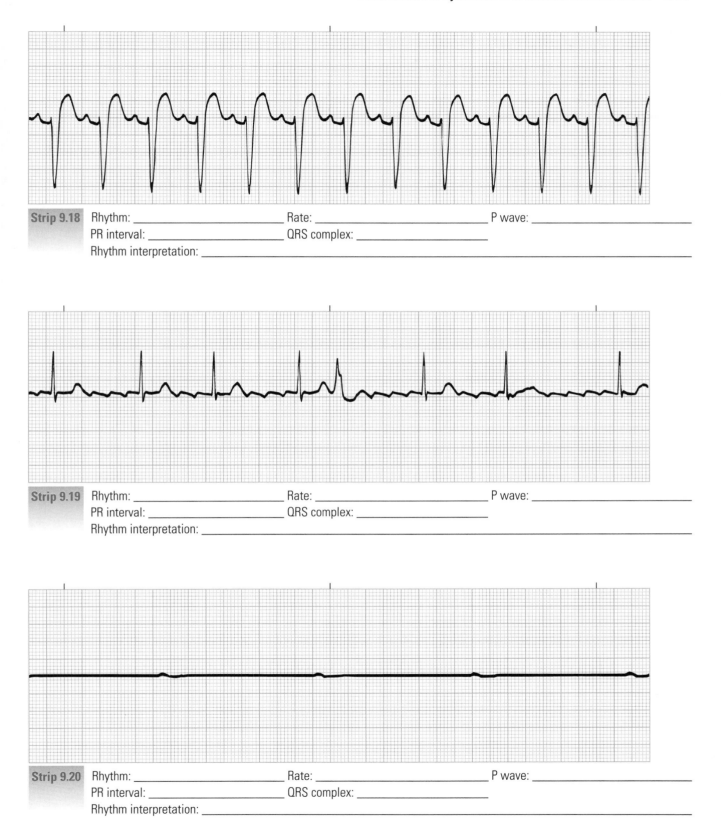

Strip 9.18 Rhythm: _____ Rate: _____ P wave: _____

PR interval: _____ QRS complex: _____

Rhythm interpretation: _____

Strip 9.19 Rhythm: _____ Rate: _____ P wave: _____

PR interval: _____ QRS complex: _____

Rhythm interpretation: _____

Strip 9.20 Rhythm: _____ Rate: _____ P wave: _____

PR interval: _____ QRS complex: _____

Rhythm interpretation: _____

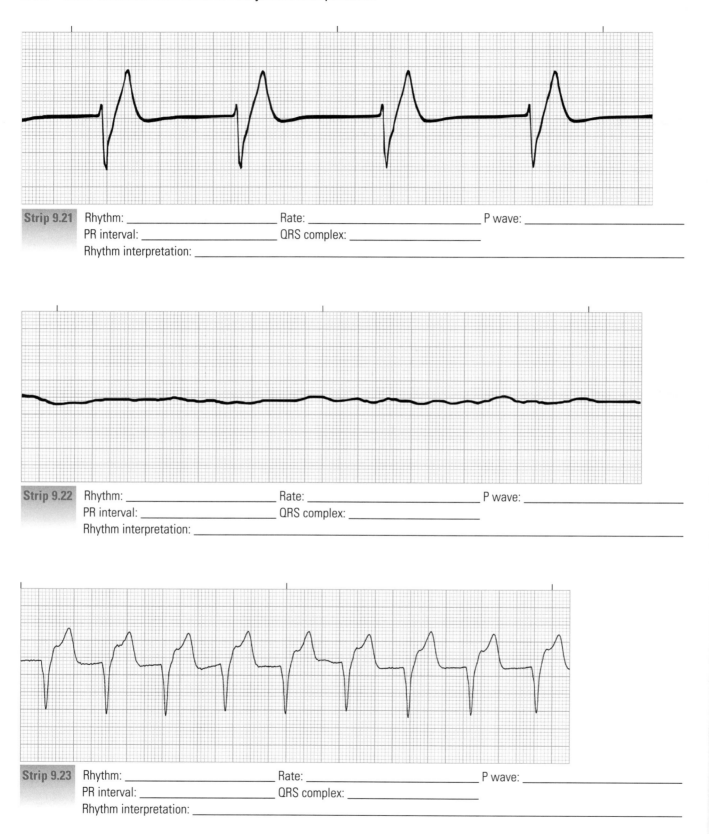

Strip 9.21 Rhythm: _____ Rate: _____ P wave: _____
PR interval: _____ QRS complex: _____
Rhythm interpretation: _____

Strip 9.22 Rhythm: _____ Rate: _____ P wave: _____
PR interval: _____ QRS complex: _____
Rhythm interpretation: _____

Strip 9.23 Rhythm: _____ Rate: _____ P wave: _____
PR interval: _____ QRS complex: _____
Rhythm interpretation: _____

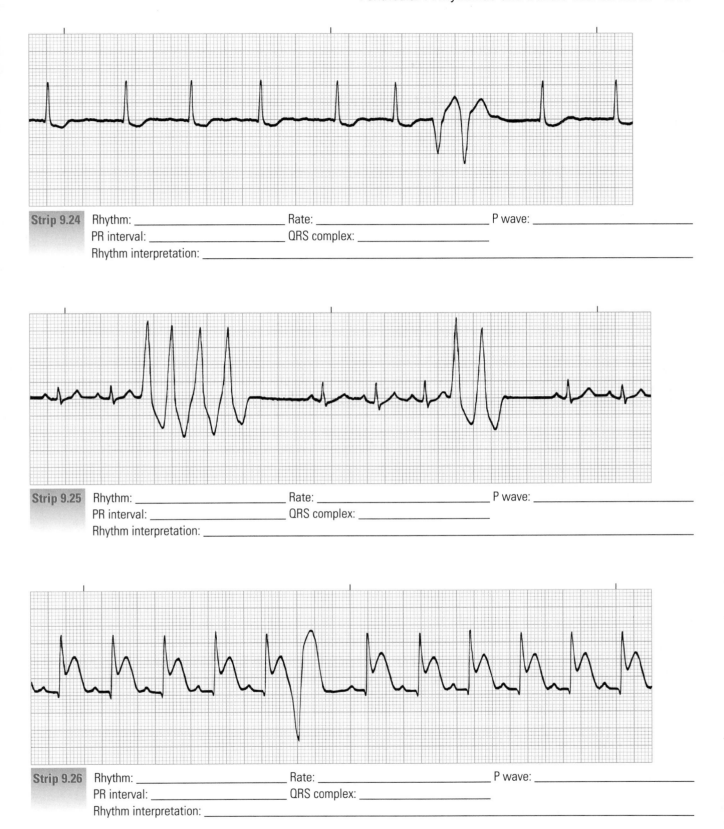

Strip 9.24 Rhythm: _____ Rate: _____ P wave: _____
PR interval: _____ QRS complex: _____
Rhythm interpretation: _____

Strip 9.25 Rhythm: _____ Rate: _____ P wave: _____
PR interval: _____ QRS complex: _____
Rhythm interpretation: _____

Strip 9.26 Rhythm: _____ Rate: _____ P wave: _____
PR interval: _____ QRS complex: _____
Rhythm interpretation: _____

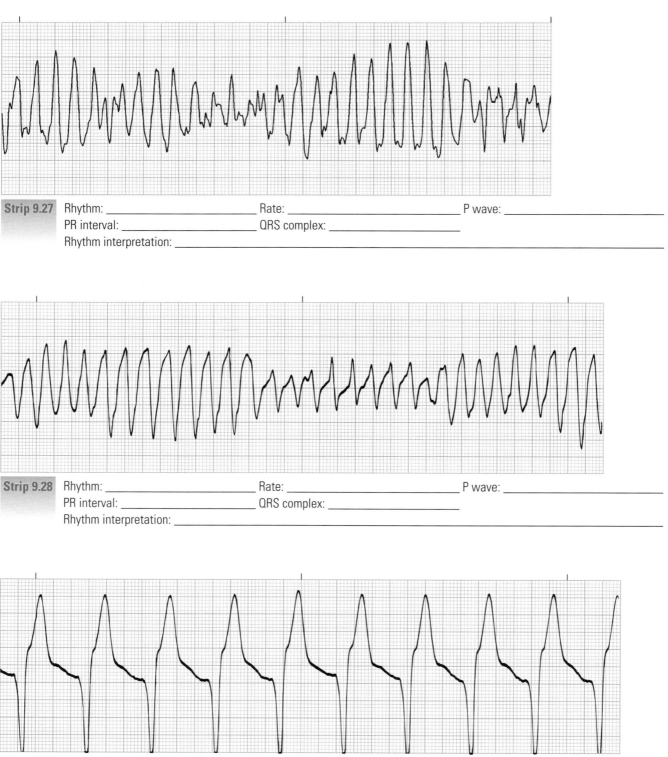

Strip 9.27 Rhythm: _____ Rate: _____ P wave: _____
PR interval: _____ QRS complex: _____
Rhythm interpretation: _____

Strip 9.28 Rhythm: _____ Rate: _____ P wave: _____
PR interval: _____ QRS complex: _____
Rhythm interpretation: _____

Strip 9.29 Rhythm: _____ Rate: _____ P wave: _____
PR interval: _____ QRS complex: _____
Rhythm interpretation: _____

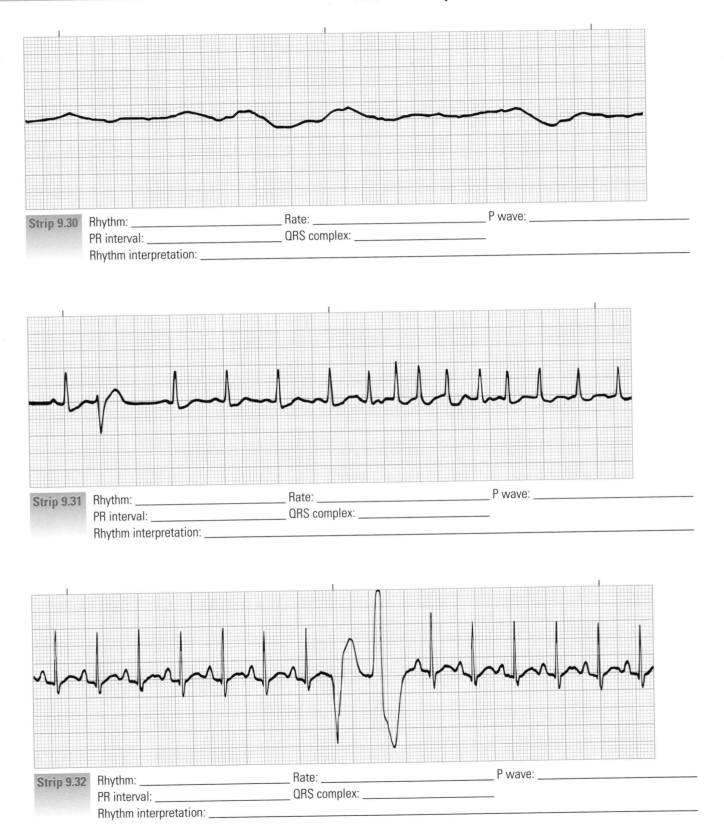

Strip 9.30 Rhythm: _____ Rate: _____ P wave: _____

PR interval: _____ QRS complex: _____

Rhythm interpretation: _____

Strip 9.31 Rhythm: _____ Rate: _____ P wave: _____

PR interval: _____ QRS complex: _____

Rhythm interpretation: _____

Strip 9.32 Rhythm: _____ Rate: _____ P wave: _____

PR interval: _____ QRS complex: _____

Rhythm interpretation: _____

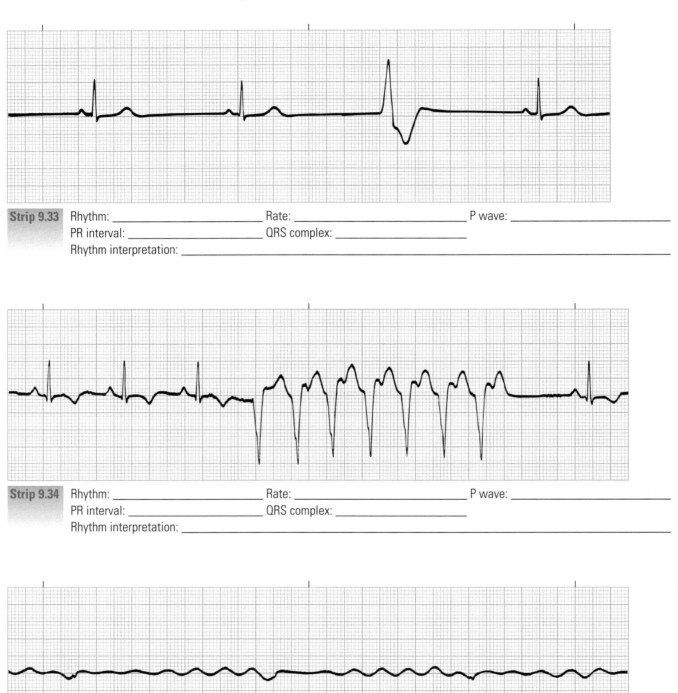

Strip 9.33 Rhythm: _____ Rate: _____ P wave: _____
PR interval: _____ QRS complex: _____
Rhythm interpretation: _____

Strip 9.34 Rhythm: _____ Rate: _____ P wave: _____
PR interval: _____ QRS complex: _____
Rhythm interpretation: _____

Strip 9.35 Rhythm: _____ Rate: _____ P wave: _____
PR interval: _____ QRS complex: _____
Rhythm interpretation: _____

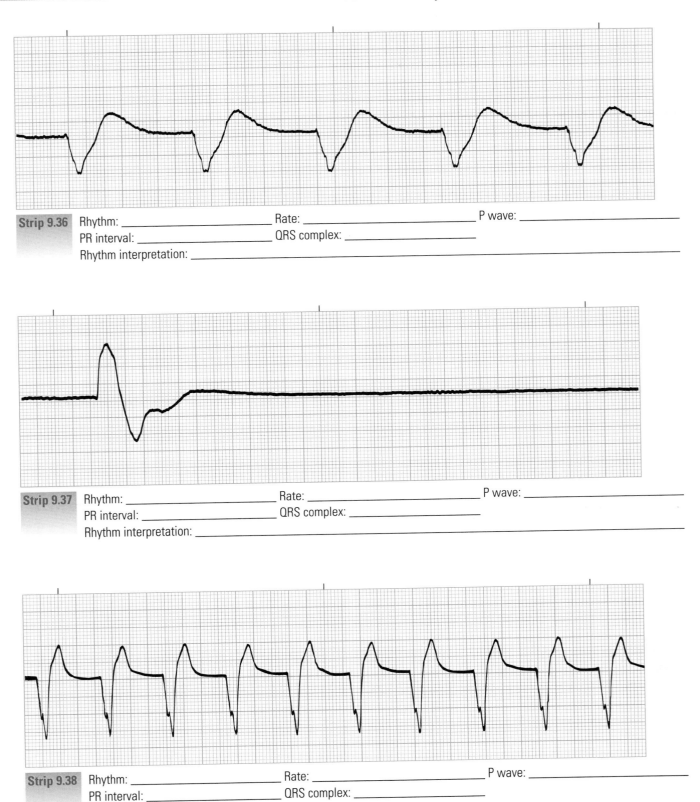

Strip 9.36   Rhythm: _____   Rate: _____   P wave: _____
PR interval: _____   QRS complex: _____
Rhythm interpretation: _____

Strip 9.37   Rhythm: _____   Rate: _____   P wave: _____
PR interval: _____   QRS complex: _____
Rhythm interpretation: _____

Strip 9.38   Rhythm: _____   Rate: _____   P wave: _____
PR interval: _____   QRS complex: _____
Rhythm interpretation: _____

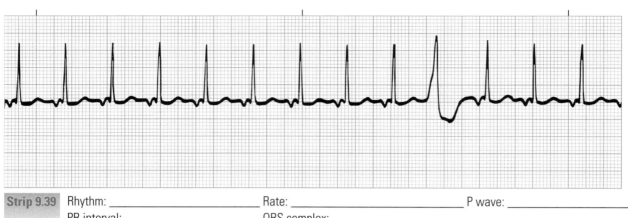

Strip 9.39	Rhythm: _____	Rate: _____	P wave: _____
	PR interval: _____	QRS complex: _____	
	Rhythm interpretation: _____		

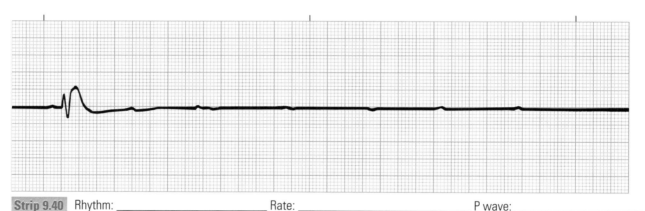

Strip 9.40	Rhythm: _____	Rate: _____	P wave: _____
	PR interval: _____	QRS complex: _____	
	Rhythm interpretation: _____		

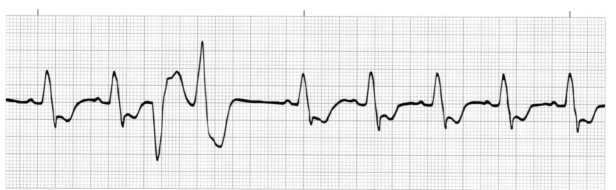

Strip 9.41	Rhythm: _____	Rate: _____	P wave: _____
	PR interval: _____	QRS complex: _____	
	Rhythm interpretation: _____		

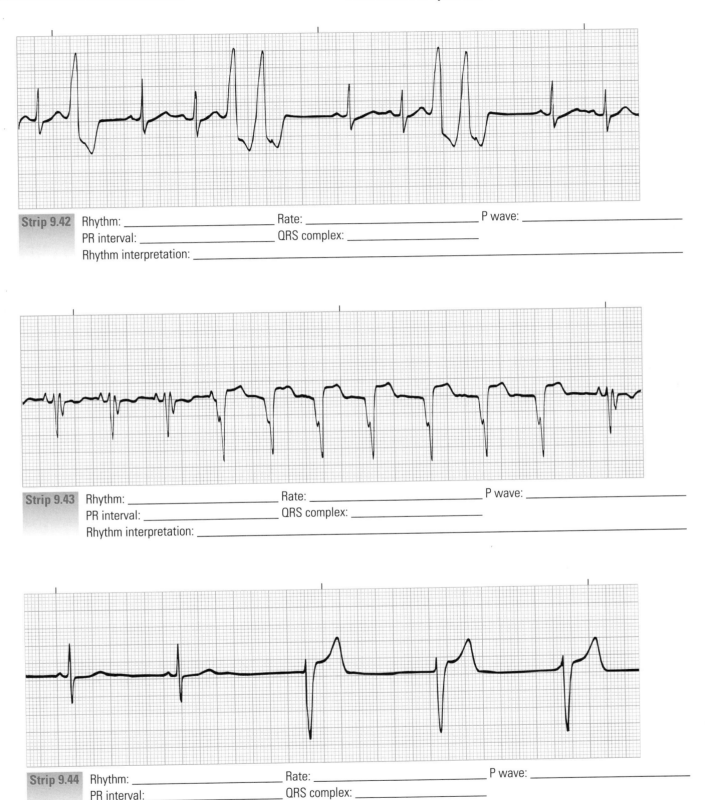

Strip 9.42 Rhythm: _____ Rate: _____ P wave: _____
PR interval: _____ QRS complex: _____
Rhythm interpretation: _____

Strip 9.43 Rhythm: _____ Rate: _____ P wave: _____
PR interval: _____ QRS complex: _____
Rhythm interpretation: _____

Strip 9.44 Rhythm: _____ Rate: _____ P wave: _____
PR interval: _____ QRS complex: _____
Rhythm interpretation: _____

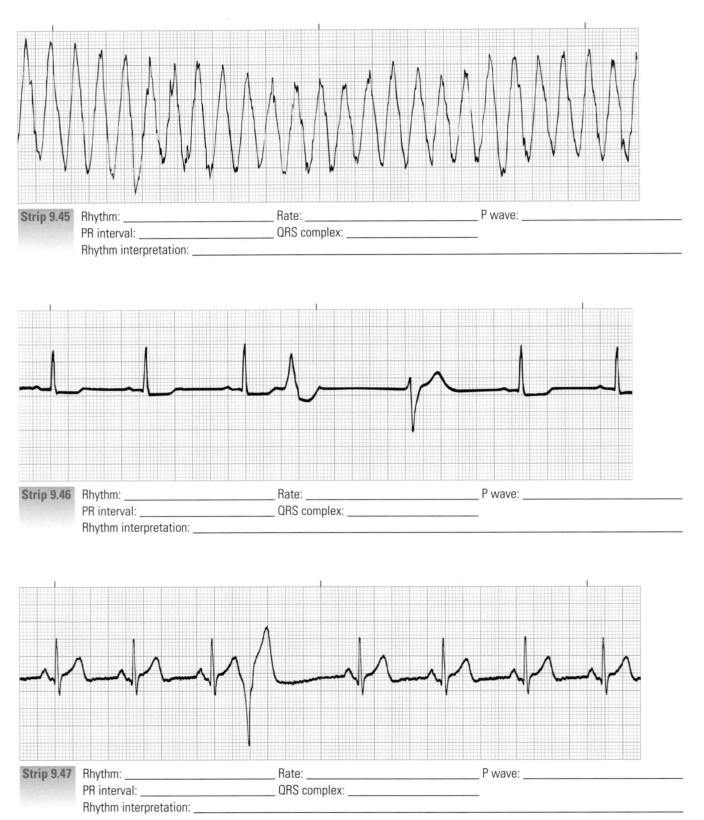

Strip 9.45 Rhythm: _____ Rate: _____ P wave: _____
PR interval: _____ QRS complex: _____
Rhythm interpretation: _____

Strip 9.46 Rhythm: _____ Rate: _____ P wave: _____
PR interval: _____ QRS complex: _____
Rhythm interpretation: _____

Strip 9.47 Rhythm: _____ Rate: _____ P wave: _____
PR interval: _____ QRS complex: _____
Rhythm interpretation: _____

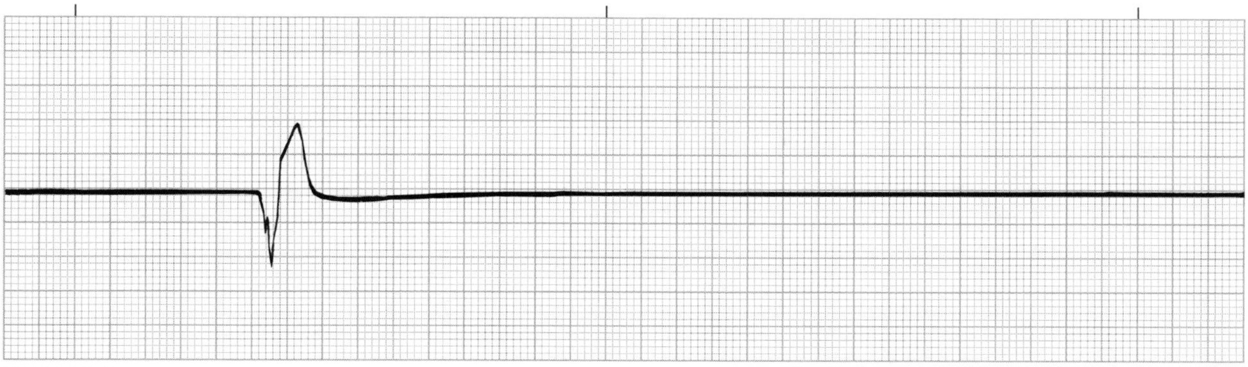

Strip 9.48 Rhythm: _____ Rate: _____ P wave: _____

PR interval: _____ QRS complex: _____

Rhythm interpretation: _____

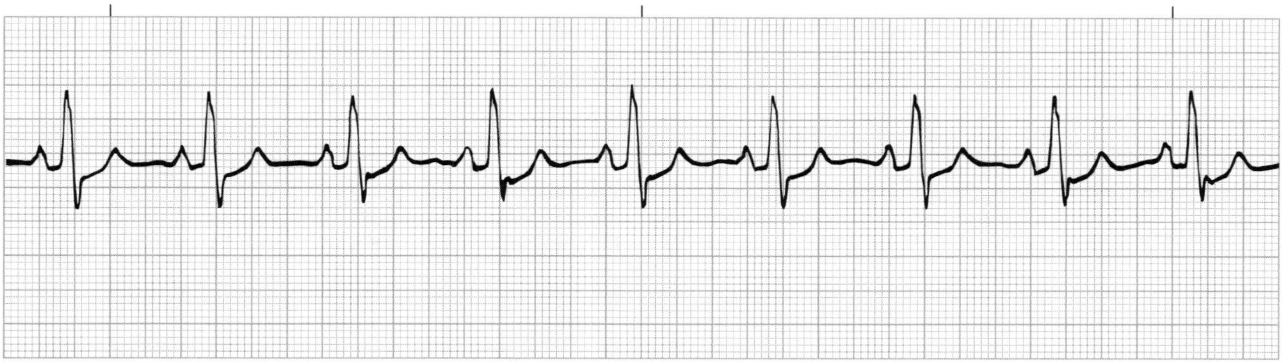

Strip 9.49 Rhythm: _____ Rate: _____ P wave: _____

PR interval: _____ QRS complex: _____

Rhythm interpretation: _____

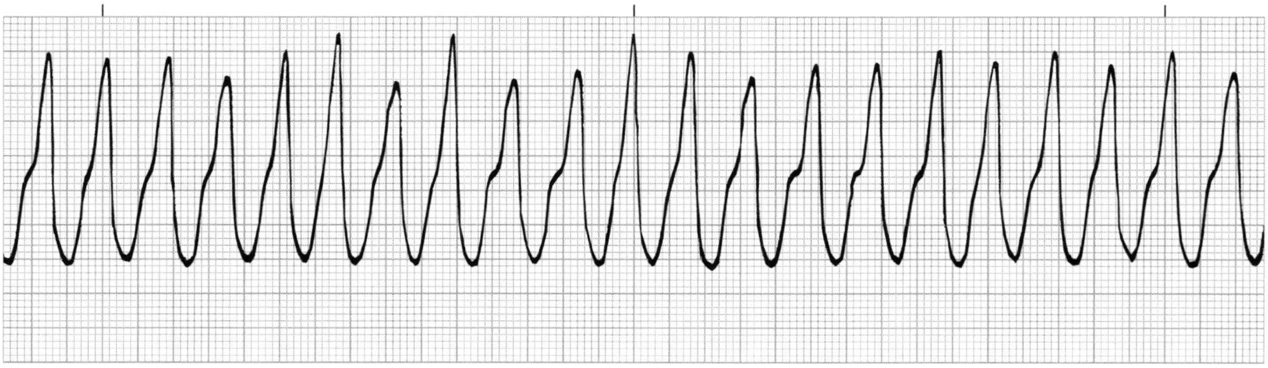

Strip 9.50 Rhythm: _____ Rate: _____ P wave: _____

PR interval: _____ QRS complex: _____

Rhythm interpretation: _____

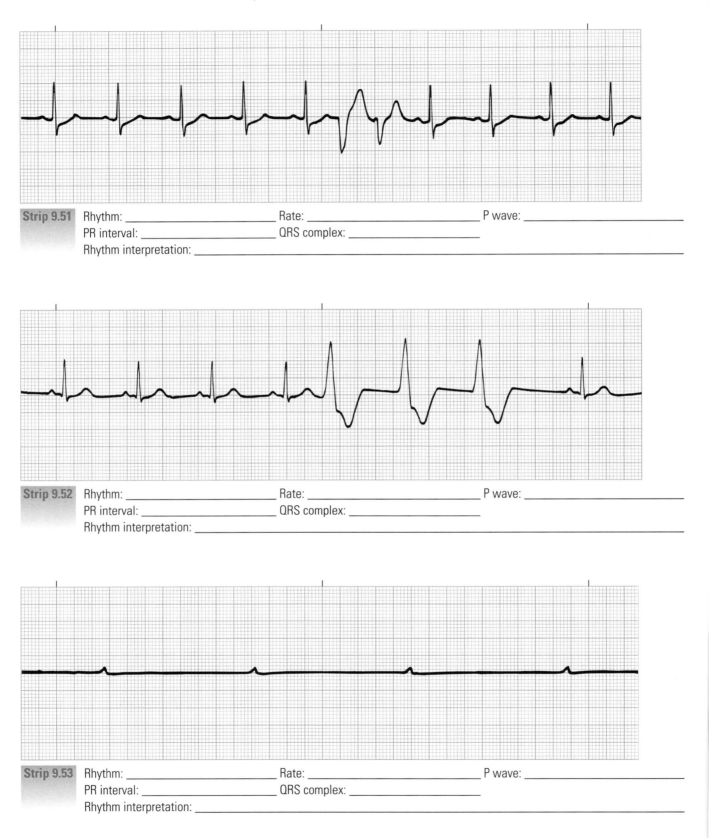

Strip 9.51 Rhythm: _____ Rate: _____ P wave: _____
PR interval: _____ QRS complex: _____
Rhythm interpretation: _____

Strip 9.52 Rhythm: _____ Rate: _____ P wave: _____
PR interval: _____ QRS complex: _____
Rhythm interpretation: _____

Strip 9.53 Rhythm: _____ Rate: _____ P wave: _____
PR interval: _____ QRS complex: _____
Rhythm interpretation: _____

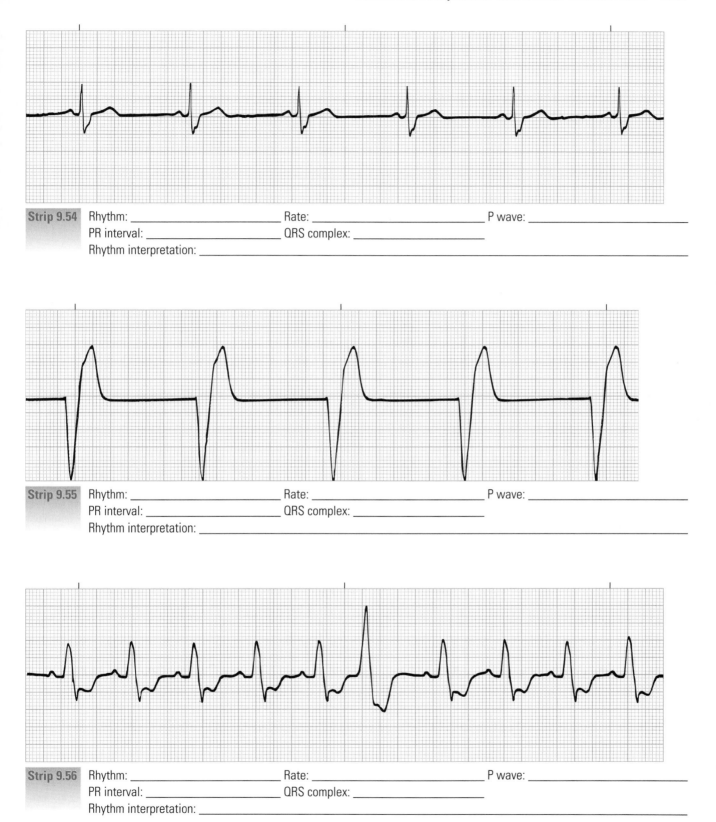

Strip 9.54 Rhythm: _____ Rate: _____ P wave: _____
PR interval: _____ QRS complex: _____
Rhythm interpretation: _____

Strip 9.55 Rhythm: _____ Rate: _____ P wave: _____
PR interval: _____ QRS complex: _____
Rhythm interpretation: _____

Strip 9.56 Rhythm: _____ Rate: _____ P wave: _____
PR interval: _____ QRS complex: _____
Rhythm interpretation: _____

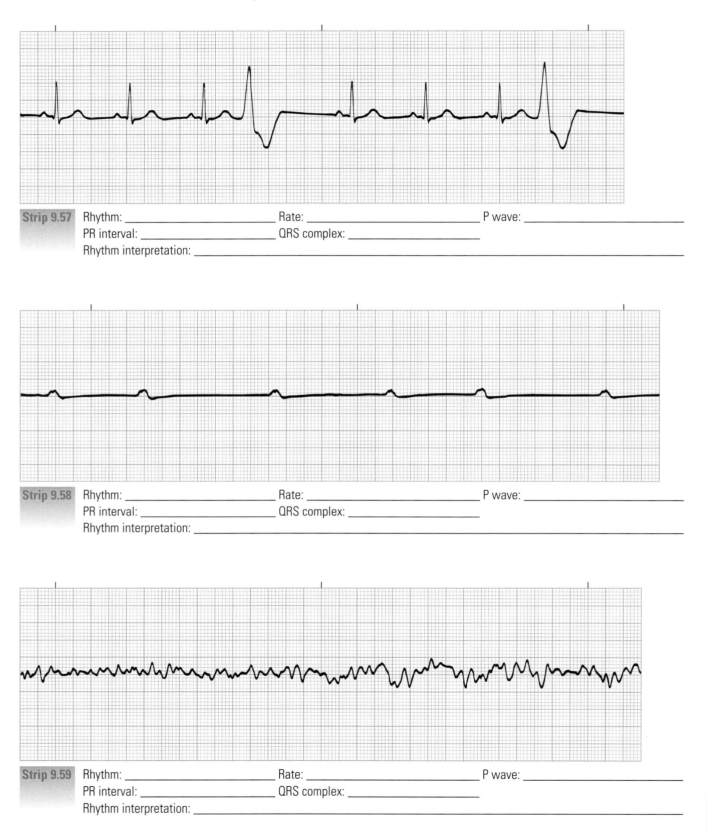

Strip 9.57 Rhythm: _____ Rate: _____ P wave: _____
PR interval: _____ QRS complex: _____
Rhythm interpretation: _____

Strip 9.58 Rhythm: _____ Rate: _____ P wave: _____
PR interval: _____ QRS complex: _____
Rhythm interpretation: _____

Strip 9.59 Rhythm: _____ Rate: _____ P wave: _____
PR interval: _____ QRS complex: _____
Rhythm interpretation: _____

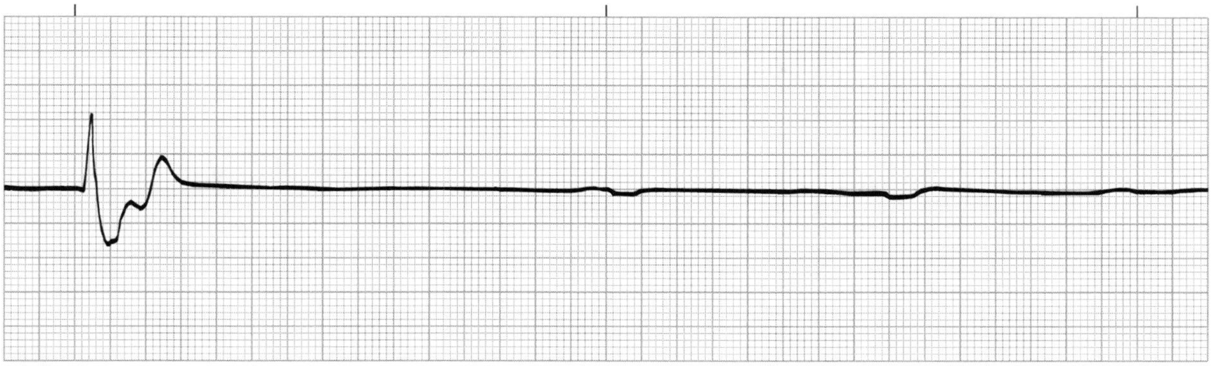

Strip 9.60 Rhythm: _____ Rate: _____ P wave: _____
PR interval: _____ QRS complex: _____
Rhythm interpretation: _____

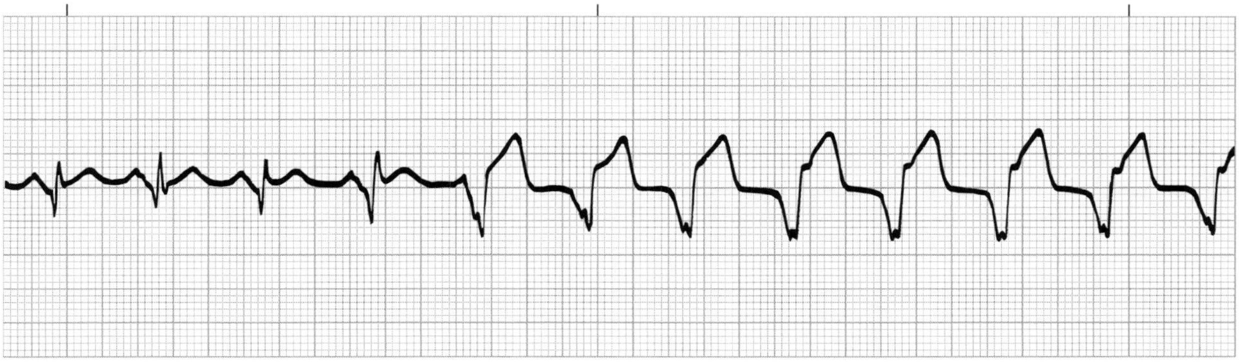

Strip 9.61 Rhythm: _____ Rate: _____ P wave: _____
PR interval: _____ QRS complex: _____
Rhythm interpretation: _____

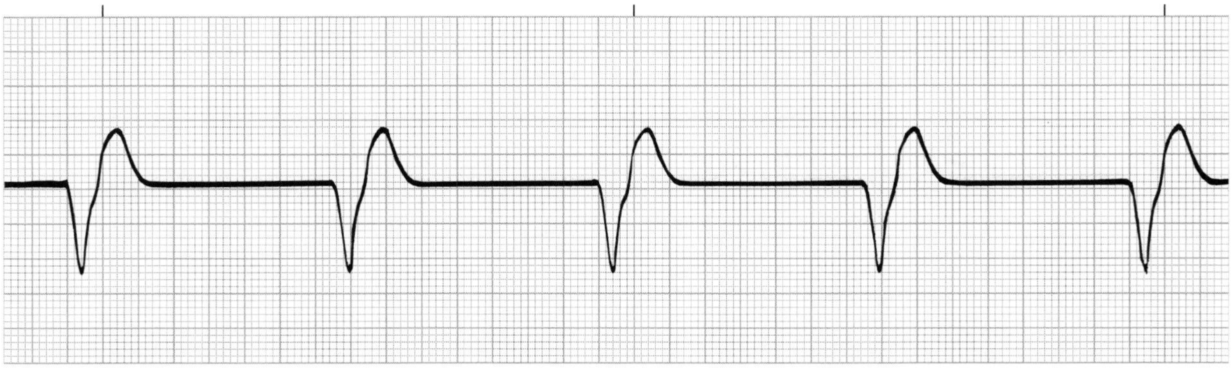

Strip 9.62 Rhythm: _____ Rate: _____ P wave: _____
PR interval: _____ QRS complex: _____
Rhythm interpretation: _____

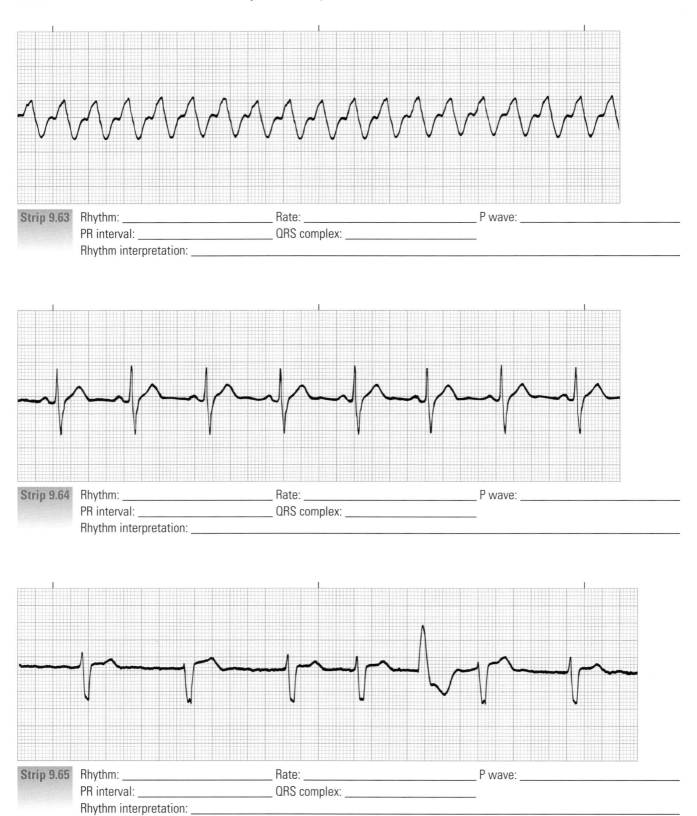

Strip 9.63 Rhythm: _____ Rate: _____ P wave: _____

PR interval: _____ QRS complex: _____

Rhythm interpretation: _____

Strip 9.64 Rhythm: _____ Rate: _____ P wave: _____

PR interval: _____ QRS complex: _____

Rhythm interpretation: _____

Strip 9.65 Rhythm: _____ Rate: _____ P wave: _____

PR interval: _____ QRS complex: _____

Rhythm interpretation: _____

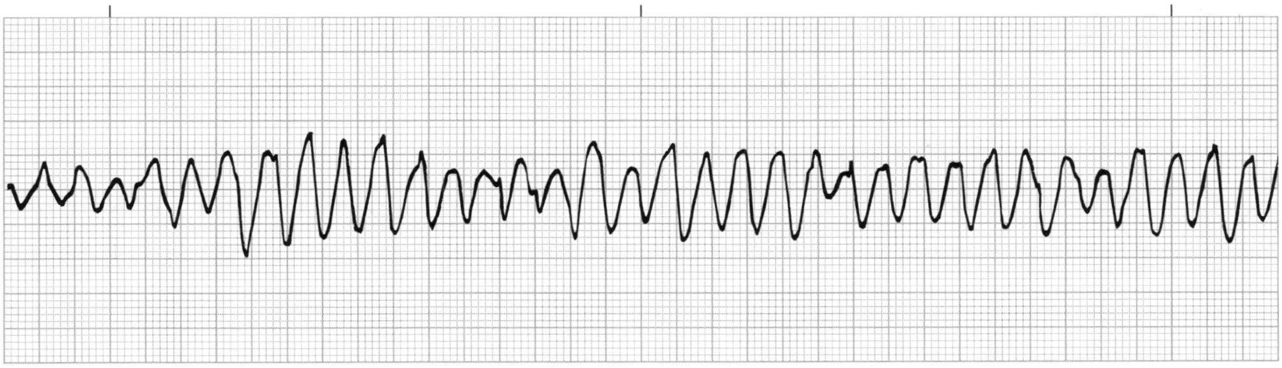

Strip 9.66 Rhythm: _____ Rate: _____ P wave: _____
PR interval: _____ QRS complex: _____
Rhythm interpretation: _____

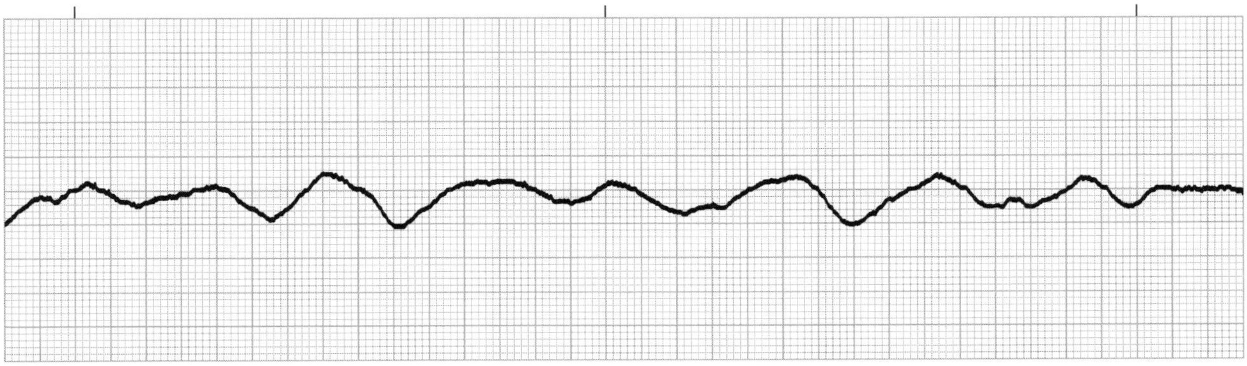

Strip 9.67 Rhythm: _____ Rate: _____ P wave: _____
PR interval: _____ QRS complex: _____
Rhythm interpretation: _____

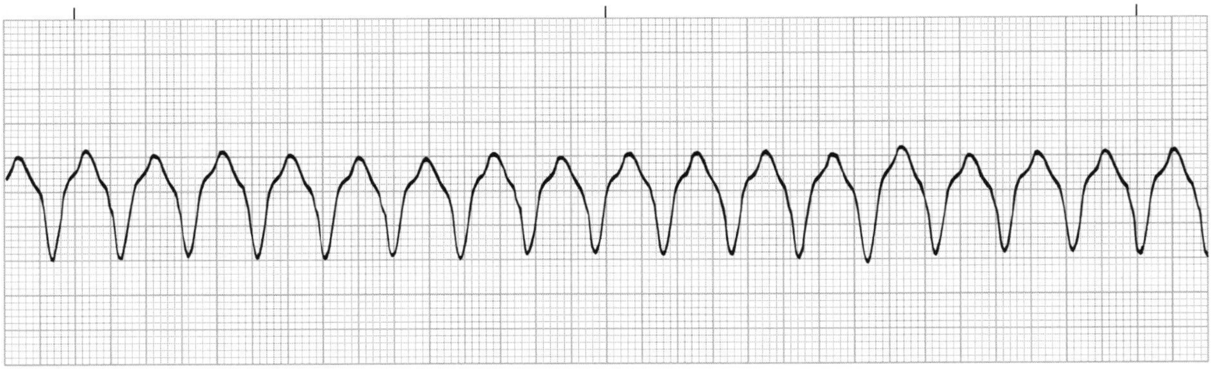

Strip 9.68 Rhythm: _____ Rate: _____ P wave: _____
PR interval: _____ QRS complex: _____
Rhythm interpretation: _____

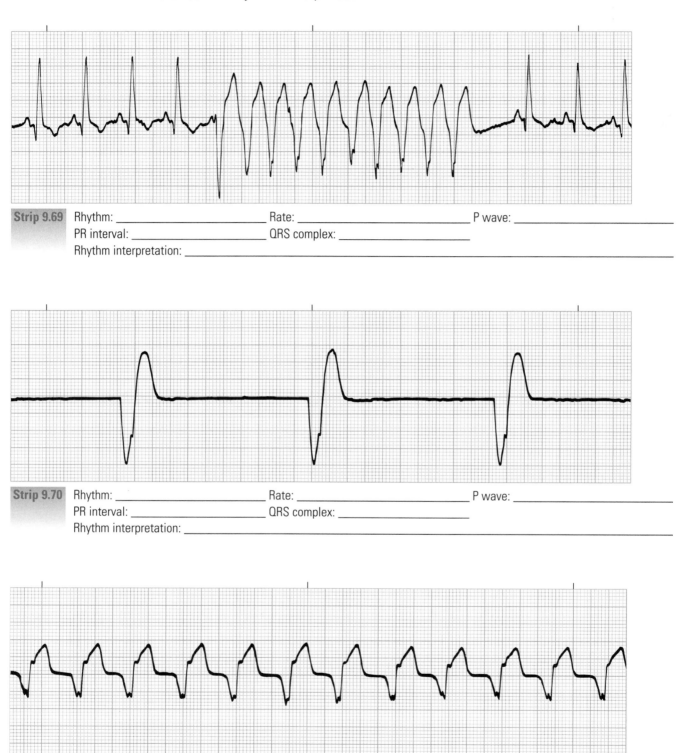

Strip 9.69 Rhythm: _____ Rate: _____ P wave: _____
PR interval: _____ QRS complex: _____
Rhythm interpretation: _____

Strip 9.70 Rhythm: _____ Rate: _____ P wave: _____
PR interval: _____ QRS complex: _____
Rhythm interpretation: _____

Strip 9.71 Rhythm: _____ Rate: _____ P wave: _____
PR interval: _____ QRS complex: _____
Rhythm interpretation: _____

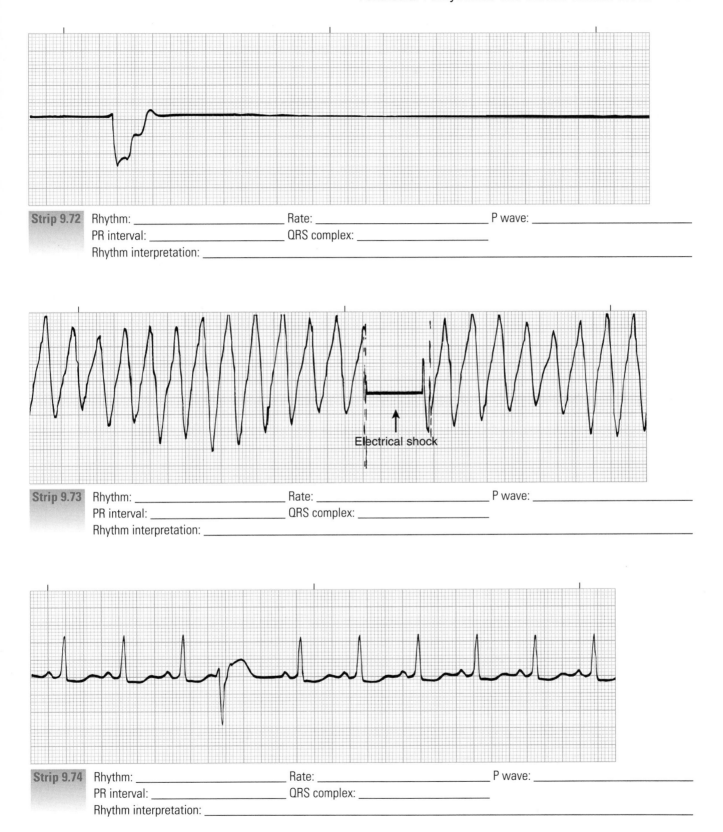

Strip 9.72 Rhythm: _____ Rate: _____ P wave: _____

PR interval: _____ QRS complex: _____

Rhythm interpretation: _____

Electrical shock

Strip 9.73 Rhythm: _____ Rate: _____ P wave: _____

PR interval: _____ QRS complex: _____

Rhythm interpretation: _____

Strip 9.74 Rhythm: _____ Rate: _____ P wave: _____

PR interval: _____ QRS complex: _____

Rhythm interpretation: _____

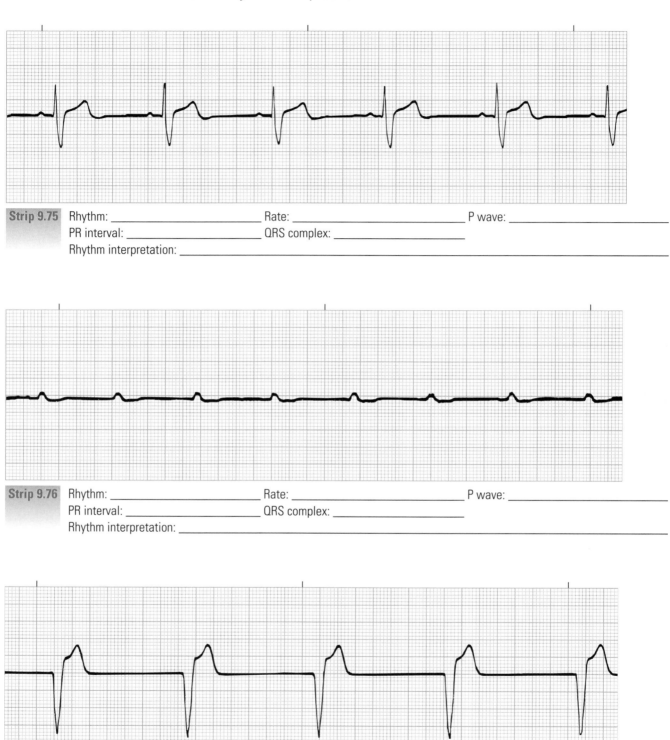

Strip 9.75   Rhythm: _____ Rate: _____ P wave: _____
PR interval: _____ QRS complex: _____
Rhythm interpretation: _____

Strip 9.76   Rhythm: _____ Rate: _____ P wave: _____
PR interval: _____ QRS complex: _____
Rhythm interpretation: _____

Strip 9.77   Rhythm: _____ Rate: _____ P wave: _____
PR interval: _____ QRS complex: _____
Rhythm interpretation: _____

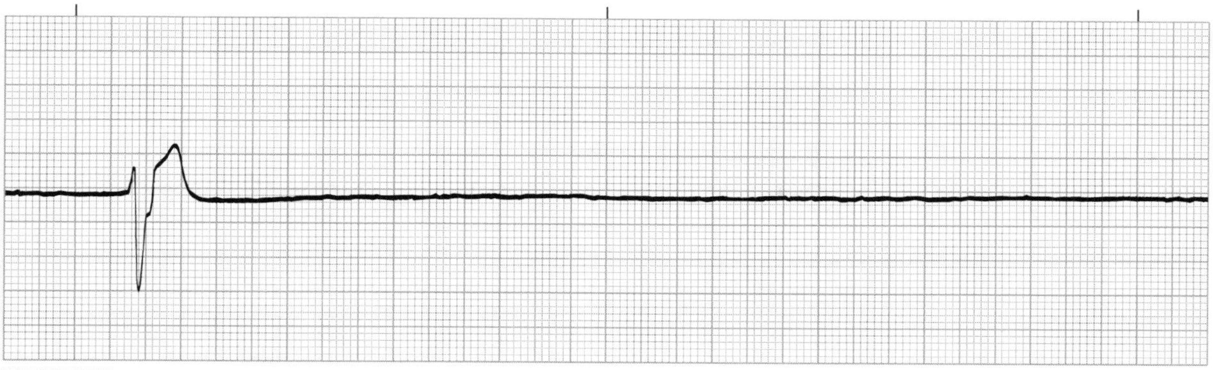

Strip 9.78 Rhythm: _____ Rate: _____ P wave: _____
PR interval: _____ QRS complex: _____
Rhythm interpretation: _____

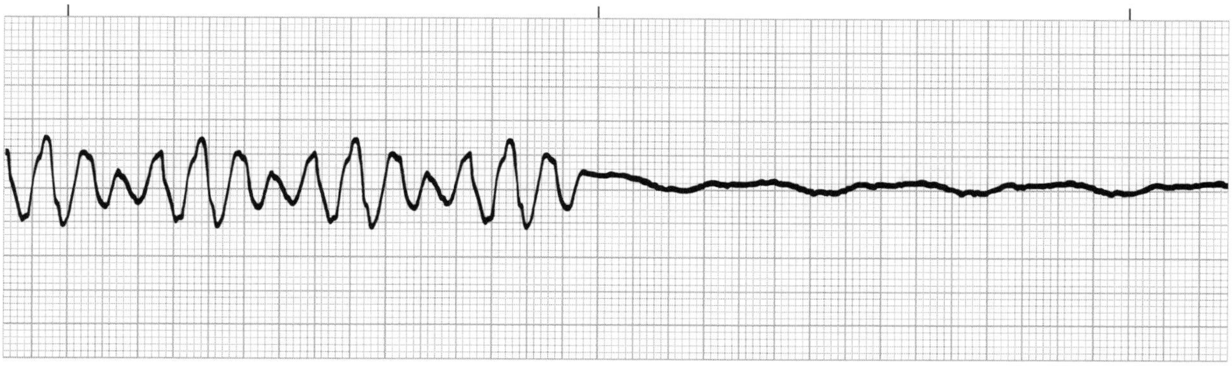

Strip 9.79 Rhythm: _____ Rate: _____ P wave: _____
PR interval: _____ QRS complex: _____
Rhythm interpretation: _____

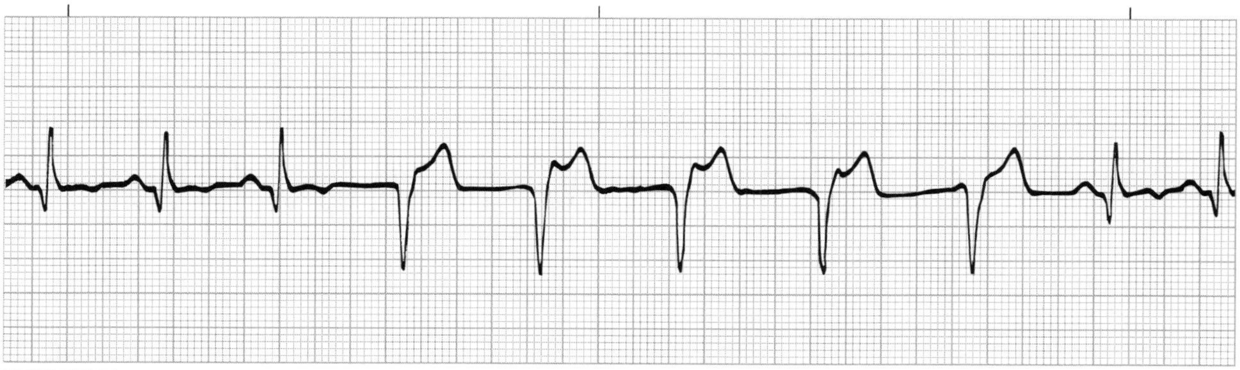

Strip 9.80 Rhythm: _____ Rate: _____ P wave: _____
PR interval: _____ QRS complex: _____
Rhythm interpretation: _____

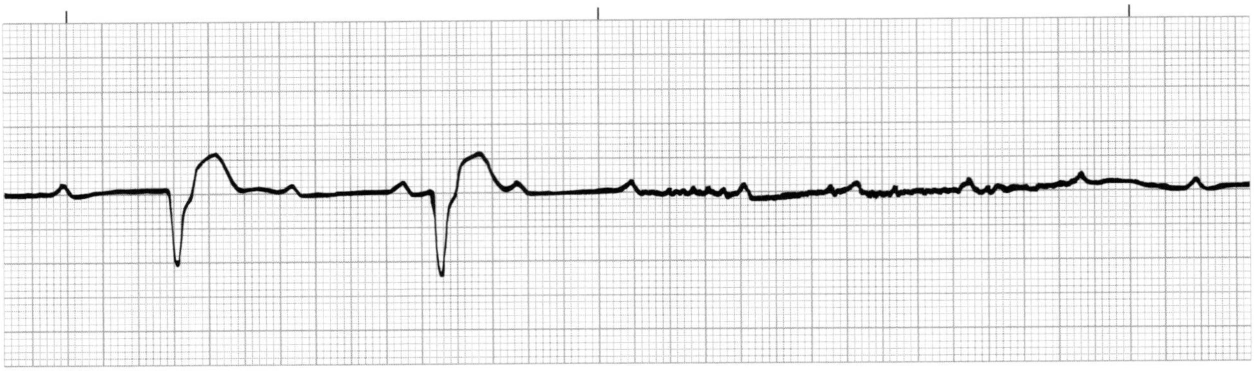

Strip 9.81 Rhythm: _____ Rate: _____ P wave: _____

PR interval: _____ QRS complex: _____

Rhythm interpretation: _____

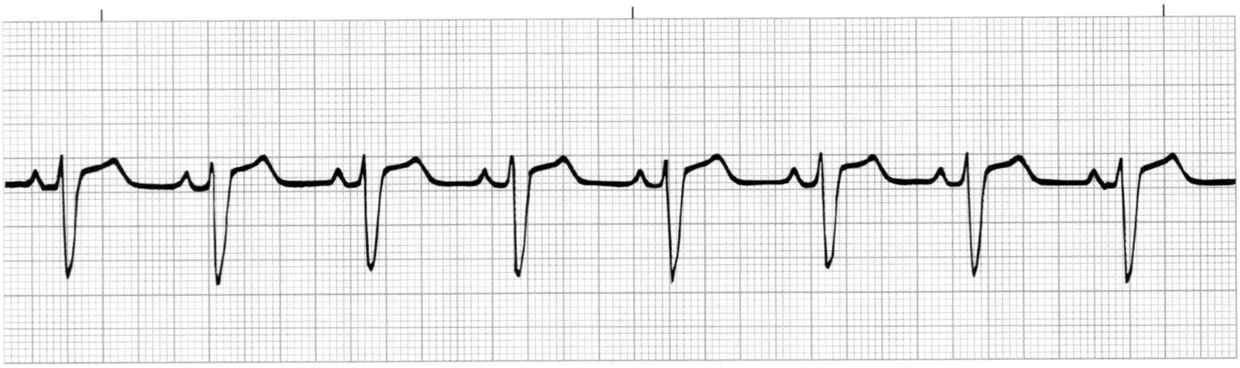

Strip 9.82 Rhythm: _____ Rate: _____ P wave: _____

PR interval: _____ QRS complex: _____

Rhythm interpretation: _____

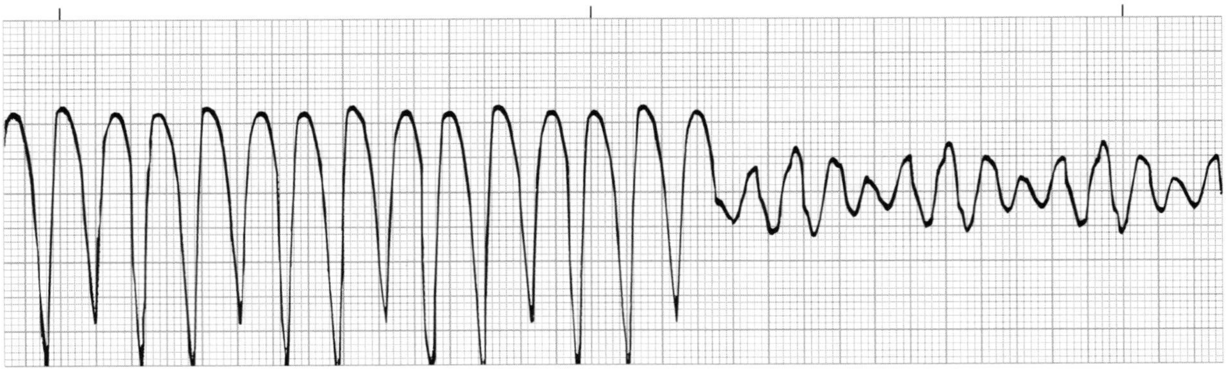

Strip 9.83 Rhythm: _____ Rate: _____ P wave: _____

PR interval: _____ QRS complex: _____

Rhythm interpretation: _____

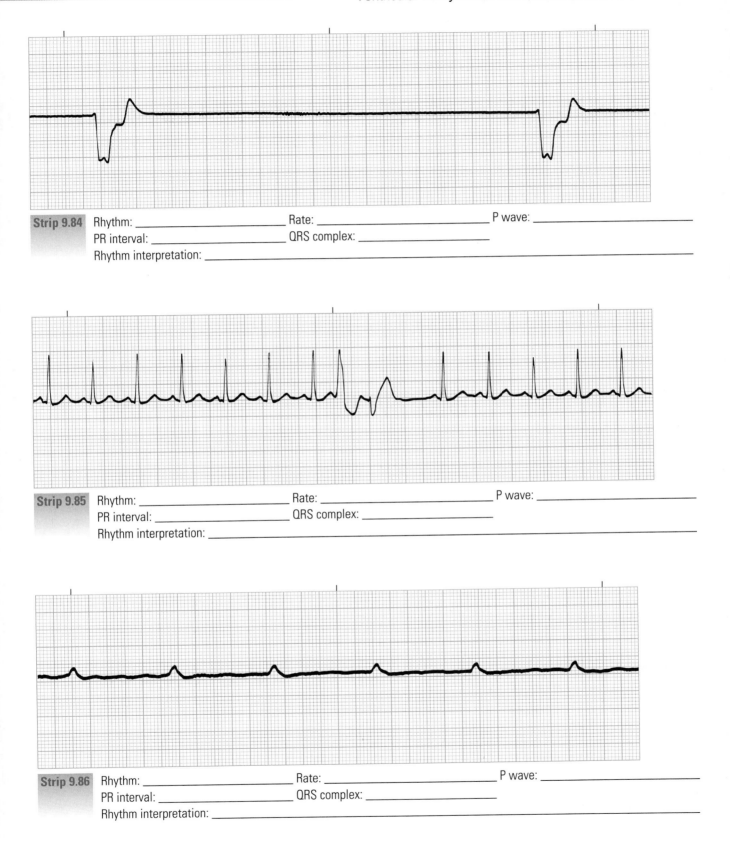

Strip 9.84 Rhythm: _____ Rate: _____ P wave: _____
PR interval: _____ QRS complex: _____
Rhythm interpretation: _____

Strip 9.85 Rhythm: _____ Rate: _____ P wave: _____
PR interval: _____ QRS complex: _____
Rhythm interpretation: _____

Strip 9.86 Rhythm: _____ Rate: _____ P wave: _____
PR interval: _____ QRS complex: _____
Rhythm interpretation: _____

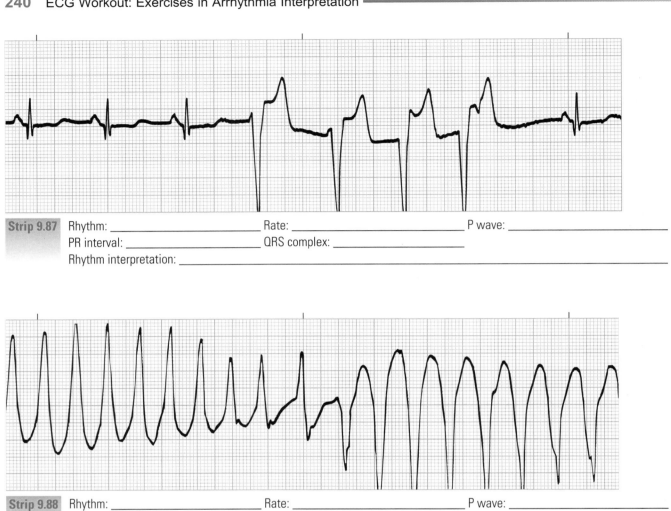

Strip 9.87 Rhythm: _____ Rate: _____ P wave: _____
PR interval: _____ QRS complex: _____
Rhythm interpretation: _____

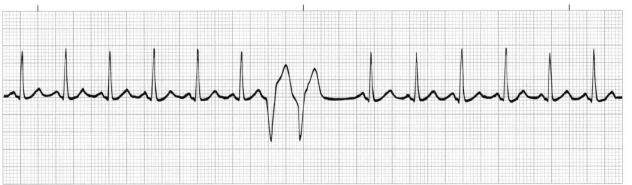

Strip 9.88 Rhythm: _____ Rate: _____ P wave: _____
PR interval: _____ QRS complex: _____
Rhythm interpretation: _____

Strip 9.89 Rhythm: _____ Rate: _____ P wave: _____
PR interval: _____ QRS complex: _____
Rhythm interpretation: _____

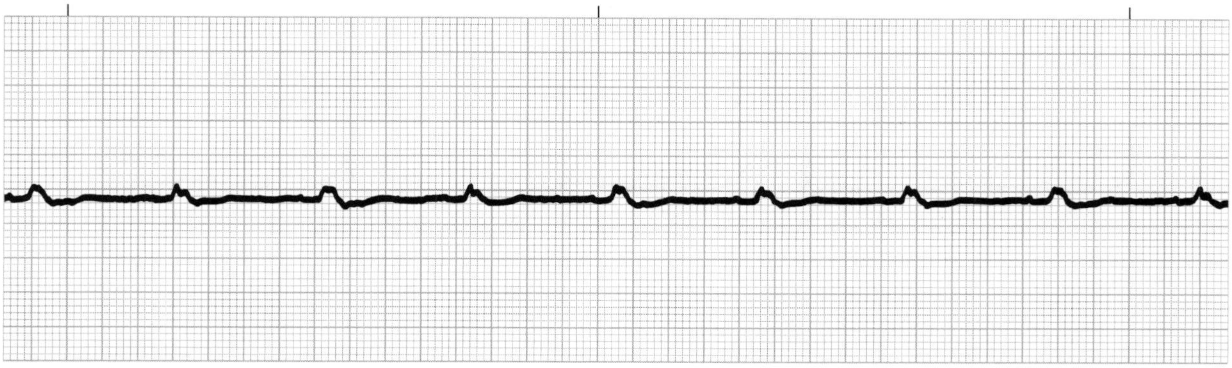

Strip 9.90 Rhythm: _____ Rate: _____ P wave: _____

PR interval: _____ QRS complex: _____

Rhythm interpretation: _____

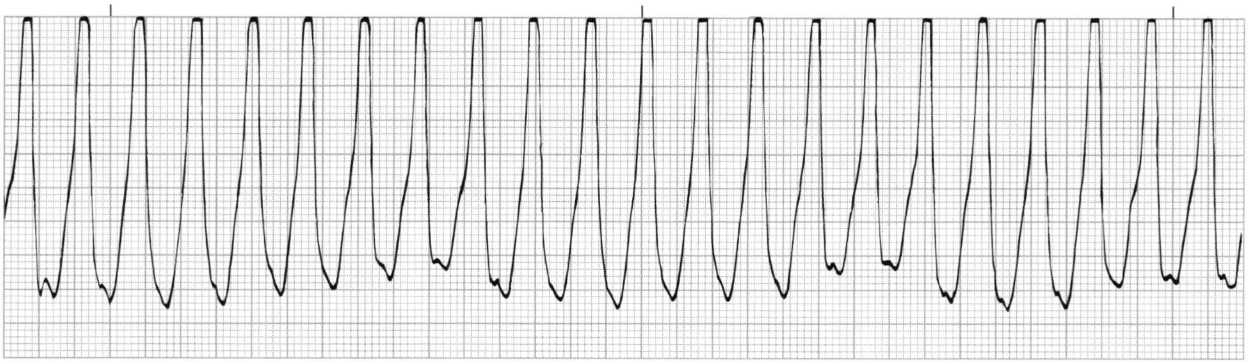

Strip 9.91 Rhythm: _____ Rate: _____ P wave: _____

PR interval: _____ QRS complex: _____

Rhythm interpretation: _____

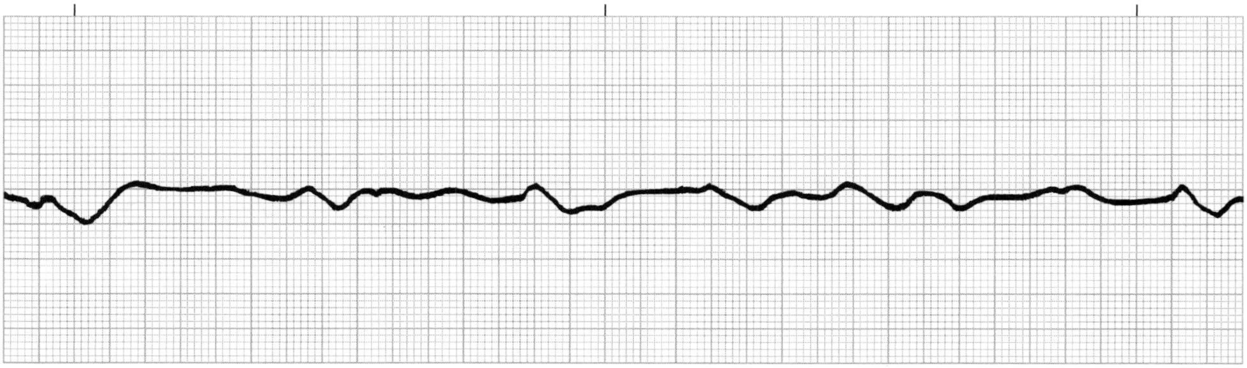

Strip 9.92 Rhythm: _____ Rate: _____ P wave: _____

PR interval: _____ QRS complex: _____

Rhythm interpretation: _____

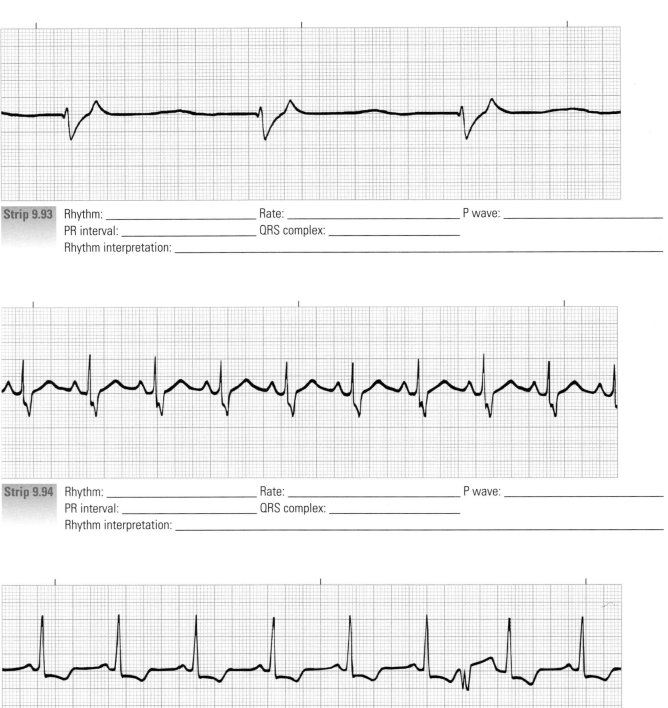

Strip 9.93   Rhythm: _____ Rate: _____ P wave: _____
PR interval: _____ QRS complex: _____
Rhythm interpretation: _____

Strip 9.94   Rhythm: _____ Rate: _____ P wave: _____
PR interval: _____ QRS complex: _____
Rhythm interpretation: _____

Strip 9.95   Rhythm: _____ Rate: _____ P wave: _____
PR interval: _____ QRS complex: _____
Rhythm interpretation: _____

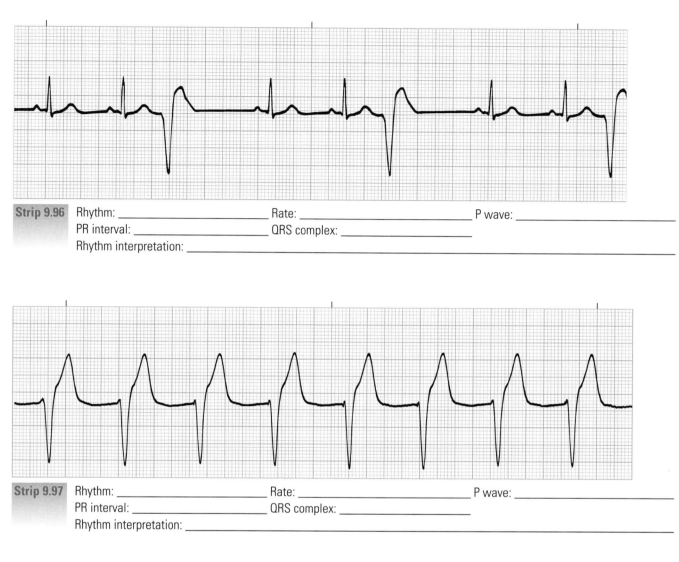

Strip 9.96 Rhythm: _____ Rate: _____ P wave: _____
PR interval: _____ QRS complex: _____
Rhythm interpretation: _____

Strip 9.97 Rhythm: _____ Rate: _____ P wave: _____
PR interval: _____ QRS complex: _____
Rhythm interpretation: _____

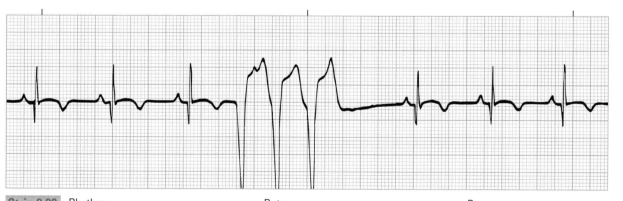

Strip 9.98 Rhythm: _____ Rate: _____ P wave: _____
PR interval: _____ QRS complex: _____
Rhythm interpretation: _____

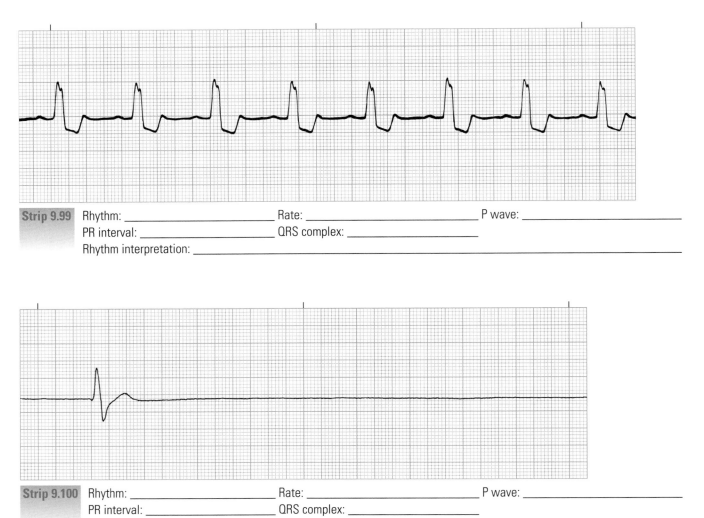

Strip 9.99 Rhythm: _____ Rate: _____ P wave: _____
PR interval: _____ QRS complex: _____
Rhythm interpretation: _____

Strip 9.100 Rhythm: _____ Rate: _____ P wave: _____
PR interval: _____ QRS complex: _____
Rhythm interpretation: _____

SKILLBUILDER PRACTICE

This section contains *mixed sinus*, *atrial*, and *junctional* and *AV block* and *ventricular rhythm strips*, allowing the student to practice differentiating between *four* rhythm groups before progressing to the posttest. As before, analyze the rhythm strips using the five-step process. Interpret the rhythm by comparing the data collected with the ECG characteristics for each rhythm. All strips are lead II, a positive lead, unless otherwise noted. Check your answers with the answer key in the appendix.

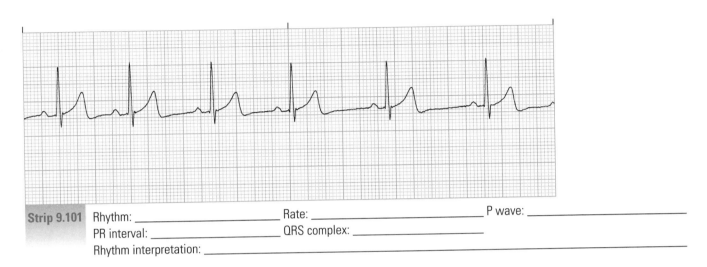

Strip 9.101	Rhythm: _____	Rate: _____	P wave: _____
	PR interval: _____	QRS complex: _____	
	Rhythm interpretation: _____		

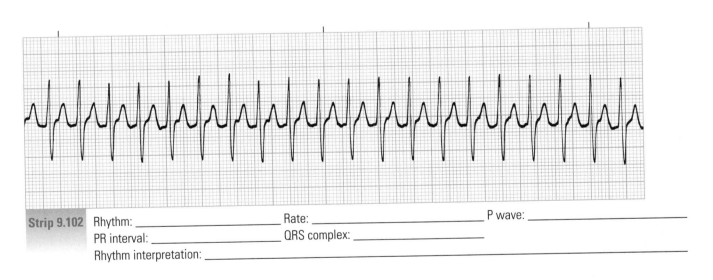

Strip 9.102	Rhythm: _____	Rate: _____	P wave: _____
	PR interval: _____	QRS complex: _____	
	Rhythm interpretation: _____		

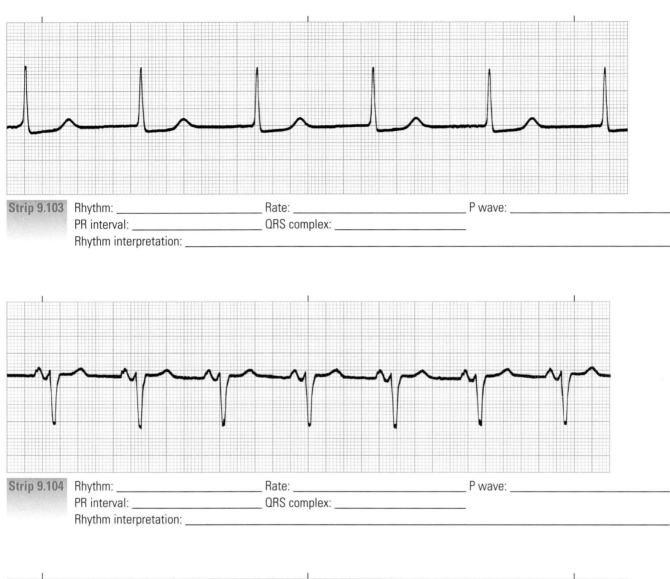

Strip 9.103 Rhythm: _____ Rate: _____ P wave: _____
PR interval: _____ QRS complex: _____
Rhythm interpretation: _____

Strip 9.104 Rhythm: _____ Rate: _____ P wave: _____
PR interval: _____ QRS complex: _____
Rhythm interpretation: _____

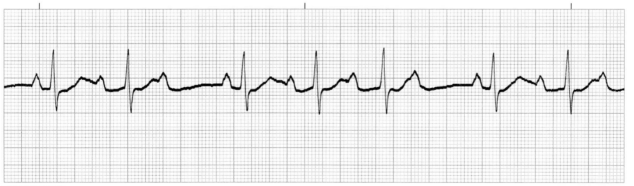

Strip 9.105 Rhythm: _____ Rate: _____ P wave: _____
PR interval: _____ QRS complex: _____
Rhythm interpretation: _____

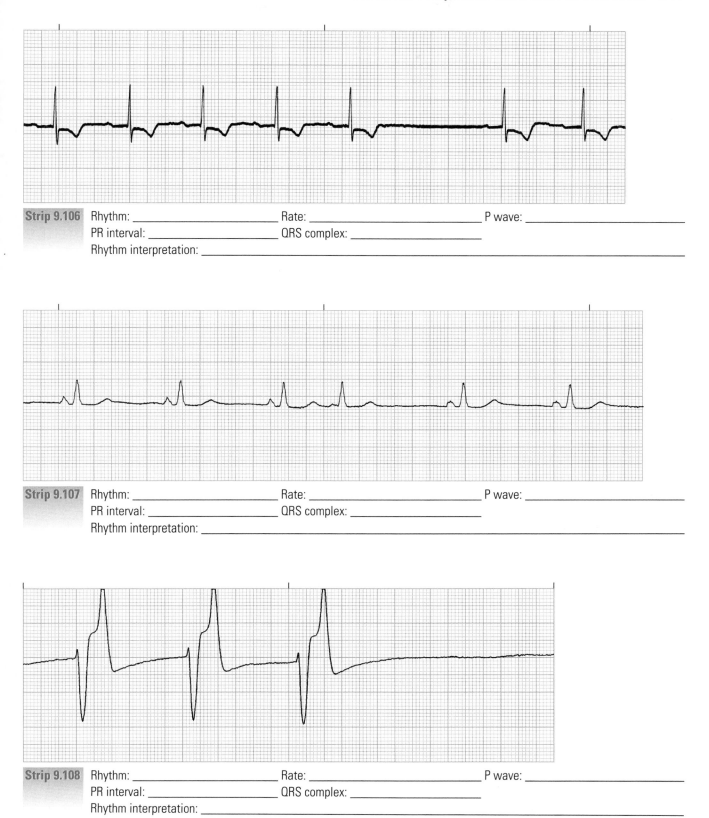

Strip 9.106 Rhythm: _____ Rate: _____ P wave: _____
PR interval: _____ QRS complex: _____
Rhythm interpretation: _____

Strip 9.107 Rhythm: _____ Rate: _____ P wave: _____
PR interval: _____ QRS complex: _____
Rhythm interpretation: _____

Strip 9.108 Rhythm: _____ Rate: _____ P wave: _____
PR interval: _____ QRS complex: _____
Rhythm interpretation: _____

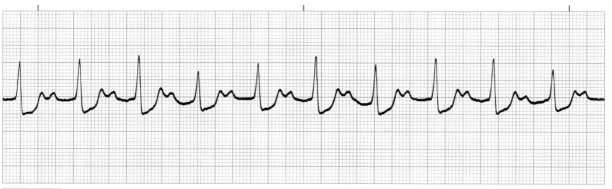

Strip 9.109   Rhythm: _____ Rate: _____ P wave: _____

PR interval: _____ QRS complex: _____

Rhythm interpretation: _____

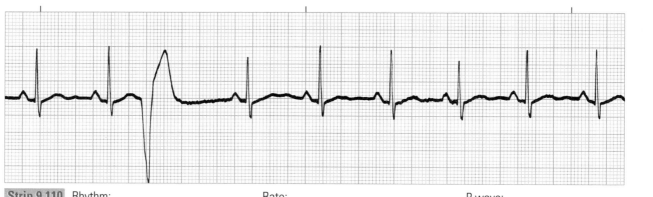

Strip 9.110   Rhythm: _____ Rate: _____ P wave: _____

PR interval: _____ QRS complex: _____

Rhythm interpretation: _____

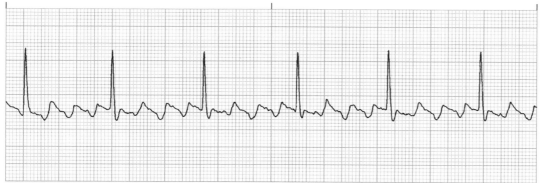

Strip 9.111   Rhythm: _____ Rate: _____ P wave: _____

PR interval: _____ QRS complex: _____

Rhythm interpretation: _____

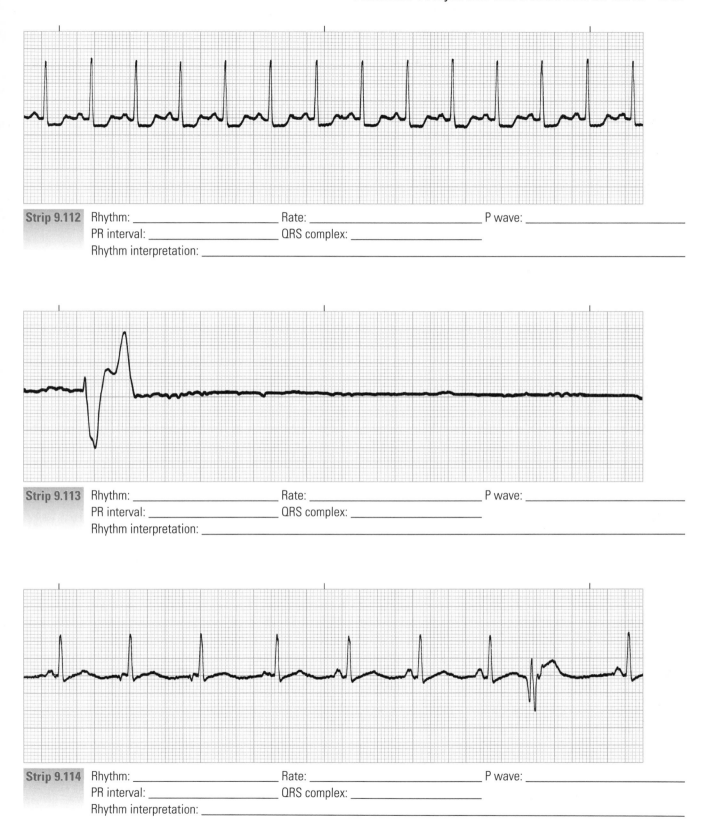

Strip 9.112 Rhythm: _____ Rate: _____ P wave: _____
PR interval: _____ QRS complex: _____
Rhythm interpretation: _____

Strip 9.113 Rhythm: _____ Rate: _____ P wave: _____
PR interval: _____ QRS complex: _____
Rhythm interpretation: _____

Strip 9.114 Rhythm: _____ Rate: _____ P wave: _____
PR interval: _____ QRS complex: _____
Rhythm interpretation: _____

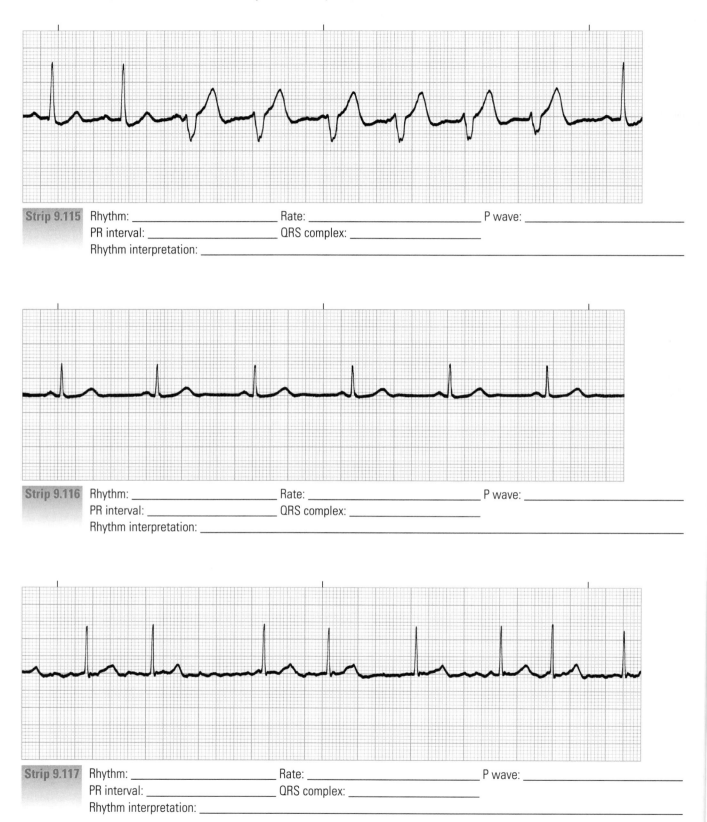

Strip 9.115   Rhythm: _____ Rate: _____ P wave: _____
PR interval: _____ QRS complex: _____
Rhythm interpretation: _____

Strip 9.116   Rhythm: _____ Rate: _____ P wave: _____
PR interval: _____ QRS complex: _____
Rhythm interpretation: _____

Strip 9.117   Rhythm: _____ Rate: _____ P wave: _____
PR interval: _____ QRS complex: _____
Rhythm interpretation: _____

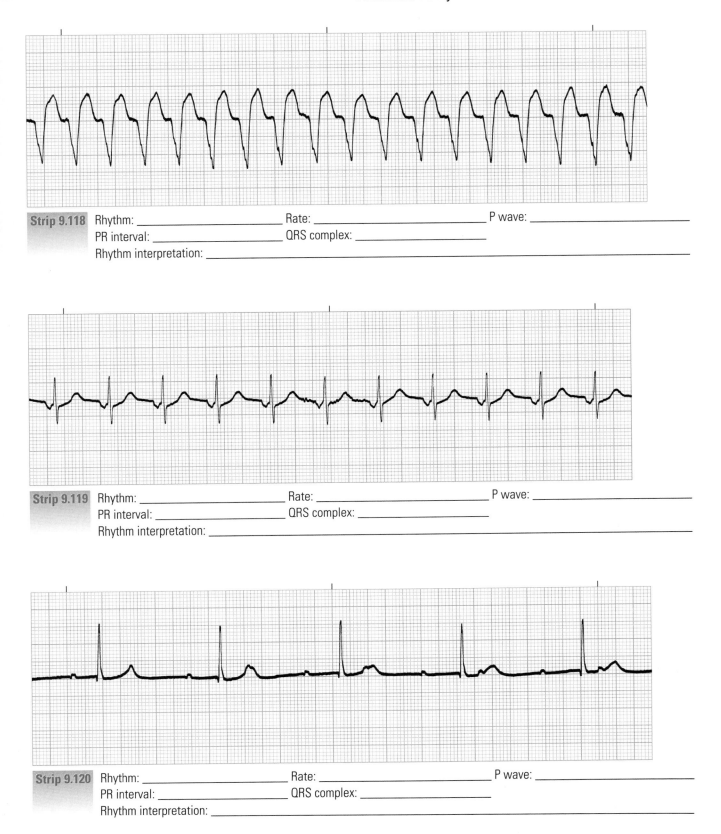

Strip 9.118   Rhythm: _____ Rate: _____ P wave: _____
PR interval: _____ QRS complex: _____
Rhythm interpretation: _____

Strip 9.119   Rhythm: _____ Rate: _____ P wave: _____
PR interval: _____ QRS complex: _____
Rhythm interpretation: _____

Strip 9.120   Rhythm: _____ Rate: _____ P wave: _____
PR interval: _____ QRS complex: _____
Rhythm interpretation: _____

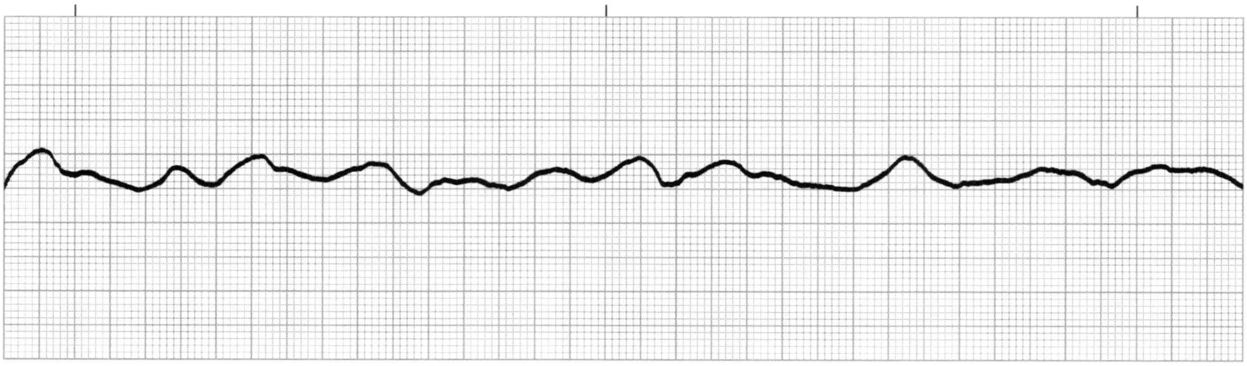

Strip 9.121 Rhythm: _____ Rate: _____ P wave: _____
PR interval: _____ QRS complex: _____
Rhythm interpretation: _____

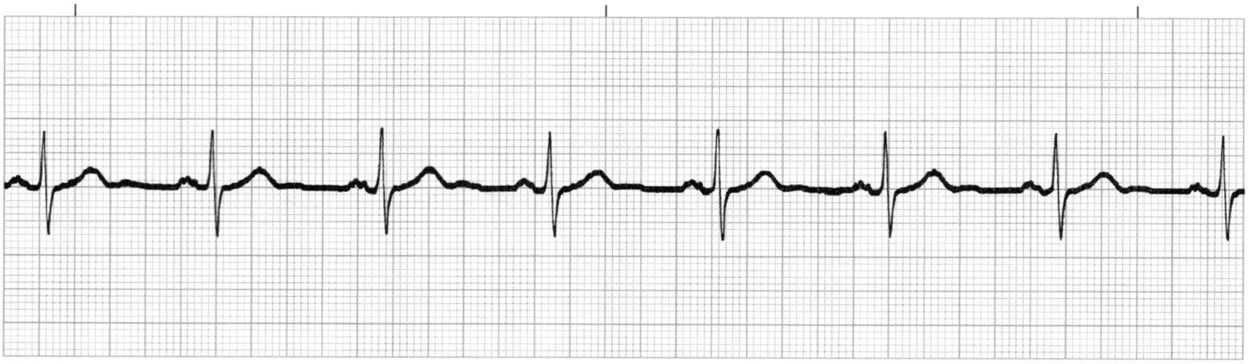

Strip 9.122 Rhythm: _____ Rate: _____ P wave: _____
PR interval: _____ QRS complex: _____
Rhythm interpretation: _____

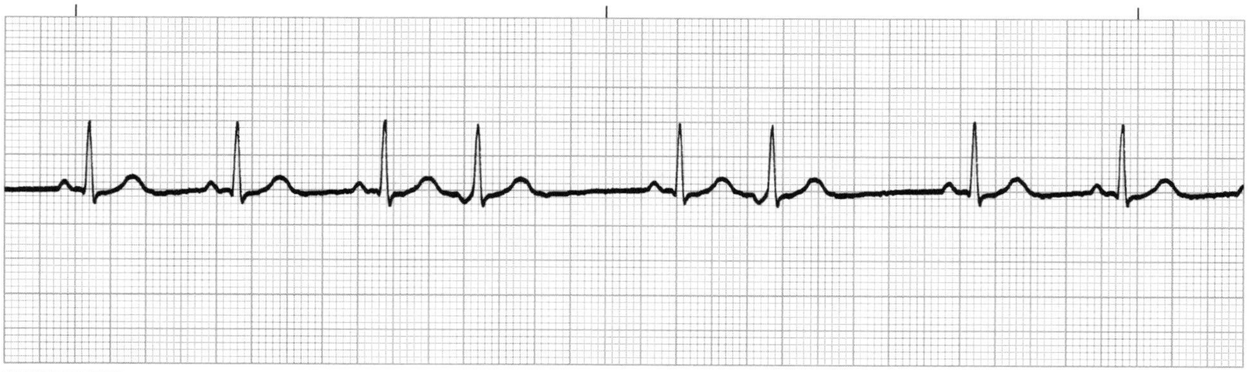

Strip 9.123 Rhythm: _____ Rate: _____ P wave: _____
PR interval: _____ QRS complex: _____
Rhythm interpretation: _____

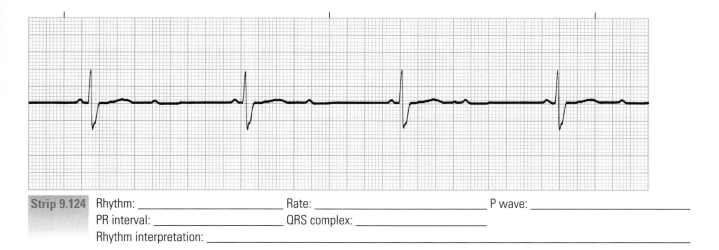

Strip 9.124   Rhythm: _____ Rate: _____ P wave: _____

PR interval: _____ QRS complex: _____

Rhythm interpretation: _____

Pacemakers

ten

Overview

An artificial pacemaker is an electronic device that generates and transmits an electrical stimulus to the atria, the ventricles, or both, resulting in depolarization, followed by muscle contraction. The use of artificial pacemakers may be necessitated when there is a significant malfunction of the heart's electrical system, usually involving the sinus node, the atria, or the atrioventricular (AV) conduction pathways. The result may be a slow, fast, or irregular rhythm, which can affect the heart's pumping ability and may lead to a decrease in cardiac output and in the quality of life. Some indications for pacing include the following:

- **Sinoatrial dysfunction**
  1. Sinus bradycardia
  2. Sinus arrest
  3. Sinus exit block
  4. Atrial flutter or fibrillation
  5. Sick sinus syndrome (rhythms in which there is marked bradycardia alternating with periods of tachycardia, especially atrial fibrillation; also called tachycardia-bradycardia syndrome)
  6. Chronotropic incompetence (sinus node is not capable of increasing its rate in response to activity)
- **AV block**
  1. Second-degree AV block, Mobitz II
  2. Third-degree AV block
- **Hypersensitive carotid sinus**—Stimulation of the carotid sinus that causes episodes of asystole resulting in recurrent syncope; turning the head from side to side or wearing a tight necktie or collar can stimulate the carotid sinus.

Pacemakers may be inserted on a temporary or permanent basis depending on the clinical situation. Temporary pacing is appropriate in emergent situations (symptomatic bradycardia or AV block associated with acute myocardial infarction, myocardial ischemia, or drug toxicity). Temporary pacing may also be used to provide prophylactic therapy for high-risk patients during cardiac catheterization or during and after cardiac surgery. Permanent pacemaker implantation is considered for unresolved rhythms or conditions in which clinical symptoms are present and for which long-term pacing is indicated.

A pacemaker system (Figure 10.1) consists of a pulse generator and a pacing lead:

- **Pulse generator**—The pulse generator houses a battery, a lead connector, electronic circuitry for pacemaker settings, and other components that generate and/or interpret impulses.
- **Pacing lead**—The pacing lead has one or two metal poles (electrodes) at the tip of the catheter that come in contact with the endocardium. A lead with only one electrode at its tip is called a unipolar pacing system. A lead with two electrodes at its tip is called a bipolar pacing system. The pacing lead serves as a transmission line between the pulse generator and the endocardium. Electrical impulses are transmitted from the pulse generator (through the pacing lead) to the endocardium, while information about electrical activity inside the heart is relayed from the electrode tip (through the pacing lead) back to the generator. If the generator responds by sending a pacing impulse to the heart, it is called triggering. If a pacing impulse is not sent to the heart, this is called inhibition. Many permanent leads are constructed with fixation devices (screws, tines, or barbs) that help guarantee long-term contact with the endocardium. Temporary pacing leads are not constructed with fixation devices so they can easily be removed when pacing is no longer required.

Pacemakers can function in a fixed-rate mode or a demand mode:

- **Fixed-rate mode (asynchronous)**—Fixed-rate pacemakers are designed to fire constantly at a preset rate without regard to the heart's electrical activity. This mode of pacing is known as asynchronous pacing because it's not synchronized to sense the patient's own rhythm. This may result in competition between the patient's natural (intrinsic) rhythm and that produced by the pacemaker. Ventricular tachycardia or ventricular fibrillation may be induced if the pacing stimulus falls during the vulnerable period of the cardiac cycle. The first pacemakers on the market were fixed rate and are uncommon today, although all pacemakers can be placed into a fixed-rate mode.
- **Demand mode (synchronous)**—Modern pacemakers are demand pacemakers. A demand pacemaker paces only when the heart fails to depolarize on its own (fires only "on demand"). Demand pacemakers are designed with a sensing mechanism that inhibits discharge when the patient's heart rate is adequate and a pacing mechanism that triggers the pacemaker to fire when no intrinsic activity occurs within a preset period. This mode of pacing is called synchronous pacing because it is synchronized to sense the patient's cardiac rhythm.

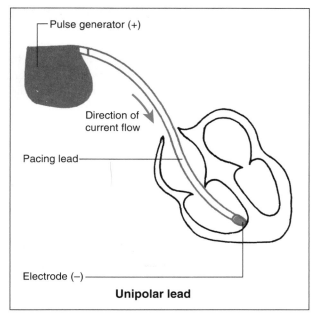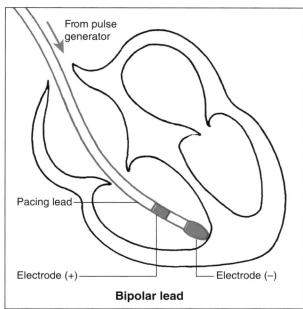

Figure 10.1 Pulse generator and pacing leads.

A pacemaker system may be single chamber or dual chamber:

- **Single chamber**—A single-chamber pacemaker system uses one lead inserted into either the right atrium or the right ventricle. This pacemaker can sense and pace only the chamber into which it is inserted.

  If a single-chamber atrial pacemaker senses a P wave, the pacemaker is inhibited from firing an electrical stimulus. If it does not sense a P wave, the pacemaker sends an electrical stimulus to the atrium. Stimulation of the atrium produces a *pacemaker spike* (a vertical line on the ECG), followed by a P wave (Figure 10.2A).

  If a single-chamber ventricular pacemaker senses a QRS complex, the pacemaker is inhibited from firing an electrical

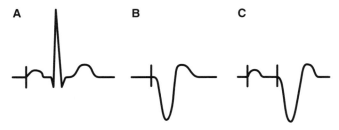

Figure 10.2 Single-chamber and dual-chamber pacing examples. **A.** The single-chamber atrial pacemaker looks for a P wave and fires into the atrium if no P wave is sensed; the pacing spike is following by a P wave. **B.** The single-chamber ventricular pacemaker looks for a QRS complex and fires into the ventricle if no QRS is sensed; the pacing spike is followed by wide QRS complex. **C.** The dual-chamber pacemaker looks for both the P wave and the QRS complex. If no P wave is sensed, the pacemaker delivers a stimulus into the atrium; the pacing spike is followed by a P wave. The pacemaker is programmed to wait, simulating an electronic PR interval (the AV interval). Then, if no QRS is sensed, the pacemaker delivers a stimulus into the ventricle; the pacing spike is followed by a wide QRS complex.

stimulus. If it does not sense a QRS complex, the pacemaker sends an electrical stimulus to the ventricle. Stimulation of the ventricle produces a pacemaker spike followed by a wide QRS complex, resembling a ventricular ectopic beat (Figure 10.2B). Single-chamber ventricular pacing is the most commonly used temporary type of pacing. Single-chamber ventricular pacing can also be used for permanent pacing, most often for chronic atrial fibrillation with a slow rate.

- **Dual chamber**—A dual-chamber pacemaker system uses two leads, one going to the right atrium and the other to the right ventricle. The dual-chamber pacemaker can sense and pace in both chambers. If a dual-chamber pacemaker senses a P wave, the pacemaker is inhibited from firing an electrical stimulus. If the pacemaker does not sense a P wave, the pacemaker sends an electrical stimulus to the atrium. Stimulation of the atrium produces a pacemaker spike, followed by a P wave. The pacemaker is programmed to wait, simulating an electronic PR interval. In pacing terminology, the artificial PR interval is called the *AV interval*. If a dual-chamber pacemaker senses a QRS complex, it is inhibited from firing an electrical stimulus. If the pacemaker does not sense a QRS complex, the pacemaker will send an electrical stimulus to the ventricle. Stimulation of the ventricle produces a pacemaker spike followed by a wide QRS complex. Figure 10.2C shows stimulation of the atria and the ventricle by a dual-chamber pacemaker.

Dual-chamber pacemakers are often called AV sequential pacemakers because of their ability to stimulate the atria and ventricles in sequence (first the atria and then the ventricles), mimicking normal heart physiology and thus preserving the atrial kick. Dual-chamber pacing is the most commonly used type of permanent pacing. Dual-chamber temporary pacing can be done, but it is difficult to place temporary atrial wires and therefore is not as reliable as single-chamber ventricular pacing.

Temporary Pacemakers

Temporary pacing can be accomplished with transcutaneous (TCP), transvenous, or epicardial methods:

- **Transcutaneous pacing (TCP)**—TCP, also known as external pacing, refers to the delivery of a pacing stimulus to the heart through pads placed on the patient's outer chest (Figure 10.3). Requirements for TCP include pacing pads, a pacing cable, and a defibrillator monitor with pacing capabilities. TCP is recommended as the initial pacing method of choice in emergent cardiac situations. External pacemakers are noninvasive, effective, quick, and easy to apply. TCP provides only ventricular pacing.

  TCP is indicated as a treatment for symptomatic bradyarrhythmias (sinus bradycardia, slow atrial flutter or fibrillation, Mobitz II second-degree AV block, or third-degree AV block). TCP is not effective in rhythms without meaningful contractile activity such as ventricular standstill and pulseless electrical activity (PEA) that occur in the setting of cardiac arrest. This is because the primary problem in these situations is the inability of the myocardium to contract when appropriately stimulated.

  External pacemakers should not be relied upon for an extended period of time. They should be used only as a temporary measure in emergency situations until transvenous access is available or the cause of the bradyarrhythmia is resolved. Transvenous pacing is still the treatment of choice for patients requiring temporary but longer period of pacemaker support.

  The technique of TCP involves:

1. **Attach pacing pads to chest**—TCP involves attaching two large pacing pads to the skin surface of the patient's chest. Multifunction pads have the capability to monitor the heart rhythm, externally pace, and defibrillate through one set of pads. The pads have conductive gel on the inner surface to help transmit the electrical current through the chest wall. The large surface area of the pad and the conductive gel also help minimize the possibility of skin burns from the procedure. If possible, excess hair should be clipped before the pads are applied to maximize contact with the skin surface.

Most manufacturers recommend the pads be placed in an anterior-posterior position (see Figure 10.3). The anterior pad (labeled "front") is placed to the left of the sternum, halfway between the xiphoid process and the left nipple. In the female patient, the anterior pad is placed under the left breast. The posterior pad (labeled "back") is placed on the left posterior chest directly behind the anterior pad.

Successful TCP requires a higher electrical current output (mA) than conventional transvenous pacing to overcome the resistance of the chest wall. Placement of the pacing pads affects the amount of current required to depolarize the ventricle. The placement that offers the most direct pathway to the heart usually requires the lowest mA in order to pace the heart. Currents of 50 mA or more may be associated with discomfort and sedation may be required.

2. **Connect pacing pads to defibrillator monitor**. Connect the pacing pads to a pacing cable and a defibrillator monitor with pacing capabilities.

3. **Initiate pacing**. Set the defibrillator monitor to pace setting. Set the pacing rate first (usually 70) and then slowly increase the mA until consistent ventricular capture is seen on the monitor (a pacing spike followed by a wide QRS complex; Figure 10.4). If capture is lost during pacing, the mA may have to be increased.

Verify that electrical capture (seen on the monitor) is associated with mechanical capture (verified by palpable pulses). Evaluate pulses on the patient's right side to avoid confusion between the presence of an actual pulse and skeletal muscle contractions caused by the external pacemaker.

- **Transvenous pacing**—Transvenous pacing refers to the delivery of a pacing stimulus to the heart through a vein (transvenous approach). Requirements for transvenous pacing include an external pulse generator, a pacing lead wire, and a bridging cable to connect the two (Figure 10.5).

  Some indications for transvenous pacing include symptomatic bradyarrhythmias (sinus bradycardia, slow atrial fibrillation or flutter, Mobitz II second-degree AV block, and third-degree AV block) and prophylactic therapy during cardiac catheterization procedures for high-risk patients. Transvenous pacing is usually not effective when

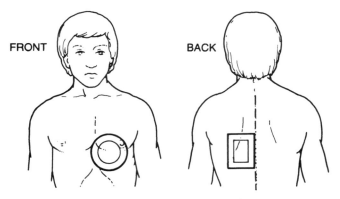

Figure 10.3 External pacing pad placement (anterior-posterior position).

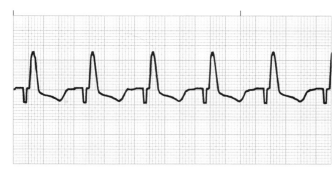

Figure 10.4 Electrical capture of the ventricle with an external pacemaker. This figure shows a square pacing spike (Zoll monitor-defibrillator with external pacemaker). Other external pacemakers may have a different pacing artifact.

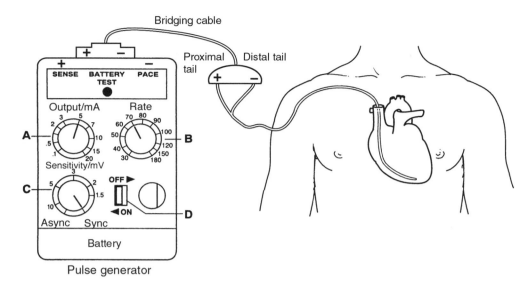

Figure 10.5   Temporary transvenous pacemaker system.

A. Output or mA dial.
   1. Controls the amount of electrical energy delivered to endocardium.
   2. Increase mA by turning dial clockwise to higher number; decrease mA by turning dial counterclockwise to lower number.
B. Rate dial.
   1. Determines the heart rate in beats/minute at which stimulus is to be delivered.
C. Sensitivity or mV dial.
   1. Controls the ability of the generator to sense the electrical activity.
   2. In maximum clockwise position (5 o'clock), provides demand (synchronous) pacing.
   3. In maximum counterclockwise position (7 o'clock), provides fixed-rate (asynchronous) pacing.
   4. Increase sensitivity (mV) by turning mV dial clockwise to lower number; decrease sensitivity by turning dial counterclockwise to higher number.
D. On/off control.
   1. Activates/inactivates the pulse generator.

meaningful contractile activity is absent (ventricular standstill and PEA). For significant unresolved rhythm or conduction disorders, permanent pacing is required.

Temporary pulse generators are externally controlled by manipulating dials on the face of the unit (see Figure 10.5). Removable batteries are contained within the generator housing. Prior to insertion of a pacing lead, prepare the equipment. Insert a new 9-volt battery into the battery compartment; set pacing rate at 100 beats per minute, the mA to 5, and the sensitivity knob to maximum clockwise position for demand (synchronous) pacing (5'clock position). Insert the end of the bridging cable into matching terminals on the pulse generator, and turn the pulse generator on to verify proper functioning of the battery and unit.

The preferred routes of access for transvenous pacing are the right internal jugular vein, the right subclavian, and the right femoral vein. The pacing lead is inserted into the vein of choice and guided into the heart using fluoroscopy. Once the wire is visualized in the right atrium, a balloon at the tip of the pacing catheter is inflated and the wire is floated through the tricuspid valve into the apex of the right ventricle for single-chamber ventricular pacing. Even though single-chamber atrial pacing and dual-chamber pacing can be done, single-chamber ventricular pacing is the most reliable and preferred choice for transvenous pacing. Once proper placement is verified, the balloon is deflated. The distal tail of the pacing catheter is connected to the negative connection of the bridging cable, and the proximal tail is connected to the positive connection of the bridging cable.

Using the dials on the external pulse generator, adjust the pacemaker settings under the direction of the cardiologist:
1. **Determine voltage threshold.** This is the smallest amount of voltage (mA) required to pace the heart. While watching the cardiac monitor, gradually turn down the mA until capture is lost (usually 0.7 to 1.0 mA) and then gradually turn up the mA until capture is regained. The point at which capture is consistently regained is the threshold. Set the mA at twice threshold level.
2. **Set pacing rate.** This is determined by the physician (usually 70 beats per minute).
3. **Set sensitivity.** Sensitivity is usually maintained at maximum clockwise position (5 o'clock on sensitivity dial).

The number of temporary transvenous pacing leads being placed is decreasing, largely because of the improved reperfusion management of acute MI and improved access to permanent pacing systems.

- *Epicardial pacing*—Epicardial pacing refers to the delivery of a pacing stimulus to the heart through wires placed on the epicardial surface of the heart during cardiac surgery. Two wires (one wire serves as a ground) are attached to the right ventricle for single-chamber ventricular pacing or two wires to the right atrium and two wires to the right ventricle for dual-chamber pacing. The wires are loosely sutured to the outer surface of the heart and pulled through the chest wall where they are attached to a bridging cable and an external pulse generator. Atrial wires usually exit to the right of the sternum and ventricular wires exit to the left. When no longer needed, the wires are gently pulled out through the wound.

Epicardial pacing is used after cardiac surgery to treat symptomatic bradyarrhythmias, as a prophylactic measure for high-risk patients, and to treat tachyarrhythmias using overdrive pacing techniques.

Permanent Pacemakers

A permanent pacemaker system (Figure 10.6) refers to an implanted generator and a lead wire (or wires) that is introduced into the heart through a central vein (often the subclavian). The implant procedure is relatively simple, usually performed in the cardiac catheterization lab using local anesthesia and conscious sedation, and lasts about 1 hour. The procedure is facilitated by fluoroscopy, which enables the cardiologist to view the passage of the lead wire. After satisfactory placement of the pacing lead is confirmed, the lead is connected to the pacemaker generator. The generator is placed in the subcutaneous tissue just below the left or right clavicle. Generally, the patient's nondominant side is chosen to minimize interference with the patient's daily activities.

The major reason for implanting a pacemaker is the presence of a symptomatic bradycardia. Symptomatic bradycardia is a term used to define a bradycardic rhythm that is directly responsible for symptoms such as syncope, transient dizziness, confusion, fatigue, exercise intolerance, congestive heart failure, dyspnea, and hypotension.

Permanent pacemaker technology has undergone major advances since pacemakers were first introduced in the 1950s. Early pacemakers paced a single chamber (the right ventricle) at a fixed rate. Today's pacemakers function as demand pacemakers, sensing the patient's natural beats and pacing the heart only when needed ("on demand"). Most of the permanent pacemakers used today are the dual-chamber demand type. Although these dual-chamber models are more expensive, they maintain AV synchrony (the atria pace first and then the ventricles), preserving the atrial kick and often providing patients with a higher quality of life. Studies have shown that unnecessary pacing of the right ventricle can lead to heart failure and an increased incidence of atrial fibrillation. The newer dual-chamber devices can keep the amount of right ventricular pacing to a minimum and thus prevent worsening of heart disease.

Permanent pacemakers are also available for specific conditions or needs:

- **Rate-responsive pacemaker**—This pacemaker has sensors that detect changes in a person's physical activity and automatically speeds up or slows down the heart rate in response to the activity. Rate-responsive pacing mimics the heart's normal rhythm, enabling patients to participate in more activities.
- **Biventricular pacemaker**—A biventricular pacemaker uses three leads: one placed in the right atrium, one placed in the right ventricle, and one placed in the left ventricle (via the coronary sinus vein). A biventricular pacemaker, also known as cardiac resynchronization therapy (CRT), stimulates both the right and left ventricles. By pacing both ventricles, the pacemaker can resynchronize a heart whose opposing walls do not contract in synchrony (a problem that occurs in 25% to 50% of heart failure patients). CRT devices have been shown to reduce mortality and improve quality of life in patients with an ejection fraction of 35% or less or in patients with heart failure symptoms.
- **Implantable cardioverter-defibrillators (ICDs)**—These devices have the ability to pace for bradycardia, overdrive pace for tachycardia (antitachycardia pacing), and deliver an electric shock if needed. They are used in the treatment of patients at risk for sudden cardiac death.

Once a permanent pacemaker is implanted, the following information is helpful to share with the patient:

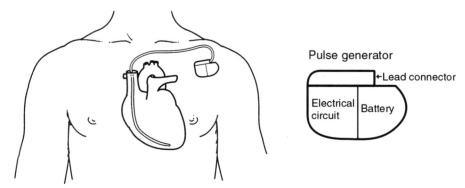

Figure 10.6 Permanent pacemaker system.

1. **Periodic pacemaker checkups**—The pacemaker is periodically checked to ensure the device is operational and performing appropriately. The status of the pacemaker can be checked or "interrogated" to provide information regarding the type of heart rhythm, the functioning of the pacemaker leads, the frequency of utilization of the pacemaker, the battery life, and the presence of any abnormal rhythms. Most present-day pacemakers are programmable, enabling adjustments to be made to the settings. Programming is usually done in an office setting.
2. **Pacemaker safety**—Built-in filters protect pacemakers from electrical interference from most devices encountered in daily life, including microwave ovens. Security devices at airports should not cause any interference to the normal operation of the pacemaker; however, they may detect the metal in the pacemaker. In this situation, the pacemaker wearer can present an ID card indicating they have a pacemaker. Cell phones do not seem to damage or affect how the pacemaker works. Any activity that involves intense magnetic fields (such as arc welding) should be avoided. Some medical procedures may disrupt a pacemaker and should be avoided: magnetic resonance imaging (MRI), shock wave lithotripsy to get rid of kidney stones, and electrocauterization to stop bleeding during surgery.
3. **Pacemaker replacement**—The life of a pacemaker is affected by how much it is utilized.

Today's pacemakers usually contain lithium-iodine batteries, which are designed to last many years. Pacemakers have a built-in indicator to signal when the battery is approaching depletion. Most reflect battery depletion by a gradual decrease in the pacing rate. The pacemaker is designed to operate for several months to allow adequate time to schedule a replacement procedure. Each person with a pacemaker should be told the rate at which their pacemaker is set and how to take their own pulse. Because the batteries are permanently sealed inside the pacemaker, the entire pacemaker is replaced when the battery runs down. Device replacement is usually a simpler procedure than the original insertion as it does not normally require leads to be replaced.

Permanent Pacemaker Identification Codes

A universal coding system is used to describe the function of single- and dual-chamber pacemakers (Table 10.1). The code is comprised of five positions. Various letters are used for each position to describe a pacemaker function or characteristic. Only one letter is used per position:

- **First position**—Identifies the chamber paced
- **Second position**—Identifies the chamber where intrinsic electrical activity is sensed
- **Third position**—Indicates how the pacemaker will respond when it senses intrinsic electrical activity
- **Fourth position**—Identifies programmable functions (simple and multiprogrammable), the capability for transmitting and receiving data (communication), and rate-responsive functions
- **Fifth position**—Identifies antitachycardia functions:
1. Antitachycardia pacing (overdrive pacing)—This function paces the heart faster than the intrinsic rate to convert the tachycardia.
2. Shock (synchronized cardioversion and defibrillation)
3. Dual—Performs both an antitachycardia pacing function and a shock function

Pacemaker Terms

Pacemaker Firing

A pacemaker produces a programmed current (stimulus) at a set rate to the myocardium. This energy travels from the pacemaker generator through the lead wires to the myocardial muscle. This is known as pacemaker firing and produces a pacemaker spike (a vertical line) on the ECG tracing.

Basic pacemaker operation consists of a closed-loop circuit in which electrical current flows between two metal poles (one negative, the other positive). The stimulating pulse is delivered through the negative electrode. Pacemaker systems may be either unipolar or bipolar. Unipolar pacing has one pole (electrode) within the heart, with the other pole being the metal case of the pulse generator. Pacemaker

table 10.1 Five-Letter Pacemaker Identification Code

First letter	Second letter	Third letter	Fourth letter	Fifth letter
Chamber paced	Chamber sensed	Response to sensing	Programmable functions	Antitachycardia functions
0 = None	0 = None	0 = None	0 = None	0 = None
A = Atrium	A = Atrium	I = Inhibits pacing	P = Simple programmable	P = Antitachycardia pacing
V = Ventricle	V = Ventricle	T = Triggers pacing	M = Multiprogrammable	S = Shock
D = Dial (A and V)	D = Dial (A and V)	D = Dial (I and T)	C = Communication	D = Dual (P and S)
			R = Rate responsive	

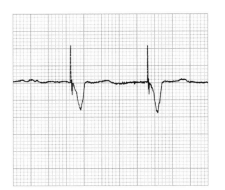
A. Unipolar pacing system (lead II)

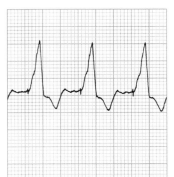
B. Bipolar pacing system (lead III)

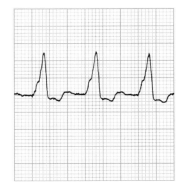
C. Bipolar pacing system (lead II)

Figure 10.7 Unipolar and bipolar pacing spikes. **A.** Large pacing spikes are seen with a unipolar pacing system. **B.** Small pacing spikes are seen with a bipolar pacing system. **C.** The electrical circuit is so small in a bipolar system that some leads may not show a pacing spike.

systems utilizing unipolar pacing involve a large electrical circuit. The circuit travels between the electrodes on the distal tip of the pacing lead in contact with the myocardium (the negative pole) to the pacemaker generator located in soft tissue (the positive pole). Because of the greater distance between the two poles, the ECG tracing will show a large, easily visible pacing spike (Figure 10.7A). Pacemaker systems utilizing bipolar pacing involve a small electrical circuit. The current travels between the electrodes on the distal tip of the pacing lead (negative pole) to the proximal electrode located a few millimeters above the distal tip (the positive pole). Because of the smaller distance between the two poles, the ECG tracing will show a small spike (Figure 10.7B) or may not be visible in some leads on an ECG tracing (Figure 10.7C).

Sensing

Sensing is the ability of the pacemaker to detect intrinsic electrical impulses (the patient's own electrical activity) or electrical impulses produced by a pacemaker (paced activity). If the pacemaker detects electrical activity, it is inhibited from delivering a stimulus. If the pacemaker does not detect electrical activity, it is triggered to initiate an electrical stimulus.

Capture

The term capture refers to the successful stimulation of the myocardium by a pacemaker stimulus, resulting in depolarization. Capture is evidenced on the ECG by a pacemaker spike followed by either a atrial complex (P wave), a ventricular complex (QRS), or both, depending on the chambers being paced. Capture beats are normal.

Atrial depolarization from a pacing stimulus results in a pacing spike followed by atrial activity (P wave). The morphology of the P waves produced may resemble that of sinus beats and be normal looking or may be abnormal in appearance and so small that they are difficult to see. The P waves may not immediately follow the atrial pacing spike. The P waves may also be associated with a long PR interval. Examples are shown in Figure 10.8.

Normal ventricular depolarization is simultaneous (both ventricles depolarize at the same time), resulting in a narrow QRS complex of 0.10 second or less in duration. Ventricular depolarization from a pacing stimulus is sequential (one ventricle depolarizes and then the other), prolonging the duration of depolarization, resulting in a wide QRS complex of 0.12 second or greater. The wide QRS complex immediately follows the pacing spike (Figure 10.9A).

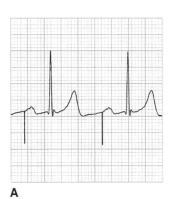
A

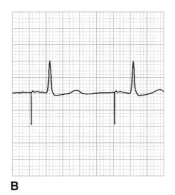
B

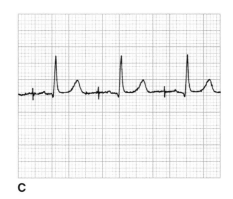
C

Figure 10.8 Examples of atrial capture. **A.** Atrial capture with normal-looking P waves conducted with long PR interval. **B.** Atrial capture with abnormal-looking P waves. **C.** Atrial capture with small, pointed P waves not immediately following the atrial spike.

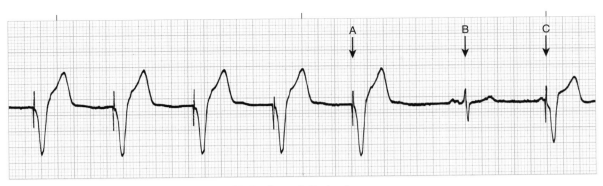

Figure 10.9 **A.** Ventricular capture beat. **B.** Native beat. **C.** Fusion beat.

Intrinsic Beat

An intrinsic beat (also called native beat) is produced by the patient's natural electrical system (Figure 10.9B). Intrinsic beats are normal.

Automatic Interval (Pacing Interval)

The automatic interval refers to the heart rate at which the pacemaker is set. This interval is measured from one pacing spike to the next consecutive pacing spike. For atrial pacing, measure from one atrial pacing spike to the next consecutive atrial pacing spike. This is called the A-A interval, analogous to the P-P interval of intrinsic waveforms. For ventricular pacing, measure from one ventricular pacing spike to the next consecutive ventricular pacing spike (Figure 10.10A). This is called the V-V interval, analogous to the R-R interval of intrinsic waveforms.

Fusion Beat

A fusion beat occurs when the pacemaker fires an electrical stimulus at the same time the patient's own electrical system fires an electrical stimulus. This results in part of the ventricle being depolarized by the pacemaker and part by the patient's own intrinsic impulse. The fusion beat is evidenced on the ECG by a pacemaker spike that occurs at the programmed rate (occurs on time), followed by a QRS that is different in height or width from the paced beats and the patient's intrinsic beats (Figures 10.9 and 10.10).

The fusion beat has characteristics of both pacemaker and patient forces, although one usually dominates the other. In Figure 10.9C, the fusion beat has more characteristics of the patient's paced beats than his intrinsic beats. In Figure 10.10B, the fusion beat has more characteristics of the patient's intrinsic beats than his paced beats. Fusion beats are normal.

Pseudofusion Beat

A pseudofusion beat occurs when the pacemaker fires an electrical stimulus after the patient's spontaneous impulse has already started depolarizing the ventricle. The pacemaker stimulus has no effect since the ventricle is already being depolarized. The pseudofusion beat is evidenced on the monitor by a pacemaker spike occurring at the programmed rate (occurs on time), along with a native QRS complex. The intrinsic QRS is not altered in height or width (Figure 10.11). Pseudofusion beats are normal.

Pacemaker Rhythm

Stimulation of the atria for one beat is called an atrial paced beat. Continuous stimulation of the atria (all P waves are pacemaker induced) is called an atrial paced rhythm (Figure 10.12). Stimulation of the ventricle for one beat is called a ventricular paced beat. Continuous stimulation of the ventricles (all QRS complexes are pacemaker induced) is called a ventricular paced rhythm (Figure 10.13). Stimulation of the atria and ventricle for one beat is called an AV paced beat. Continuous stimulation of the atria and ventricles (all P waves and QRS complexes are pacemaker

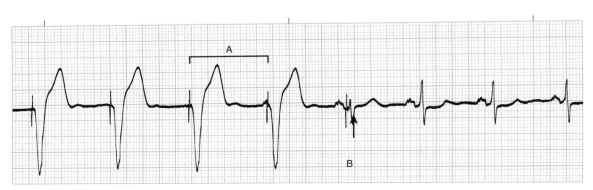

Figure 10.10 **A**. Automatic interval. **B**. Fusion beat.

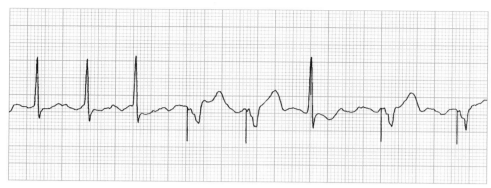

Figure 10.11   Pseudofusion beat (6th complex). The pacing spike occurs within a native QRS complex—the native QRS is not altered in height or width.

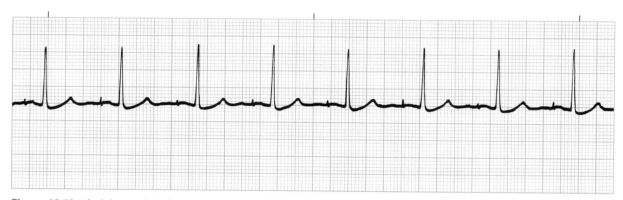

Figure 10.12   Atrial paced rhythm.

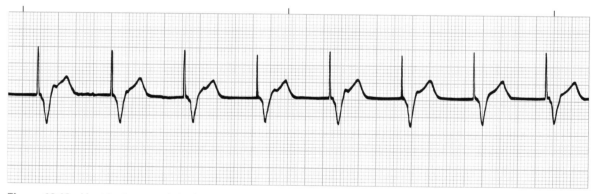

Figure 10.13   Ventricular paced rhythm.

induced) is called an AV paced rhythm (Figure 10.14). Figure 10.15 shows atrial pacing with one AV paced beat.

Pacemaker Malfunctions

Basic functions of all pacemaker include the ability to fire (stimulus release), to sense electrical activity (intrinsic and paced), and to capture (depolarize the chambers being paced). Most malfunctions can be traced to problems with the generator (parameter settings, battery failure), the lead (problems at the interface between the catheter tip and the endocardium, fracture in the lead or its insulating surface), or a disconnection in the system.

This section includes a description of pacemaker malfunctions, common causes, and interventions. It is directed primarily toward temporary transvenous ventricular demand pacemakers since nurses can interact more directly with them than with permanent pacemakers. The same concepts apply to permanent pacemakers, but most cases are resolved by interrogation of the pacemaker system to find the specific cause and reprogramming of the pacemaker settings. Some malfunctions associated with permanent pacemakers may require surgical intervention.

The external pulse generator should always be secured away from the patient to prevent manipulation of the generator controls and disconnection of the bridging cable.

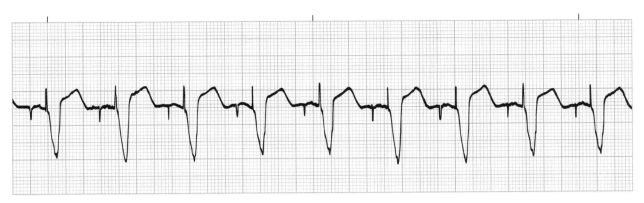

Figure 10.14 AV paced rhythm.

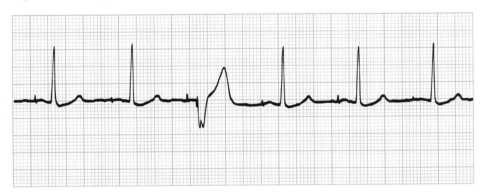

Figure 10.15 Atrial paced rhythm with one AV paced beat.

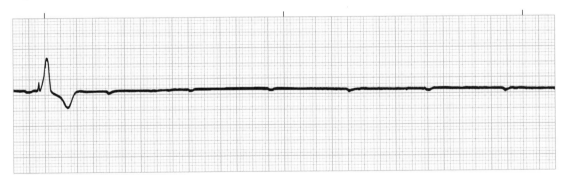

Figure 10.16 Failure to fire.

Failure to Fire

With failure to fire, the pacemaker does not discharge a stimulus to the myocardium. Failure to fire will be evidenced on the ECG by an absence of a pacemaker spike where expected (Figure 10.16). Failure to fire is abnormal.

Causes and interventions for failure to fire (for temporary transvenous ventricular demand pacemakers):

1. **The pacemaker is turned off**—Check on/off switch on generator (see Figure 10.5D).
2. **Battery depletion**—Replace the battery.
3. **Disconnection in the system**—Check the connections between the generator, bridging cable, and lead; reconnect or tighten connections.
4. **Fracture of lead or lead insulation**—Do an overpenetrated chest x-ray to detect fractures; have the physician replace the lead.

5. **Electromagnetic interference**—Exposure of a pacing unit to such sources as electrocautery devices or MRI may result in inhibition of the pacing stimulus. Avoid exposure.

Failure to Capture

With failure to capture, the pacemaker delivers a pacing stimulus, but electrical stimulation of the myocardium (depolarization) does not occur. This is evidenced on the ECG by pacemaker spikes that occur at the programmed rate, but are not followed by a QRS. Figure 10.17 shows loss of capture with ventricular pacing. Loss of capture is abnormal.

Causes and interventions for failure to capture (for temporary transvenous ventricular demand pacemakers):

1. **mA output is too low**—Increase the mA on the generator by turning the mA dial clockwise to a higher number (see Figure 10.5A). Over a period of days, inflammation or

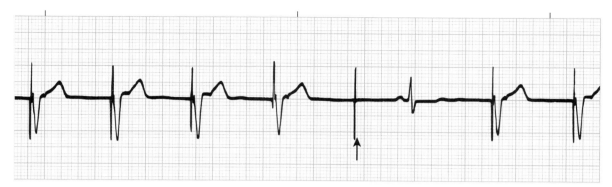

Figure 10.17 Loss of capture.

fibrin formation at the catheter tip may raise the stimulation threshold, requiring a higher mA output.

2. **Lead is out of position or lying in infarcted tissue**—The electrode tip must be in contact with the endocardium for the electrical stimulus to cause depolarization. Infarcted tissue does not respond to a stimulus. Do an overpenetrated chest x-ray to determine the catheter position. If the catheter is out of position, a temporary maneuver is to turn the patient on his left side (gravity may allow the catheter to contact the endocardium). A physician will have to reposition the lead.

3. **Electrolyte imbalance**—Electrolyte imbalances can alter the ability of the heart to respond to a pacing stimulus. Check serum electrolyte levels and replace if needed.

Sensing Failure

Sensing failure occurs when the pacemaker either does not sense myocardial electrical activity or the pacemaker oversenses the wrong signals. Sensing failure falls into two categories: undersensing and oversensing.

Undersensing

The most common cause of sensing failure is undersensing. The pacemaker does not sense (does not "see") myocardial electrical activity (either intrinsic or paced) and fires earlier than it should. Undersensing is recognized on the ECG by a pacing spike that occurs earlier than expected. It can occur with capture (Figure 10.18B and C) or without capture (Figure 10.18A).

Causes and interventions for undersensing (for temporary transvenous ventricular demand pacemakers):

1. **Sensitivity set too low**—Increase sensitivity by turning sensitivity dial on generator clockwise to a lower number (see Figure 10.5C).

2. **Pacing catheter out of position or lying in infarcted tissue**—The electrode tip must be in contact with the endocardium to sense appropriately. Infarcted tissue does not have the ability to sense. Do an overpenetrated chest x-ray to determine catheter position. If the catheter is out of position, a temporary maneuver is to turn the patient on his left side, which may allow migration of the catheter into a better position. A physician will have to reposition the lead.

3. **Pacemaker set on asynchronous (fixed-rate) mode**—With asynchronous pacing, the sensing circuit is off. Turn the sensitivity dial on the generator to synchronous (demand) pacing mode (see Figure 10.5C).

Oversensing

The pacemaker is too sensitive ("sees" too much) and is sensing the wrong signals (large P waves, large T waves, muscle movement, etc.), causing the pacemaker to fire later than it should. Oversensing is recognized on the ECG by a paced beat that occurs later than expected (see Figure 10.19).

Causes and interventions for oversensing (for temporary transvenous ventricular demand pacemakers):

1. **Sensitivity set too high**—Decrease the sensitivity by turning the sensitivity dial on the generator counterclockwise to a higher number (see Figure 10.5C).

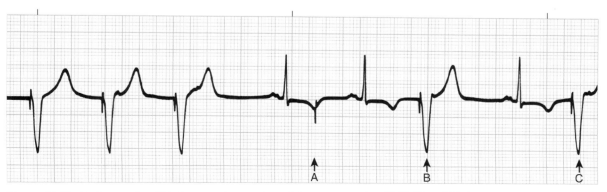

Figure 10.18 Undersensing. **(A)** shows undersensing without capture (no QRS). **(B and C)** show undersensing with capture (has QRS).

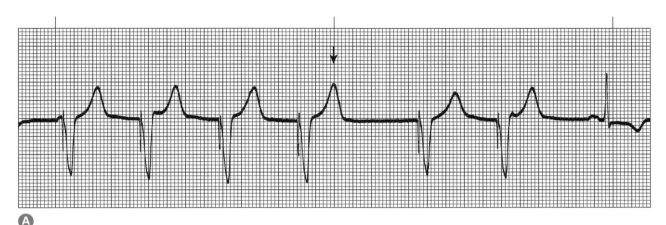

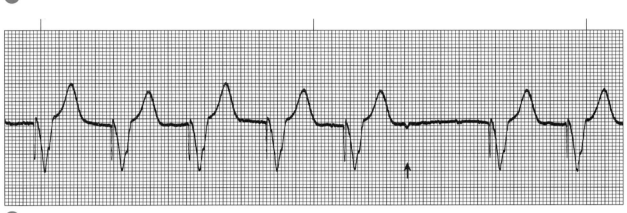

Figure 10.19   Oversensing.
Example A: Pacemaker is sensing a large T wave.
Example B: Pacemaker is sensing a low waveform artifact. *Note*: Using the automatic interval marks on index card, place right mark on spike of late paced beat. The left mark will match whatever pacemaker is sensing.

Analyzing Pacemaker Strips (Ventricular Demand Type)

Most pacemaker strips have a mixture of pacemaker-induced beats as well as the patient's own beats. It is helpful to follow steps in analyzing pacemaker strips just as you do with rhythm strips:

- **Step one**—Identify patient's intrinsic beats: The patient's beats do not need analyzing, but you need to be able to identify them from the paced beats.
- **Step two**—Measure the automatic interval—Place an index card above two consecutive pacing spikes and mark on index card. "Left mark" and "right mark" in steps below refer to marks on index card. The automatic interval measurement will assist you in determining if the pacemaker fired on time, fired too early, fired too late, or did not fire.
- **Step three**—Starting on left side of strip, analyze each pacing spike one at a time—Place left mark on pacing spike of complex just before pacing spike being analyzed; if complex doesn't have a pacing spike, use R wave of a native QRS.
- **Step four**—Observe where right mark falls in relation to pacing spike being analyzed:

  ○ Does pacing spike match right mark?
  ○ Does pacing spike occur earlier than right mark?
  ○ Does pacing spike occur later than right mark?
  ○ Does pacing spike not occur at all?
  (See Table 10.2 for answers.)

Review Figures 10.20 through 10.25. These strips have been analyzed for you.

table 10.2   Using Automatic Interval Measurement to Identify Pacemaker Malfunctions

Spike occurs on time (spike matches right mark)	Spike occurs too early (spike earlier than right mark)
• Ventricular capture beat (normal) • Fusion beat (normal) • Pseudofusion beat (normal) • Failure to capture (abnormal)	• Undersensing (abnormal)

Spike doesn't occur	Spike occurs too late (spike later than right mark)
• Failure to fire (abnormal)	• Oversensing (abnormal)

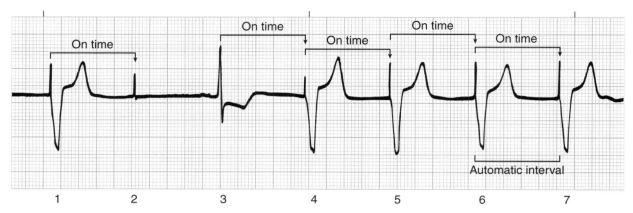

Figure 10.20   Pacemaker analysis strip #1.

- #3 is a native beat.
- The automatic interval can be measured from #6 to #7. Mark automatic interval on index card. Left mark and right mark in steps below refer to marks on index card.
- #2 can be analyzed by placing left mark on spike of paced beat just before it; #2 matches right mark; #2 occurs on time, but does not cause ventricular depolarization (no QRS), so it indicates failure to capture.
- #4 can be analyzed by placing left mark on R wave of native beat just before it; #4 matches right mark; #4 occurs on time and causes ventricular depolarization (QRS present) indicating ventricular capture beat.
- #5, #6, and #7 can be analyzed by placing left mark on spikes of paced beats just before it; all occur on time and cause ventricular depolarization indicating ventricular capture beats.

Interpretation: Ventricular paced rhythm with one native beat and one episode of failure to capture (abnormal pacemaker function).

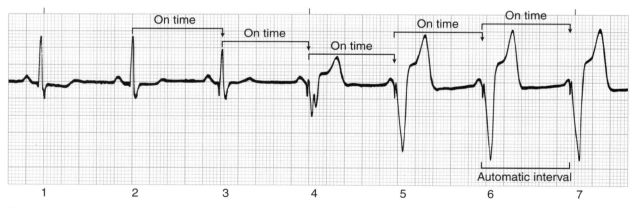

Figure 10.21   Pacemaker analysis strip #2.

- #1 and #2 are native beats.
- The automatic interval can be measured from #6 to #7. Mark automatic interval on index card. Left mark and right mark in steps below refer to marks on index card.
- #3 has spike at beginning of QRS so it needs analyzing. Place left mark on R wave of native beat just before it; #3 matches right mark; #3 occurs on time, but is different in height and/or width from both the native and paced beats, so this represent a fusion beat. This fusion beat has more characteristics of the native beats.
- #4 can be analyzed by placing left mark on spike of fusion beat just before it; #4 matches right mark; #4 occurs on time, but is different in height and/or width from both the native and paced beats, so this represents a fusion beat. This fusion beat has more characteristics of the paced beats.
- #5 can be analyzed by placing left mark on spike of fusion beat just before it; #5 matches right mark; #5 occurs on time and causes ventricular depolarization (QRS present), indicating ventricular capture beat.
- #6 and #7 can be analyzed by placing left mark on spikes of the paced beats just before it; both match right mark; both occur on time and cause ventricular depolarization, indicating ventricular capture beats.

Interpretation: Ventricular paced rhythm with two native beats and two fusion beats (normal pacemaker function).

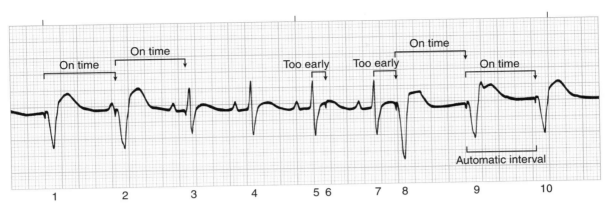

Figure 10.22 Pacemaker analysis strip #3.

- #4, #5, and #7 are native beats.
- The automatic interval can be measured from #9 to #10. Mark automatic interval on index card. Left mark and right mark in steps below refer to marks on index card.
- #2 can be analyzed by placing left mark on spike of paced beat just before it; #2 matches right mark; #2 occurs on time and causes ventricular depolarization (QRS present), indicating ventricular capture beat.
- #3 has spike at beginning of R wave so it needs analyzing. Place left mark on spike of paced beat just before it; #3 matches right mark; #3 occurs on time, but differs in height and/or width from both the native and paced beats, so this represents a fusion beat. This fusion beat has more characteristics of the native beats.
- #6 can be analyzed by placing left mark on R wave of native beat just before it; #6 occurs earlier than right mark; #6 indicates that the pacemaker did not sense the preceding beat and represents an undersensing problem. This undersensing problem occurred without capture (no QRS).
- #8 can be analyzed by placing left mark on R wave of native beat just before it; #8 occurs earlier than right mark; #8 indicates that the pacemaker did not sense the preceding beat and represents an undersensing problem. This undersensing problem occurred with capture (has QRS).
- #9 and #10 can be analyzed by placing left mark on pacing spikes of beats just before it; both match right mark; both occur on time and cause ventricular depolarization, indicating capture beats.

Interpretation: Ventricular paced rhythm with three native beats, one fusion beat and two episodes of undersensing (abnormal pacemaker function).

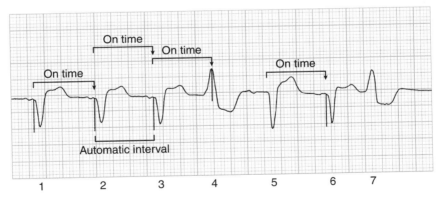

Figure 10.23 Pacemaker analysis strip #4.

- #5 and #7 are native beats (each coming from a different focus).
- The automatic interval can be measured from #2 to #3. Mark automatic interval on index card. Left mark and right mark in steps below refer to marks on index card.
- #2 can be analyzed by placing left mark on spike of paced beat just before it; #2 matches right mark; #2 occurs on time and causes ventricular depolarization (QRS present) indicating ventricular capture beat.
- #3 can be analyzed by placing left mark on spike of paced beat just before it; #3 matches right mark; #3 match occurs on time and causes ventricular depolarization (QRS present) indicating ventricular capture beat.
- Complex #4 has spike in it, so it needs analyzing. Place left mark on spike of paced beat just before it; #4 matches right mark; #4 occurs on time and is not altered in height or width from native beat #7, so this represents a pseudofusion beat.
- #6 can be analyzed by placing left mark at beginning of QS complex just before it (no R wave with this complex). #6 matches right mark; #6 occurs on time and causes ventricular depolarization (QRS present), indicating a ventricular capture beat.

Interpretation: Ventricular paced rhythm with two native beats and one pseudofusion beat (normal pacemaker function).

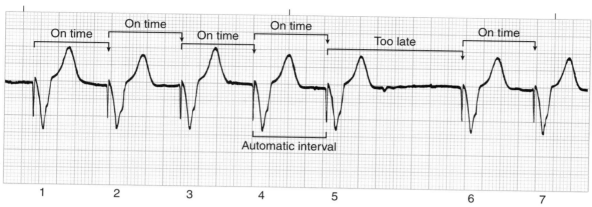

Figure 10.24 **Pacemaker analysis strip #5.**

- No native beats are seen.
- The automatic interval can be measured from #4 to #5. Mark automatic interval on index card. Left mark and right mark in steps below refer to marks on index card.
- #2, #3, #4, and #5 can be analyzed by placing left mark on spikes of the paced beat just before it; all match right mark; all occur on time and cause ventricular depolarization (QRS present) indicating ventricular capture.
- #6 can be analyzed by placing left mark on spike of paced beat just before it; #6 occurs later than right mark; #6 indicates the pacemaker sensed baseline artifact or a waveform that caused pacemaker to fire later than it should. If you place the right mark on the spike of complex #6, the left mark will match what pacemaker is sensing (in this case, a low waveform artifact).
- #7 can be analyzed by placing left mark on spike of paced beat just before it; #7 matches right mark; #7 occurs on time and causes ventricular depolarization, indicating ventricular capture.

Interpretation: Ventricular paced rhythm with one episode of oversensing (abnormal pacemaker function).

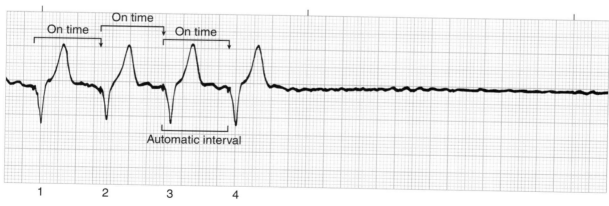

Figure 10.25 **Pacemaker analysis strip #6.**

- No native beats are seen.
- The automatic interval can be measured from #3 to #4. Mark automatic interval on index card. Left mark and right mark in steps below refer to marks on index card.
- #2, #3, and #4 can be analyzed by placing left mark on spikes of paced beats just before it; all match right mark; all occur on time and cause ventricular depolarization (QRS present) indicating ventricular capture beats. After 4th complex, no spikes or QRS complexes are seen.

Interpretation: Ventricular paced rhythm with failure to fire, resulting in ventricular asystole (abnormal pacemaker function).

RHYTHM STRIP PRACTICE: PACEMAKERS

Follow the four basic steps for analyzing pacemaker strips as discussed on page 265. Refer to Table 10.2 and to Figures 10.20 through 10.25 which have been analyzed for you. All pacemaker strips are lead II, a positive lead, unless otherwise noted. Check your answers with the answer keys in the appendix.

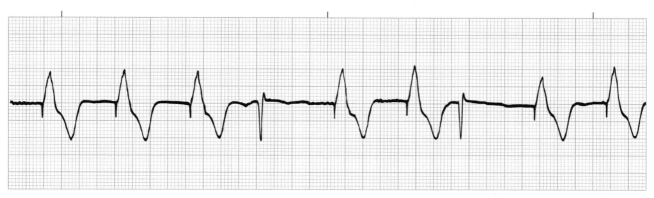

Strip 10.1 Analysis: _____

Interpretation: _____

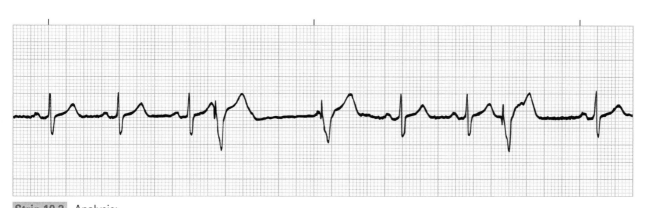

Strip 10.2 Analysis: _____

Interpretation: _____

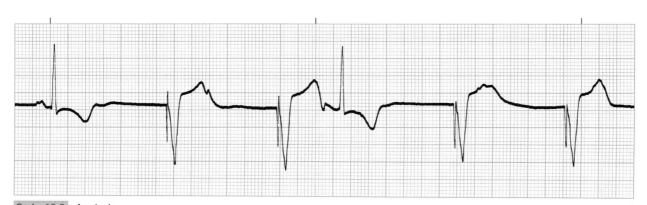

Strip 10.3 Analysis: _____

Interpretation: _____

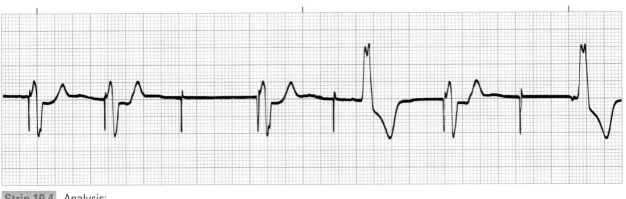

Strip 10.4 Analysis: _____

Interpretation: _____

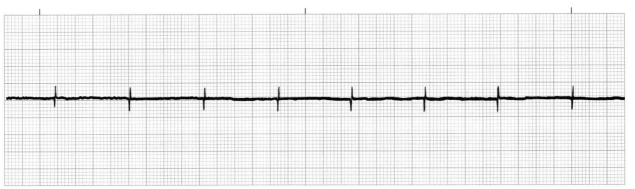

Strip 10.5 Analysis: _____

Interpretation: _____

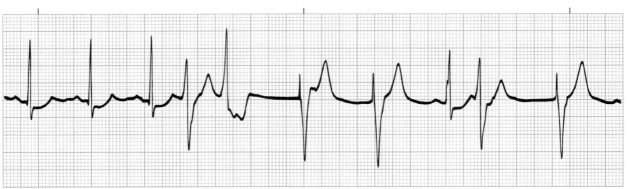

Strip 10.6 Analysis: _____

Interpretation: _____

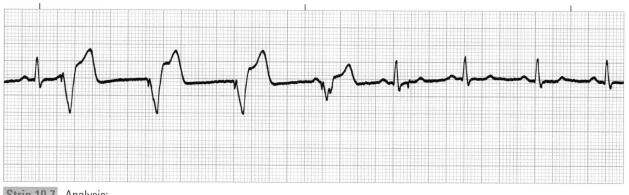

Strip 10.7 Analysis: _____

Interpretation: _____

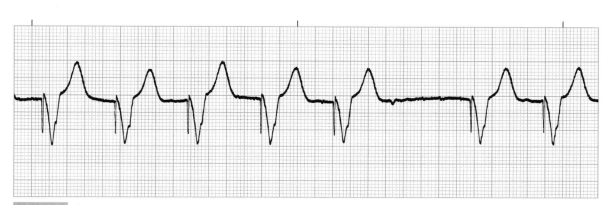

Strip 10.8 Analysis: _____

Interpretation: _____

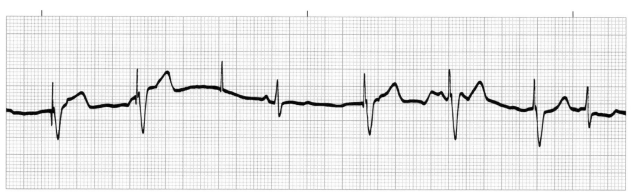

Strip 10.9 Analysis: _____

Interpretation: _____

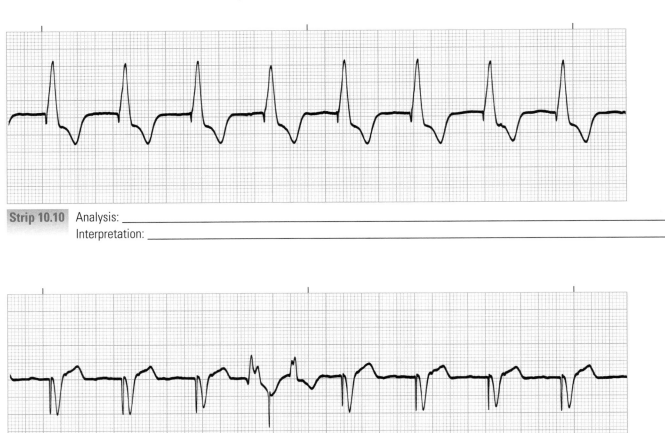

Strip 10.10   Analysis: _____

Interpretation: _____

Strip 10.11   Analysis: _____

Interpretation: _____

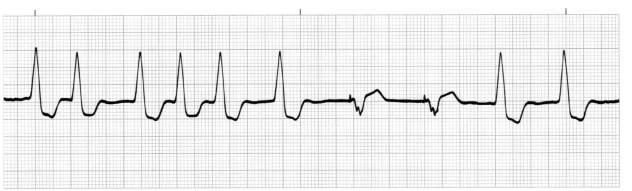

Strip 10.12   Analysis: _____

Interpretation: _____

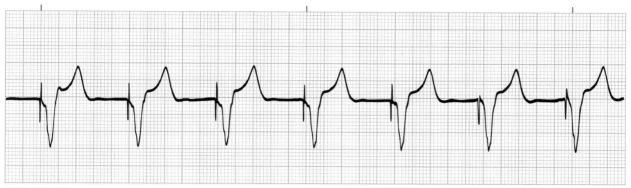

Strip 10.13 Analysis: _____

Interpretation: _____

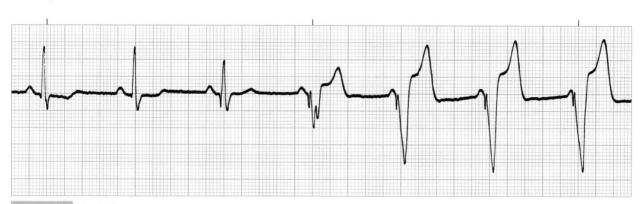

Strip 10.14 Analysis: _____

Interpretation: _____

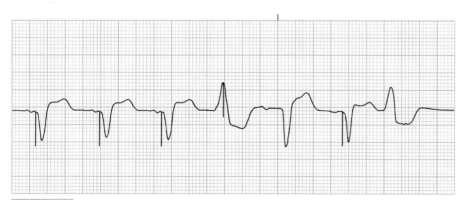

Strip 10.15 Analysis: _____

Interpretation: _____

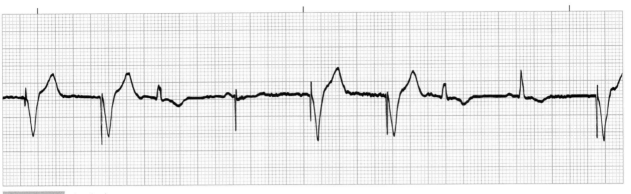

Strip 10.16 Analysis: _____

Interpretation: _____

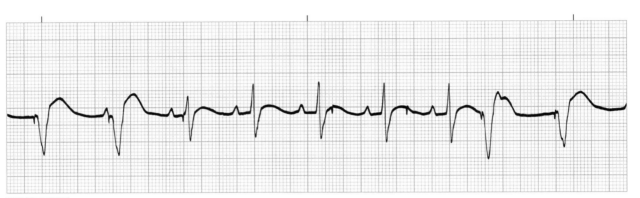

Strip 10.17 Analysis: _____

Interpretation: _____

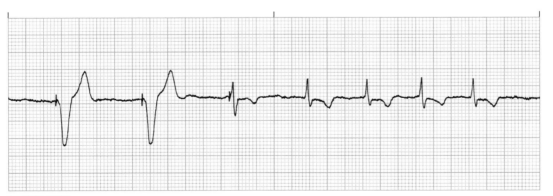

Strip 10.18 Analysis: _____

Interpretation: _____

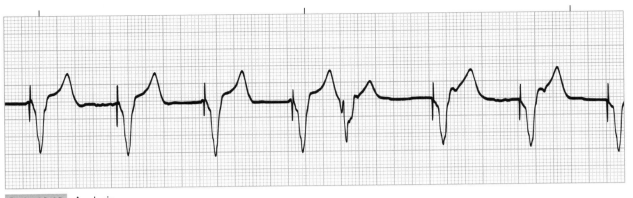

Strip 10.19   Analysis: _____

Interpretation: _____

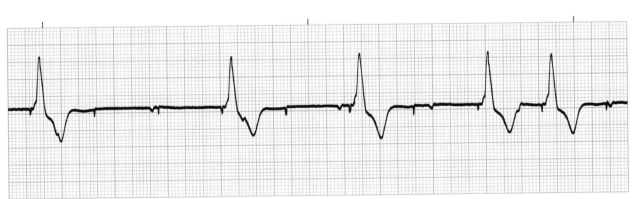

Strip 10.20   Analysis: _____

Interpretation: _____

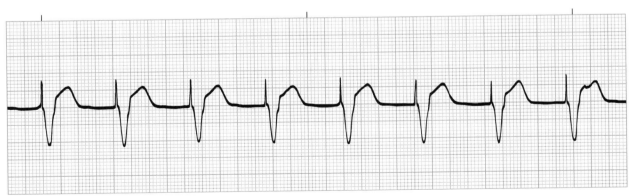

Strip 10.21   Analysis: _____

Interpretation: _____

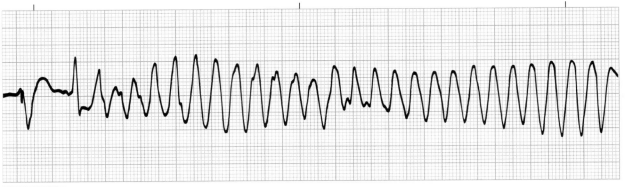

Strip 10.22 Analysis: _____

Interpretation: _____

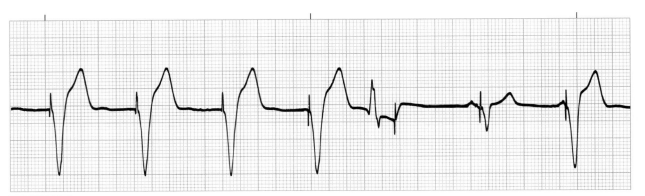

Strip 10.23 Analysis: _____

Interpretation: _____

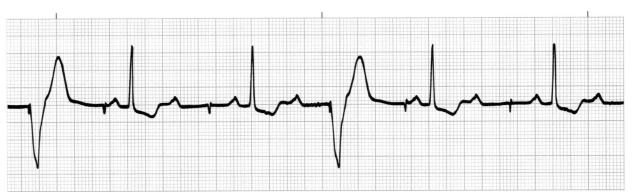

Strip 10.24 Analysis: _____

Interpretation: _____

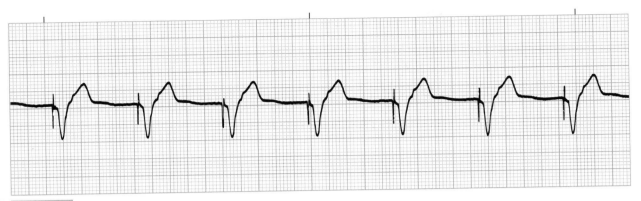

Strip 10.25 Analysis: _____

Interpretation: _____

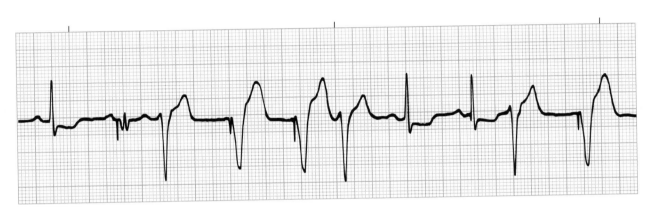

Strip 10.26 Analysis: _____

Interpretation: _____

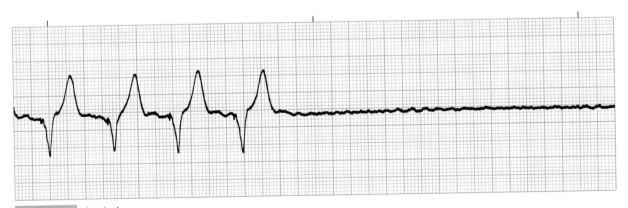

Strip 10.27 Analysis: _____

Interpretation: _____

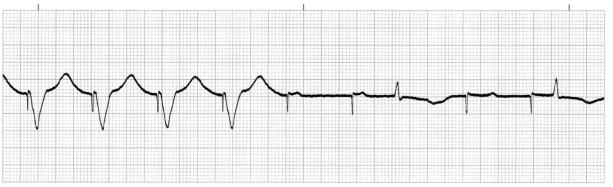

Strip 10.28 Analysis: _____

Interpretation: _____

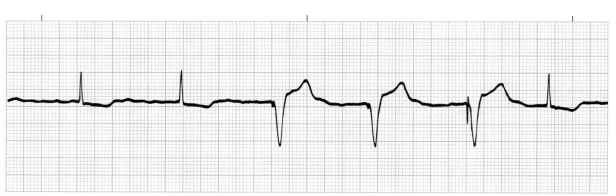

Strip 10.29 Analysis: _____

Interpretation: _____

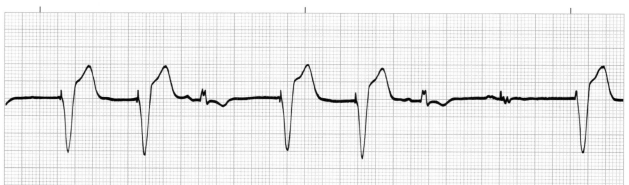

Strip 10.30 Analysis: _____

Interpretation: _____

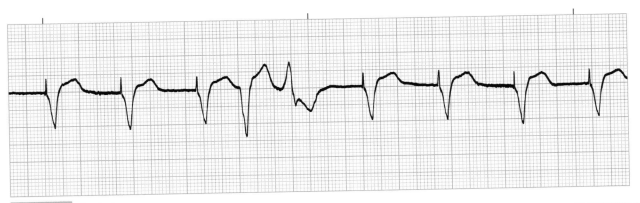

Strip 10.31 Analysis: _____

Interpretation: _____

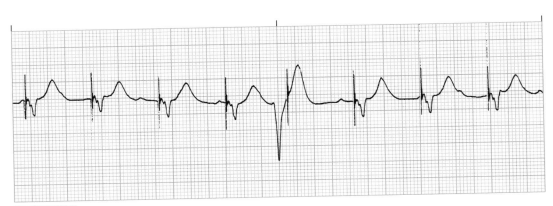

Strip 10.32 Analysis: _____

Interpretation: _____

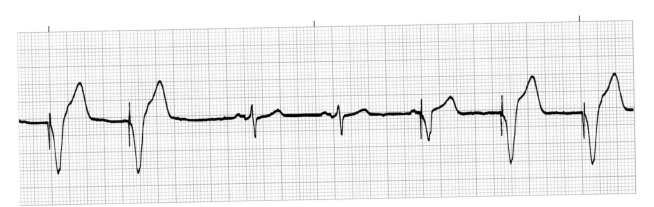

Strip 10.33 Analysis: _____

Interpretation: _____

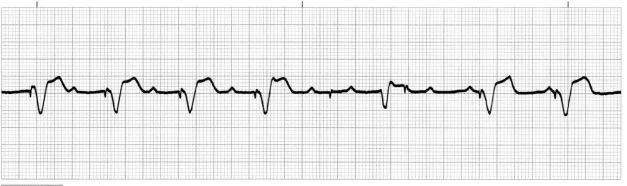

Strip 10.34   Analysis: _____

Interpretation: _____

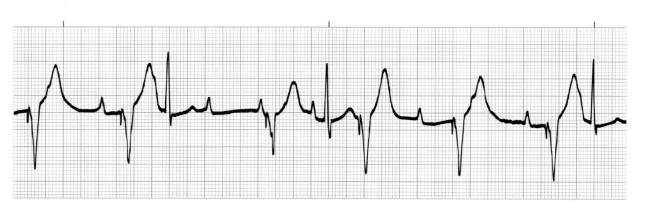

Strip 10.35   Analysis: _____

Interpretation: _____

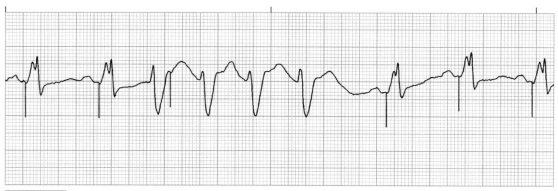

Strip 10.36   Analysis: _____

Interpretation: _____

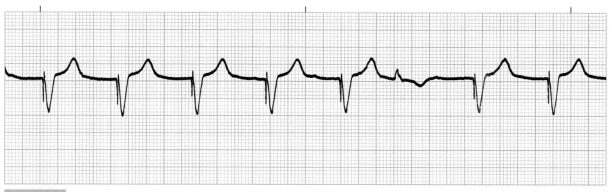

Strip 10.37 Analysis: _____

Interpretation: _____

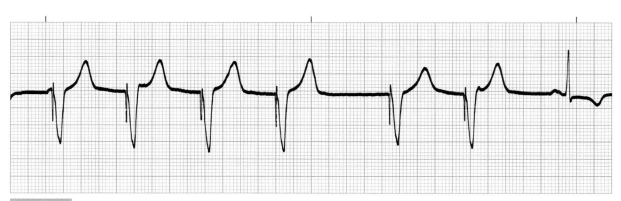

Strip 10.38 Analysis: _____

Interpretation: _____

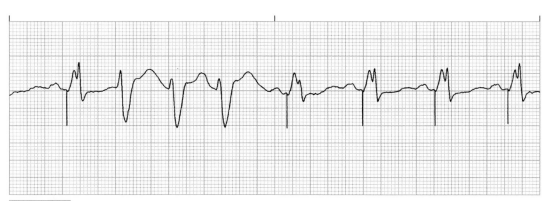

Strip 10.39 Analysis: _____

Interpretation: _____

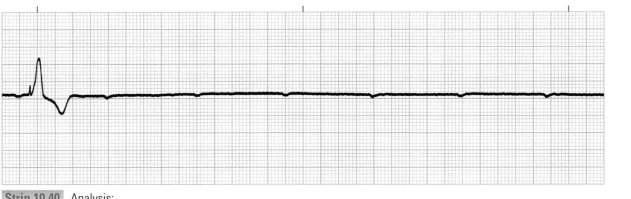

Strip 10.40 Analysis: _____

Interpretation: _____

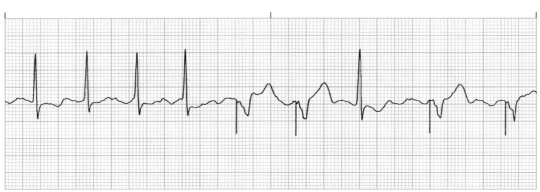

Strip 10.41 Analysis: _____

Interpretation: _____

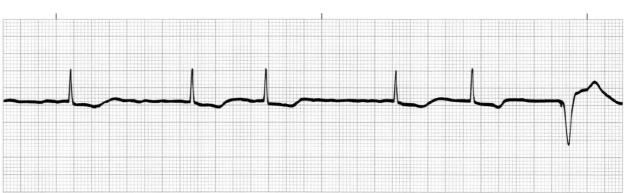

Strip 10.42 Analysis: _____

Interpretation: _____

eleven

Posttest

Posttest: Arrhythmia Strips

Follow the five basic steps in analyzing a rhythm strip.
Interpret the rhythm by comparing this data with the ECG
characteristics for each rhythm.

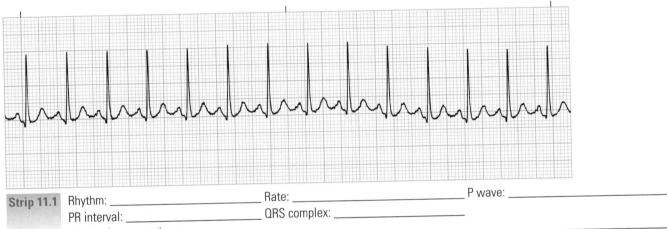

Strip 11.1 Rhythm: _____ Rate: _____ P wave: _____
PR interval: _____ QRS complex: _____
Rhythm interpretation: _____

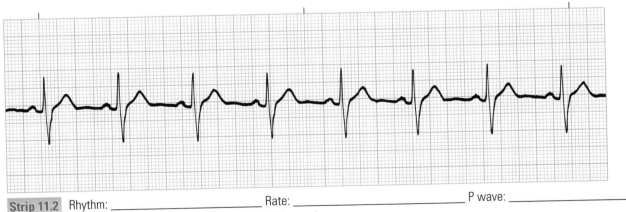

Strip 11.2 Rhythm: _____ Rate: _____ P wave: _____
PR interval: _____ QRS complex: _____
Rhythm interpretation: _____

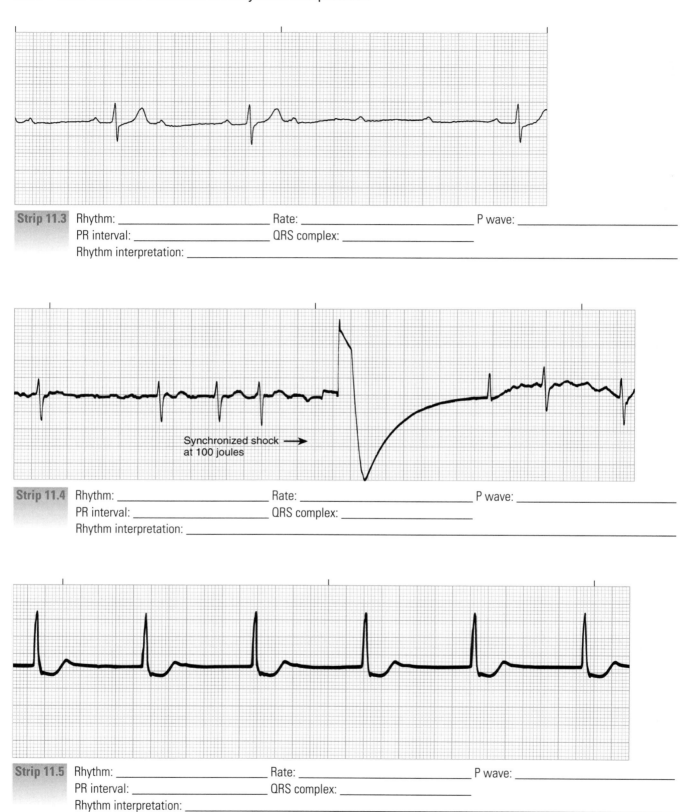

Strip 11.3 Rhythm: _____ Rate: _____ P wave: _____
PR interval: _____ QRS complex: _____
Rhythm interpretation: _____

Strip 11.4 Rhythm: _____ Rate: _____ P wave: _____
PR interval: _____ QRS complex: _____
Rhythm interpretation: _____

Strip 11.5 Rhythm: _____ Rate: _____ P wave: _____
PR interval: _____ QRS complex: _____
Rhythm interpretation: _____

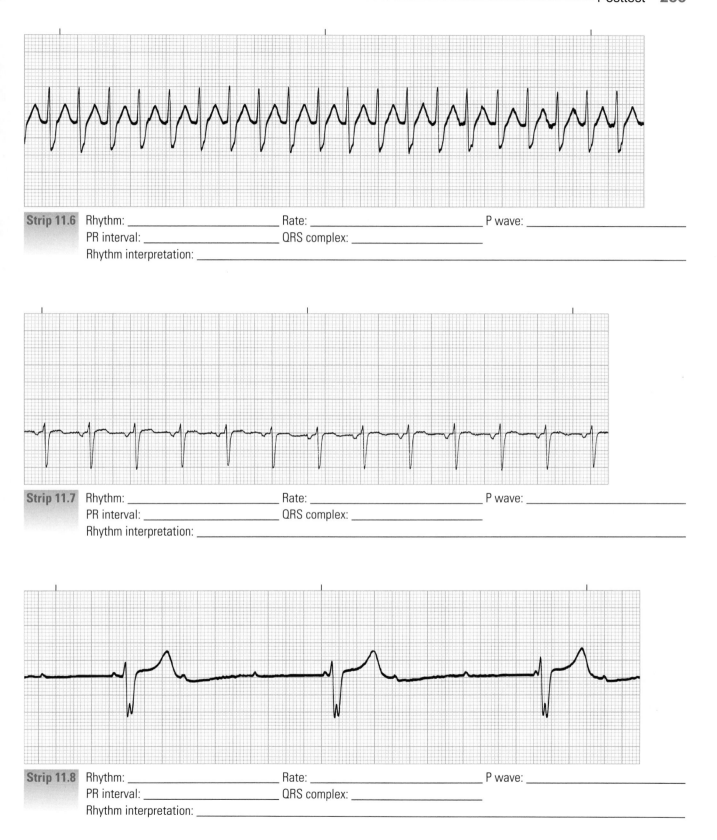

Strip 11.6 Rhythm: _____ Rate: _____ P wave: _____
PR interval: _____ QRS complex: _____
Rhythm interpretation: _____

Strip 11.7 Rhythm: _____ Rate: _____ P wave: _____
PR interval: _____ QRS complex: _____
Rhythm interpretation: _____

Strip 11.8 Rhythm: _____ Rate: _____ P wave: _____
PR interval: _____ QRS complex: _____
Rhythm interpretation: _____

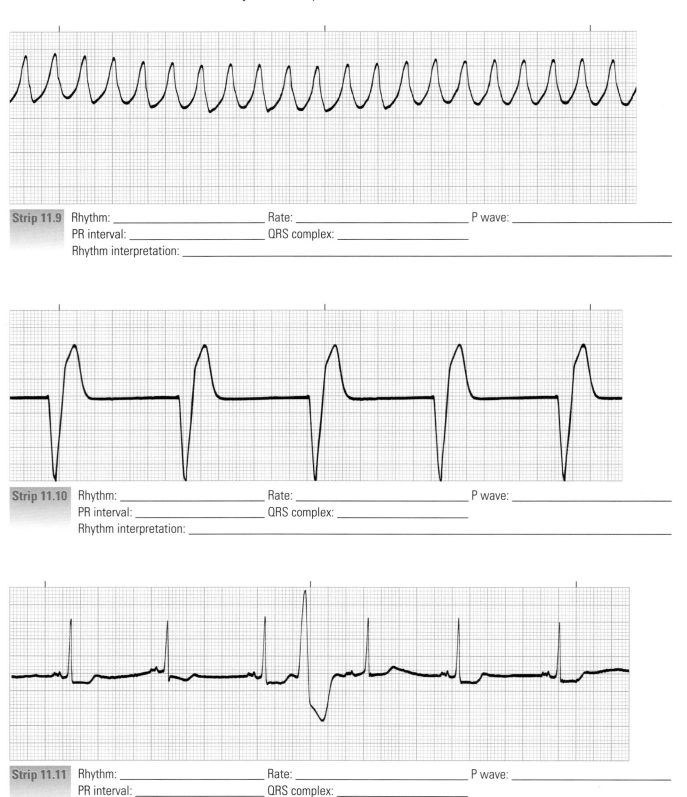

Strip 11.9   Rhythm: _____ Rate: _____ P wave: _____
PR interval: _____ QRS complex: _____
Rhythm interpretation: _____

Strip 11.10   Rhythm: _____ Rate: _____ P wave: _____
PR interval: _____ QRS complex: _____
Rhythm interpretation: _____

Strip 11.11   Rhythm: _____ Rate: _____ P wave: _____
PR interval: _____ QRS complex: _____
Rhythm interpretation: _____

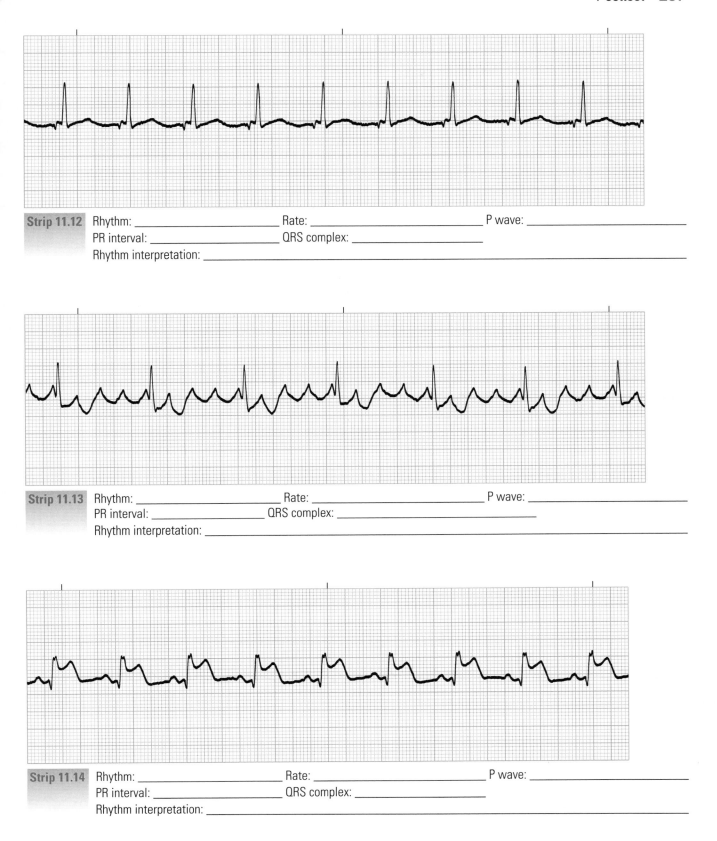

Strip 11.12 Rhythm: _____ Rate: _____ P wave: _____
PR interval: _____ QRS complex: _____
Rhythm interpretation: _____

Strip 11.13 Rhythm: _____ Rate: _____ P wave: _____
PR interval: _____ QRS complex: _____
Rhythm interpretation: _____

Strip 11.14 Rhythm: _____ Rate: _____ P wave: _____
PR interval: _____ QRS complex: _____
Rhythm interpretation: _____

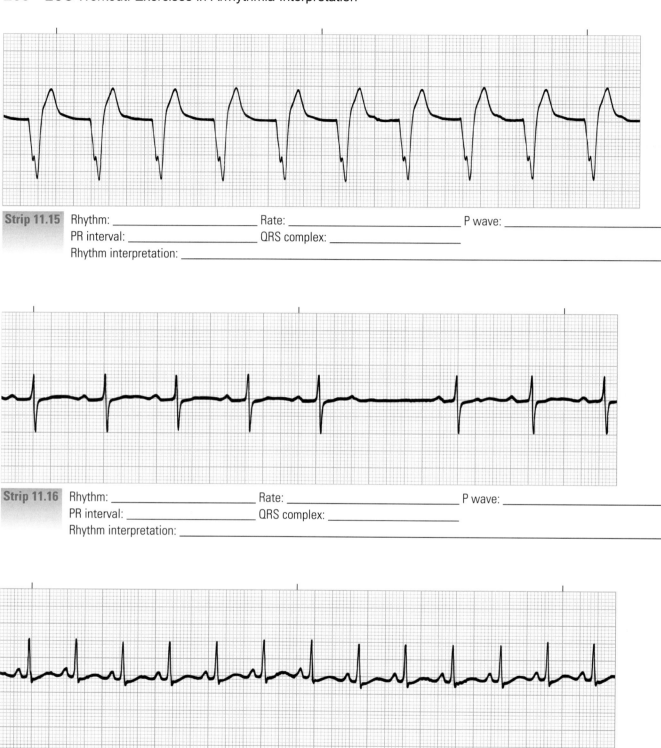

Strip 11.15   Rhythm: _____ Rate: _____ P wave: _____
PR interval: _____ QRS complex: _____
Rhythm interpretation: _____

Strip 11.16   Rhythm: _____ Rate: _____ P wave: _____
PR interval: _____ QRS complex: _____
Rhythm interpretation: _____

Strip 11.17   Rhythm: _____ Rate: _____ P wave: _____
PR interval: _____ QRS complex: _____
Rhythm interpretation: _____

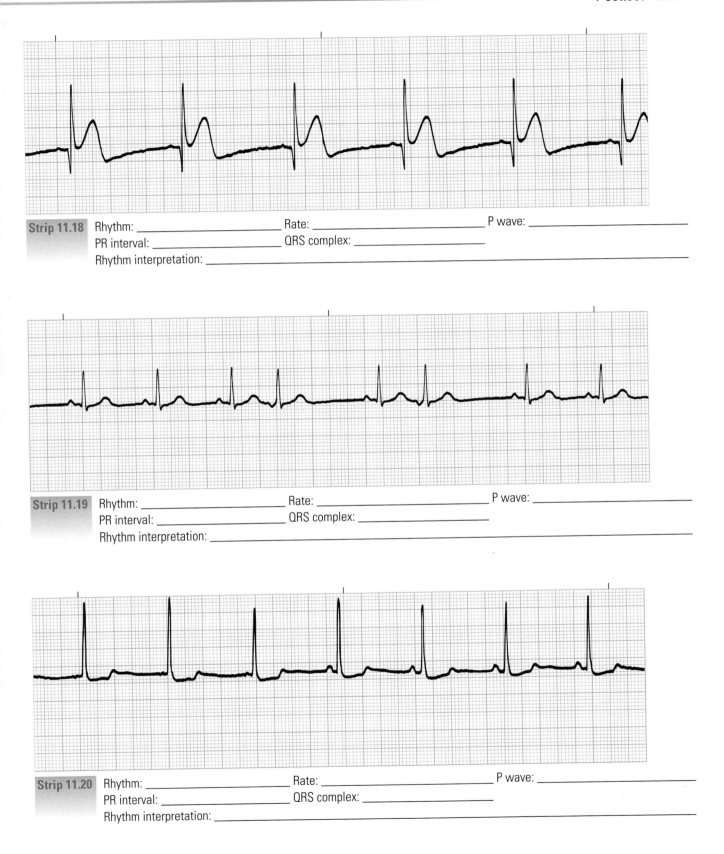

Strip 11.18 Rhythm: _____ Rate: _____ P wave: _____
PR interval: _____ QRS complex: _____
Rhythm interpretation: _____

Strip 11.19 Rhythm: _____ Rate: _____ P wave: _____
PR interval: _____ QRS complex: _____
Rhythm interpretation: _____

Strip 11.20 Rhythm: _____ Rate: _____ P wave: _____
PR interval: _____ QRS complex: _____
Rhythm interpretation: _____

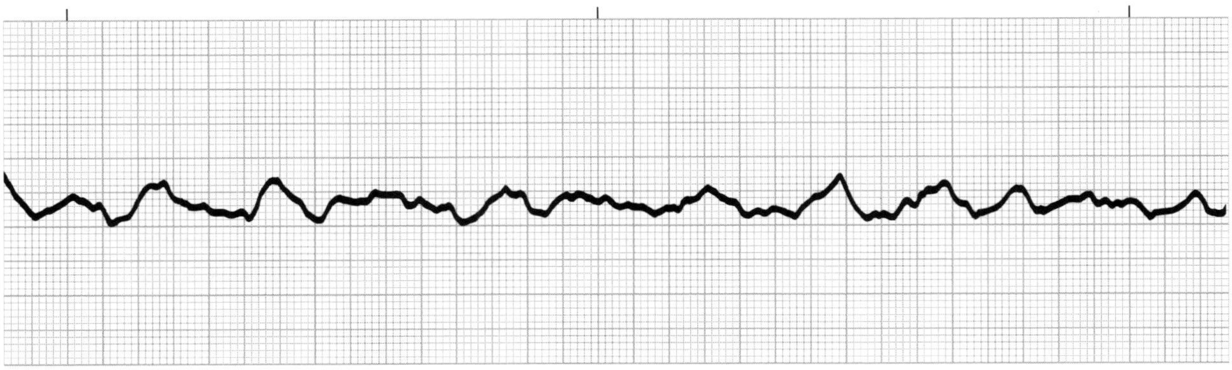

Strip 11.21 Rhythm: _____ Rate: _____ P wave: _____

PR interval: _____ QRS complex: _____

Rhythm interpretation: _____

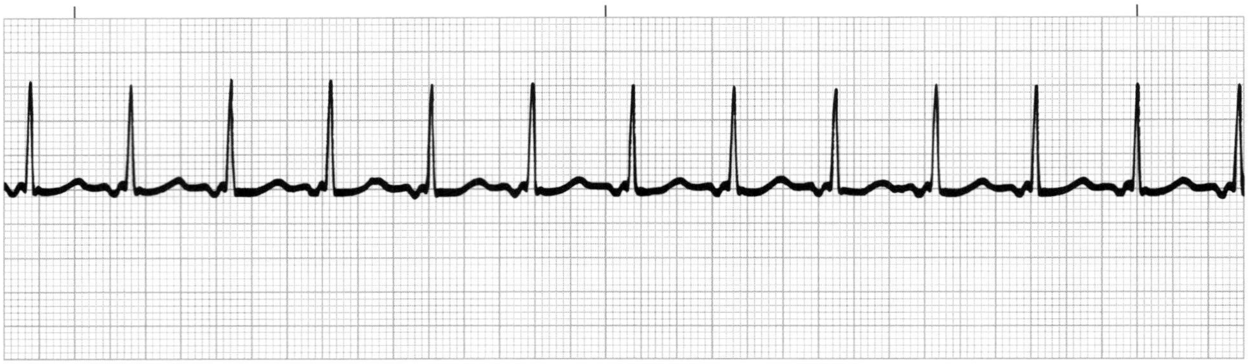

Strip 11.22 Rhythm: _____ Rate: _____ P wave: _____

PR interval: _____ QRS complex: _____

Rhythm interpretation: _____

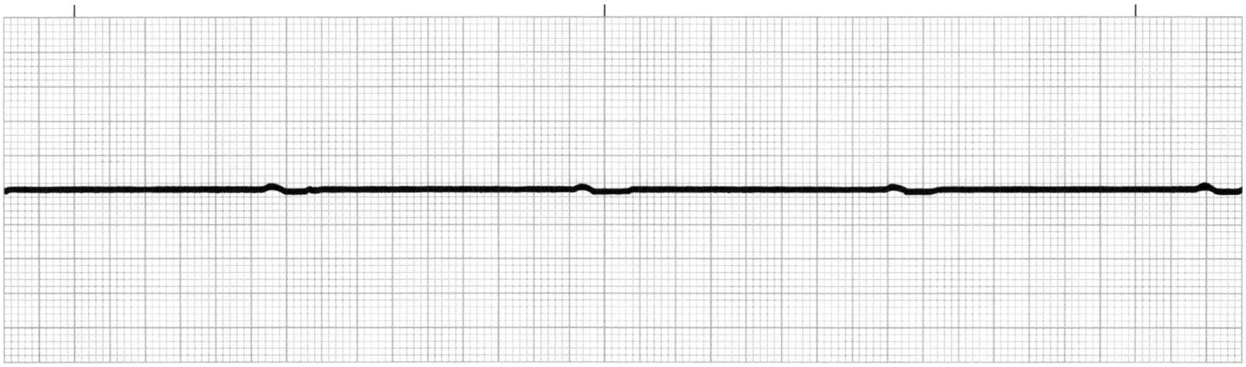

Strip 11.23 Rhythm: _____ Rate: _____ P wave: _____

PR interval: _____ QRS complex: _____

Rhythm interpretation: _____

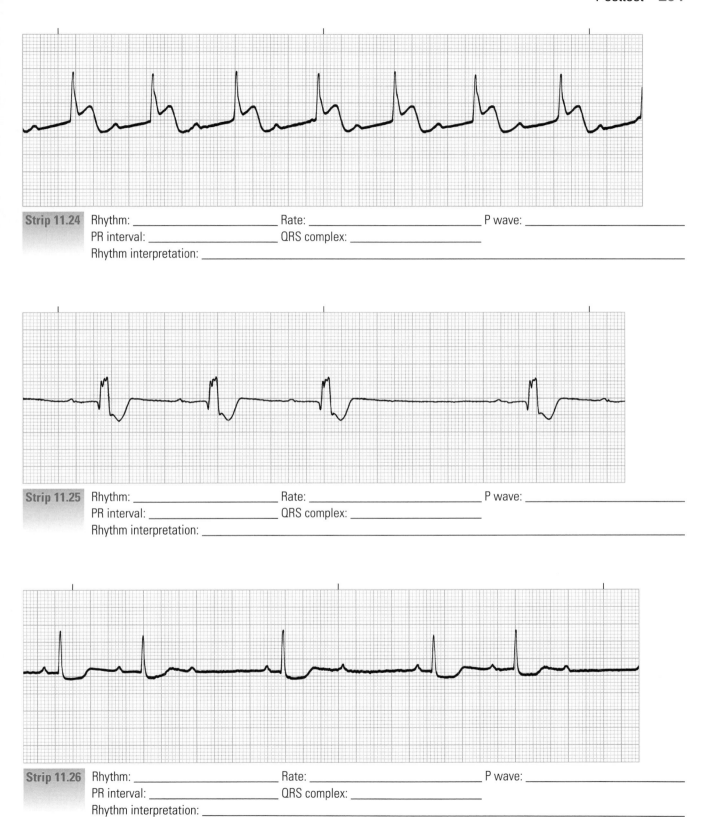

Strip 11.24 Rhythm: _____ Rate: _____ P wave: _____
PR interval: _____ QRS complex: _____
Rhythm interpretation: _____

Strip 11.25 Rhythm: _____ Rate: _____ P wave: _____
PR interval: _____ QRS complex: _____
Rhythm interpretation: _____

Strip 11.26 Rhythm: _____ Rate: _____ P wave: _____
PR interval: _____ QRS complex: _____
Rhythm interpretation: _____

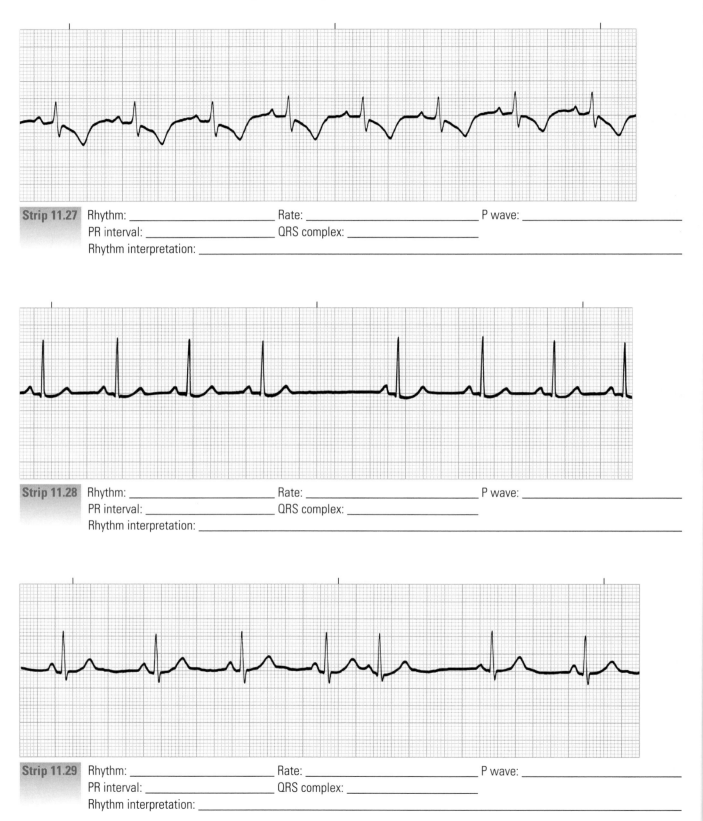

Strip 11.27
Rhythm: _____ Rate: _____ P wave: _____

PR interval: _____ QRS complex: _____

Rhythm interpretation: _____

Strip 11.28
Rhythm: _____ Rate: _____ P wave: _____

PR interval: _____ QRS complex: _____

Rhythm interpretation: _____

Strip 11.29
Rhythm: _____ Rate: _____ P wave: _____

PR interval: _____ QRS complex: _____

Rhythm interpretation: _____

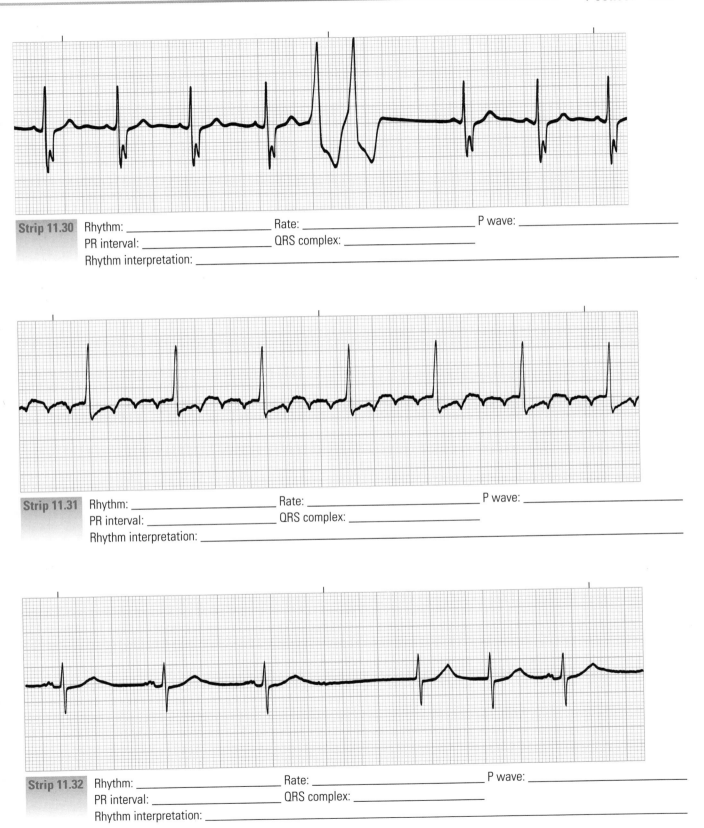

Strip 11.30 Rhythm: _____ Rate: _____ P wave: _____
PR interval: _____ QRS complex: _____
Rhythm interpretation: _____

Strip 11.31 Rhythm: _____ Rate: _____ P wave: _____
PR interval: _____ QRS complex: _____
Rhythm interpretation: _____

Strip 11.32 Rhythm: _____ Rate: _____ P wave: _____
PR interval: _____ QRS complex: _____
Rhythm interpretation: _____

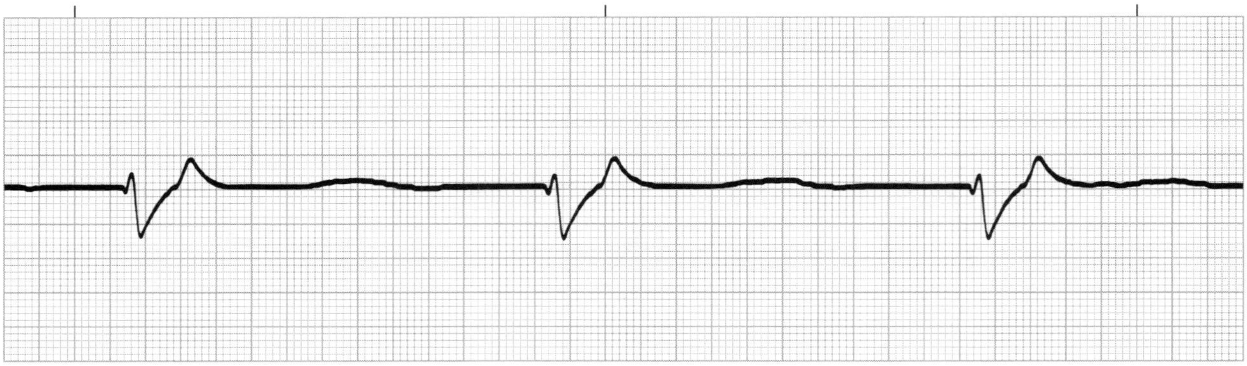

Strip 11.33 Rhythm: _____ Rate: _____ P wave: _____
PR interval: _____ QRS complex: _____
Rhythm interpretation: _____

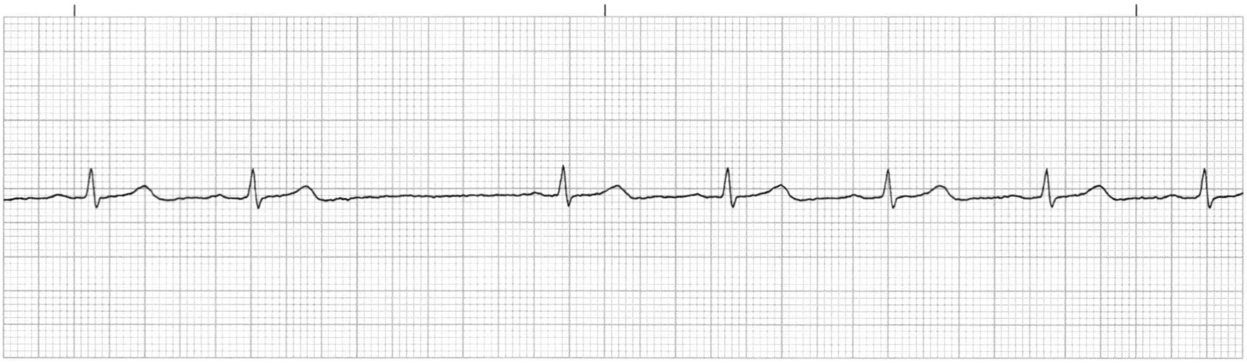

Strip 11.34 Rhythm: _____ Rate: _____ P wave: _____
PR interval: _____ QRS complex: _____
Rhythm interpretation: _____

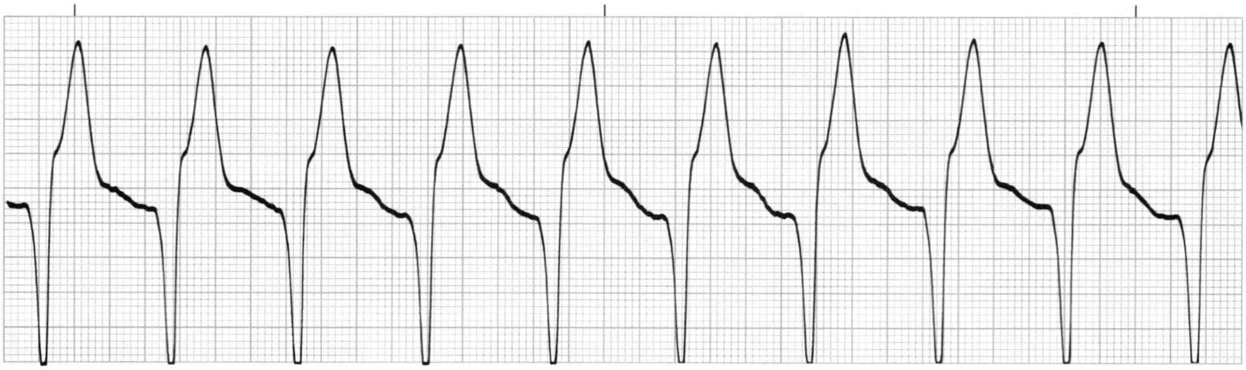

Strip 11.35 Rhythm: _____ Rate: _____ P wave: _____
PR interval: _____ QRS complex: _____
Rhythm interpretation: _____

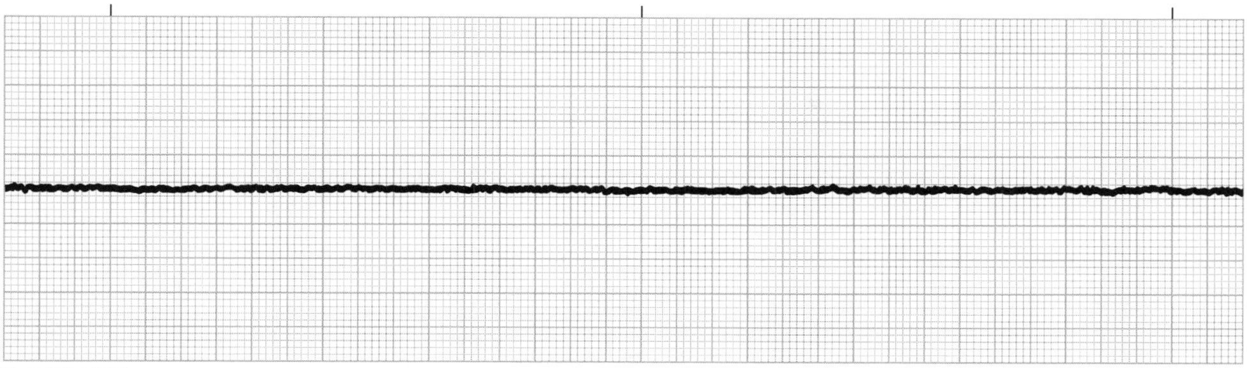

Strip 11.36 Rhythm: _____ Rate: _____ P wave: _____
PR interval: _____ QRS complex: _____
Rhythm interpretation: _____

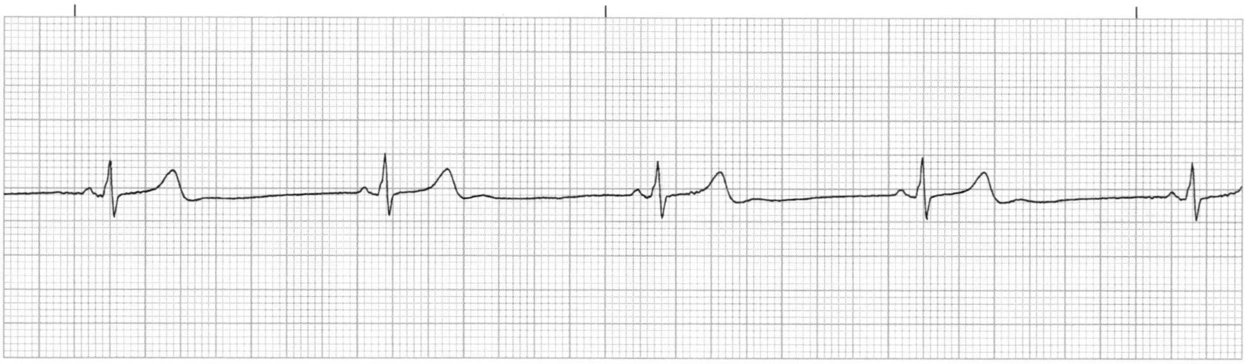

Strip 11.37 Rhythm: _____ Rate: _____ P wave: _____
PR interval: _____ QRS complex: _____
Rhythm interpretation: _____

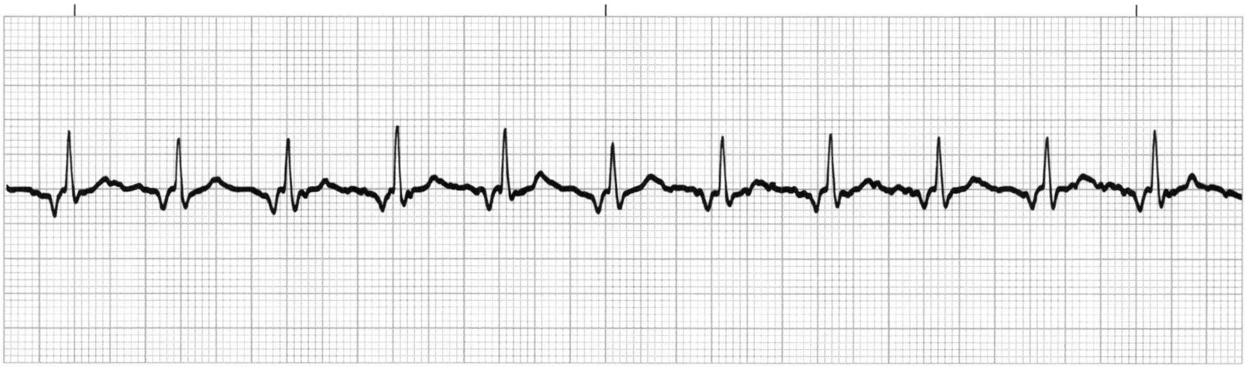

Strip 11.38 Rhythm: _____ Rate: _____ P wave: _____
PR interval: _____ QRS complex: _____
Rhythm interpretation: _____

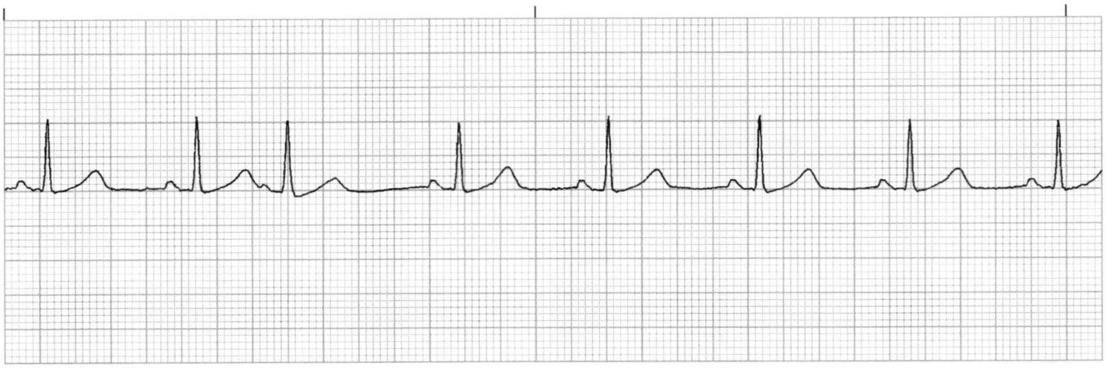

Strip 11.39
Rhythm: _____ Rate: _____ P wave: _____
PR interval: _____ QRS complex: _____
Rhythm interpretation: _____

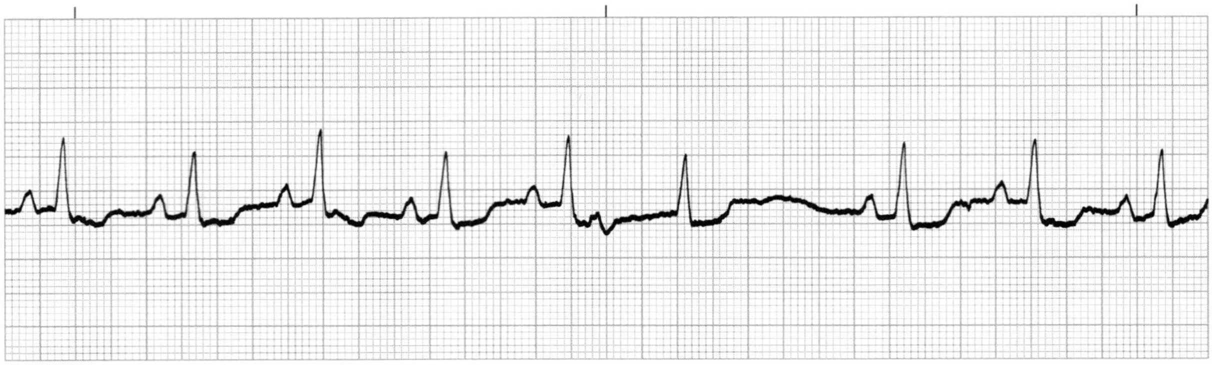

Strip 11.40
Rhythm: _____ Rate: _____ P wave: _____
PR interval: _____ QRS complex: _____
Rhythm interpretation: _____

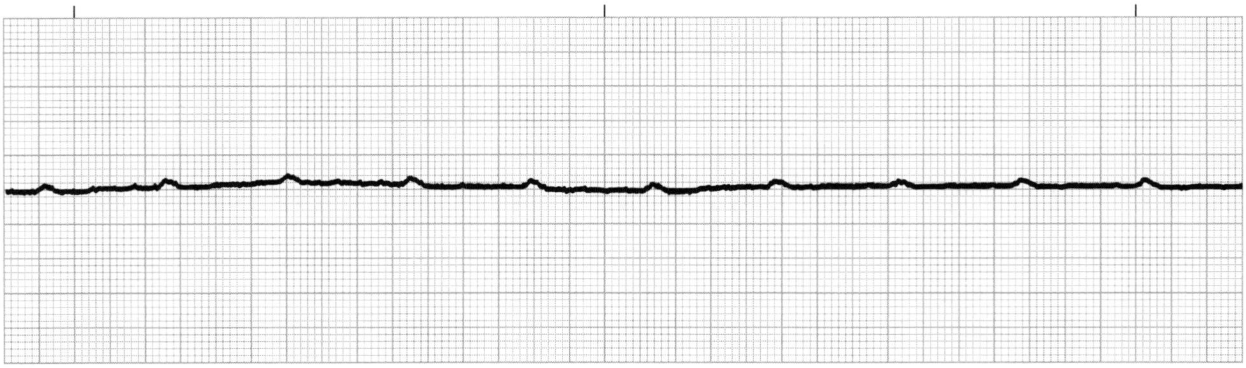

Strip 11.41
Rhythm: _____ Rate: _____ P wave: _____
PR interval: _____ QRS complex: _____
Rhythm interpretation: _____

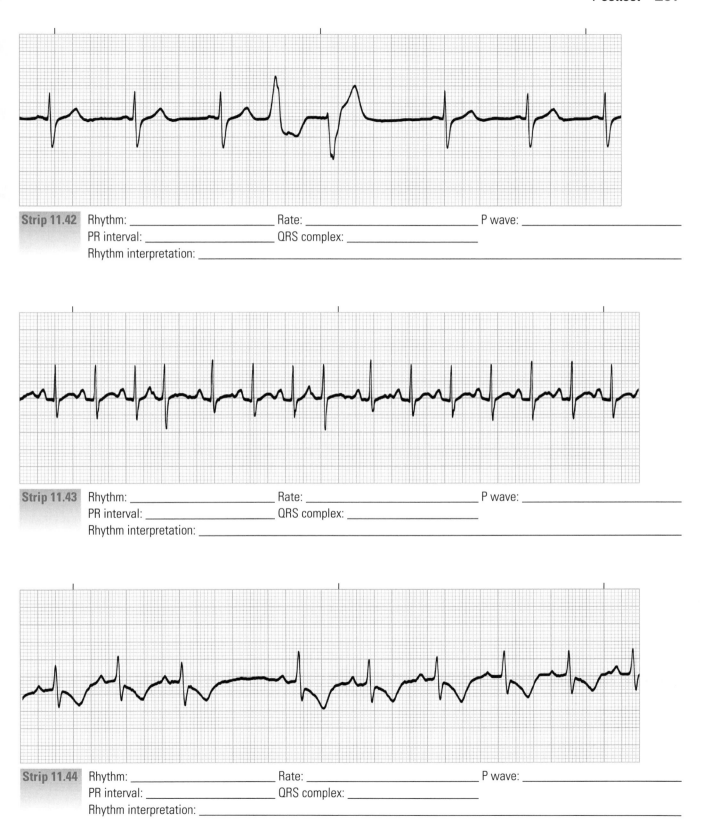

Strip 11.42 Rhythm: _____ Rate: _____ P wave: _____
PR interval: _____ QRS complex: _____
Rhythm interpretation: _____

Strip 11.43 Rhythm: _____ Rate: _____ P wave: _____
PR interval: _____ QRS complex: _____
Rhythm interpretation: _____

Strip 11.44 Rhythm: _____ Rate: _____ P wave: _____
PR interval: _____ QRS complex: _____
Rhythm interpretation: _____

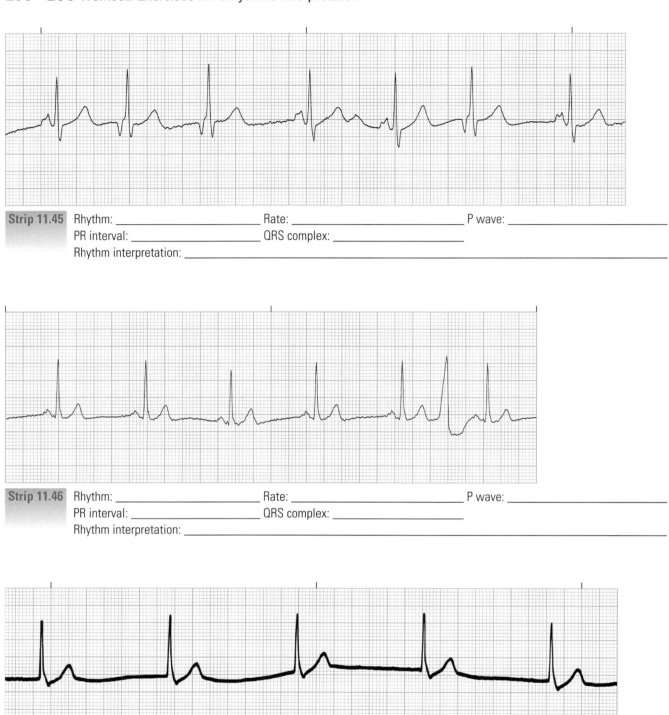

Strip 11.45 Rhythm: _____ Rate: _____ P wave: _____
PR interval: _____ QRS complex: _____
Rhythm interpretation: _____

Strip 11.46 Rhythm: _____ Rate: _____ P wave: _____
PR interval: _____ QRS complex: _____
Rhythm interpretation: _____

Strip 11.47 Rhythm: _____ Rate: _____ P wave: _____
PR interval: _____ QRS complex: _____
Rhythm interpretation: _____

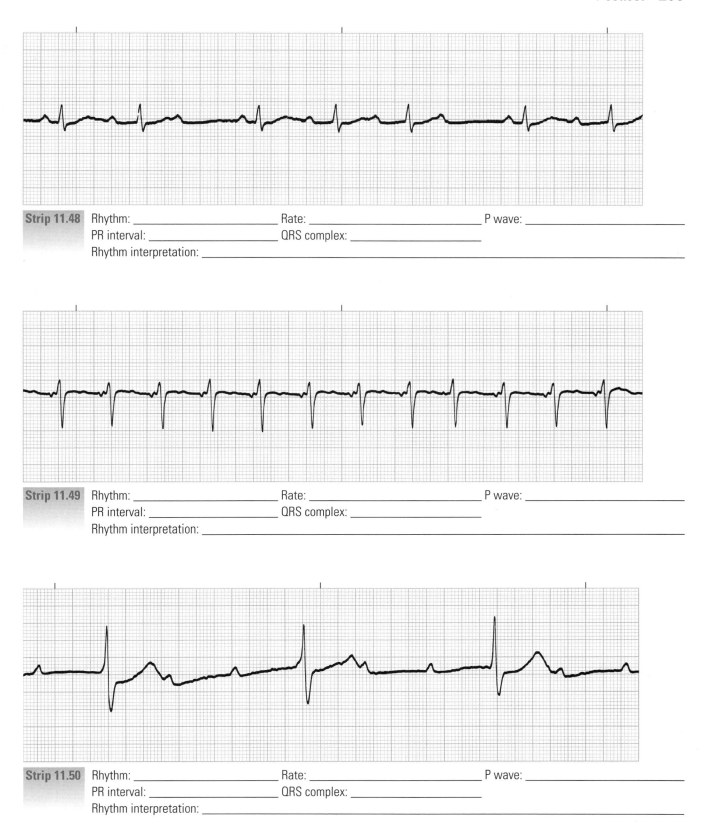

Strip 11.48 Rhythm: _____ Rate: _____ P wave: _____
PR interval: _____ QRS complex: _____
Rhythm interpretation: _____

Strip 11.49 Rhythm: _____ Rate: _____ P wave: _____
PR interval: _____ QRS complex: _____
Rhythm interpretation: _____

Strip 11.50 Rhythm: _____ Rate: _____ P wave: _____
PR interval: _____ QRS complex: _____
Rhythm interpretation: _____

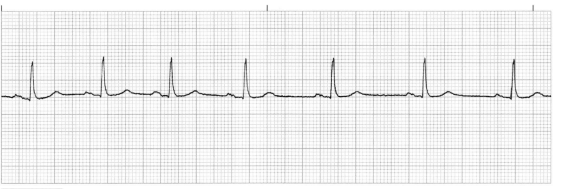

Strip 11.51   Rhythm: _____ Rate: _____ P wave: _____
PR interval: _____ QRS complex: _____
Rhythm interpretation: _____

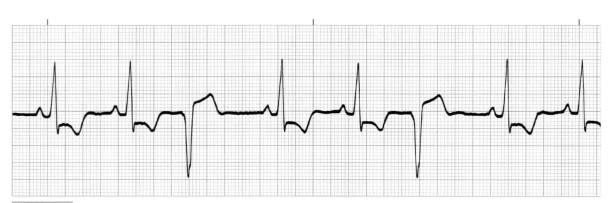

Strip 11.52   Rhythm: _____ Rate: _____ P wave: _____
PR interval: _____ QRS complex: _____
Rhythm interpretation: _____

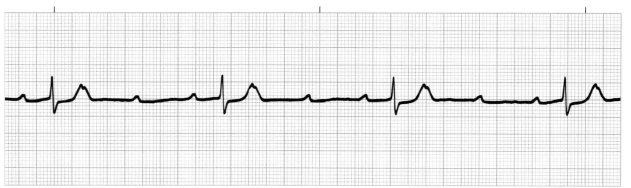

Strip 11.53   Rhythm: _____ Rate: _____ P wave: _____
PR interval: _____ QRS complex: _____
Rhythm interpretation: _____

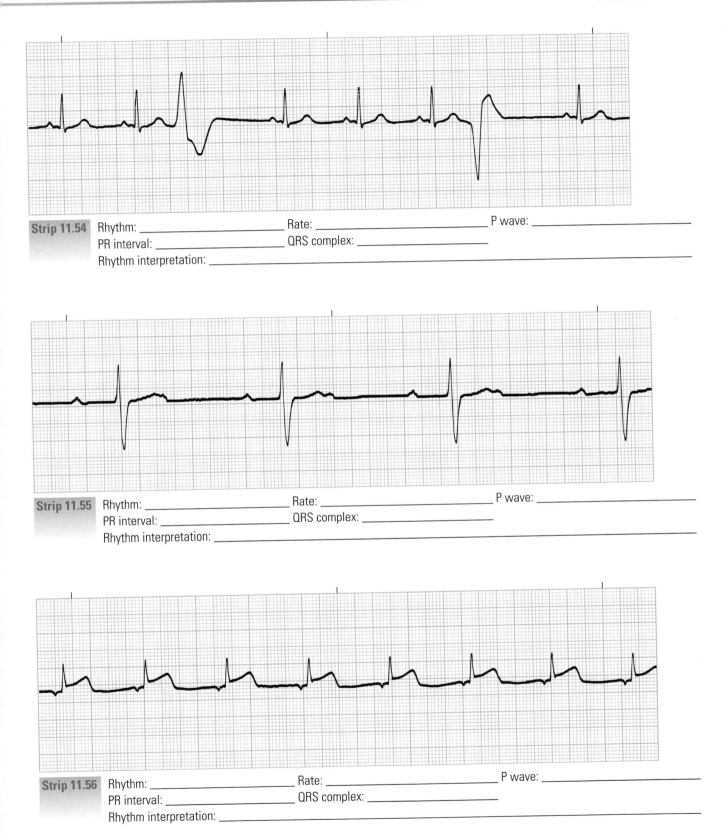

Strip 11.54   Rhythm: _____   Rate: _____   P wave: _____
PR interval: _____   QRS complex: _____
Rhythm interpretation: _____

Strip 11.55   Rhythm: _____   Rate: _____   P wave: _____
PR interval: _____   QRS complex: _____
Rhythm interpretation: _____

Strip 11.56   Rhythm: _____   Rate: _____   P wave: _____
PR interval: _____   QRS complex: _____
Rhythm interpretation: _____

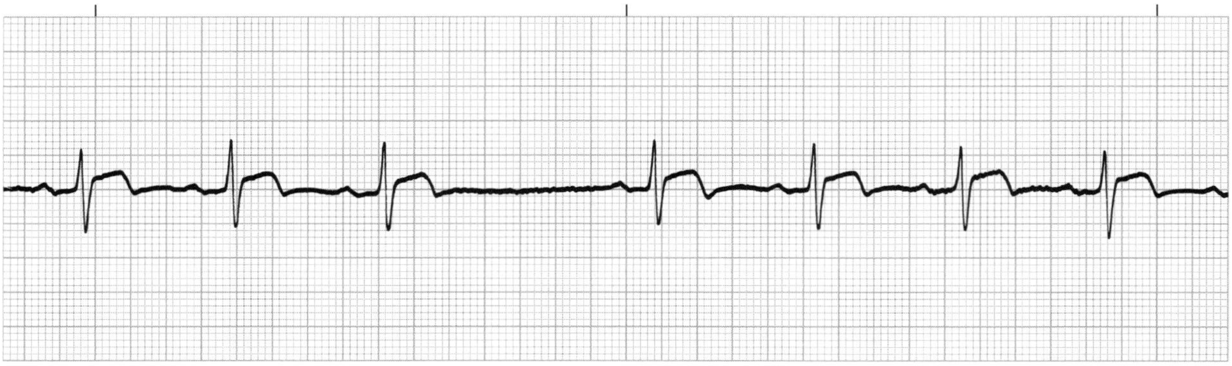

Strip 11.57 Rhythm: _____ Rate: _____ P wave: _____
PR interval: _____ QRS complex: _____
Rhythm interpretation: _____

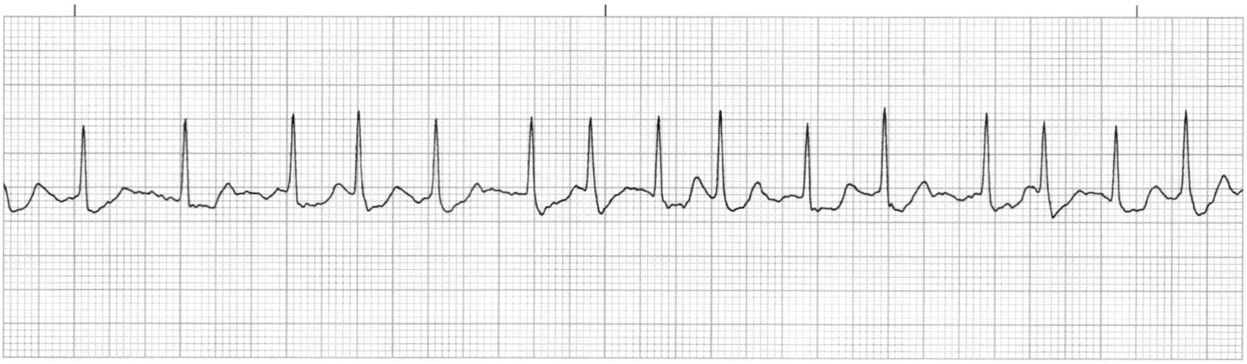

Strip 11.58 Rhythm: _____ Rate: _____ P wave: _____
PR interval: _____ QRS complex: _____
Rhythm interpretation: _____

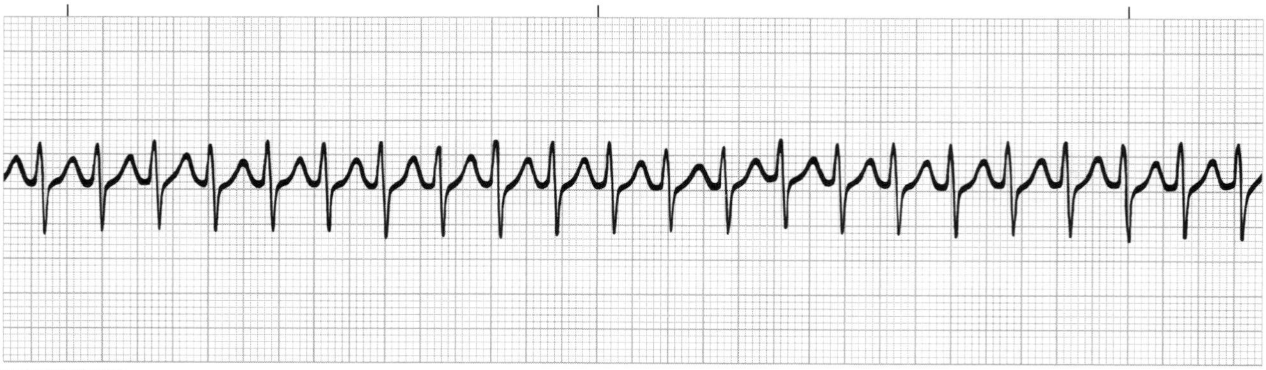

Strip 11.59 Rhythm: _____ Rate: _____ P wave: _____
PR interval: _____ QRS complex: _____
Rhythm interpretation: _____

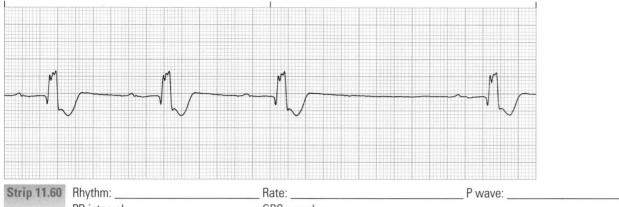

Strip 11.60 Rhythm: _____ Rate: _____ P wave: _____

PR interval: _____ QRS complex: _____

Rhythm interpretation: _____

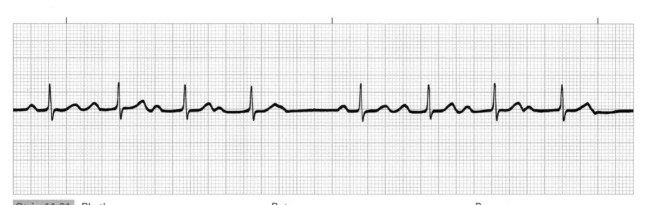

Strip 11.61 Rhythm: _____ Rate: _____ P wave: _____

PR interval: _____ QRS complex: _____

Rhythm interpretation: _____

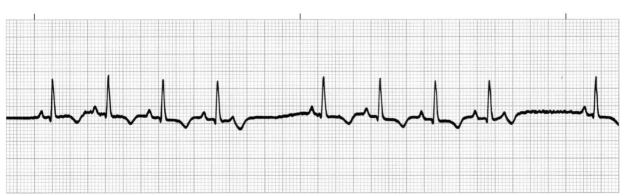

Strip 11.62 Rhythm: _____ Rate: _____ P wave: _____

PR interval: _____ QRS complex: _____

Rhythm interpretation: _____

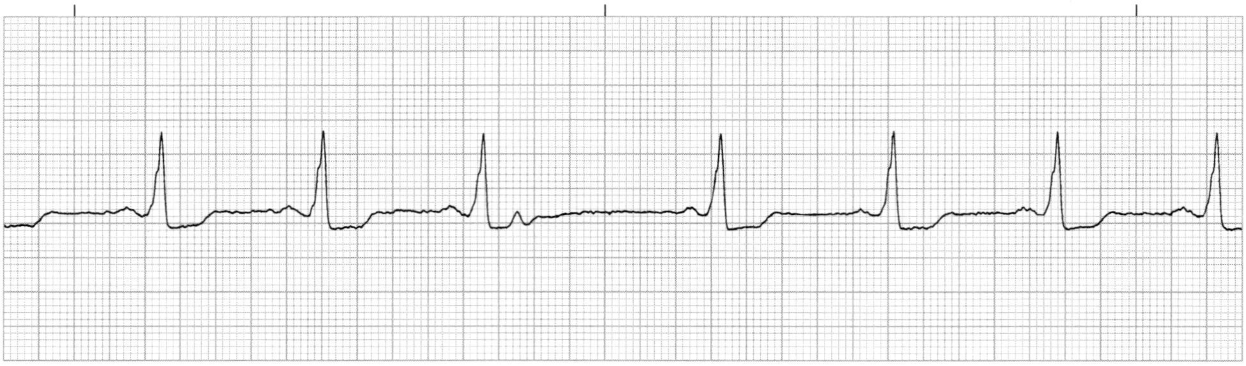

Strip 11.63 Rhythm: _____ Rate: _____ P wave: _____

PR interval: _____ QRS complex: _____

Rhythm interpretation: _____

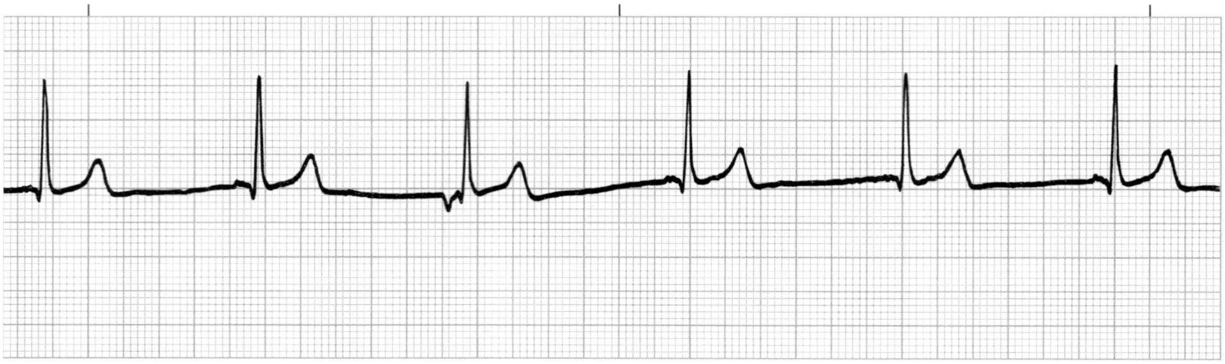

Strip 11.64 Rhythm: _____ Rate: _____ P wave: _____

PR interval: _____ QRS complex: _____

Rhythm interpretation: _____

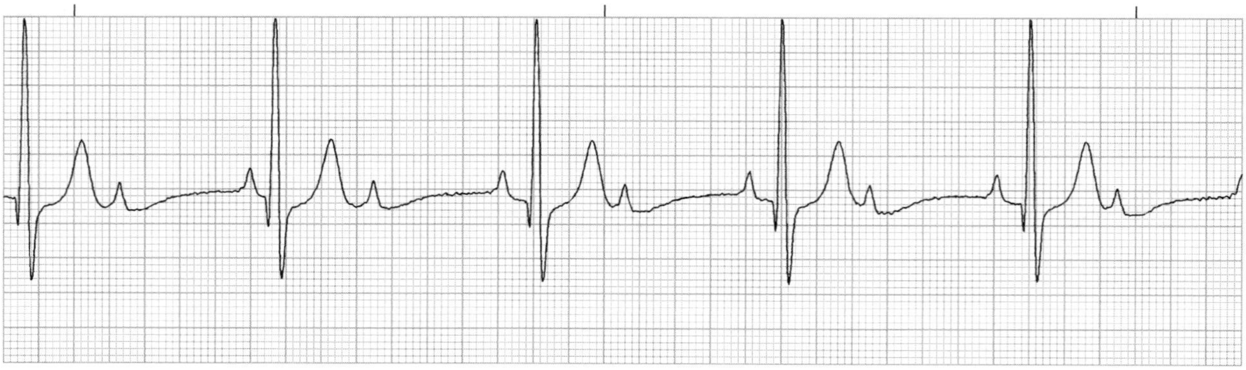

Strip 11.65 Rhythm: _____ Rate: _____ P wave: _____

PR interval: _____ QRS complex: _____

Rhythm interpretation: _____

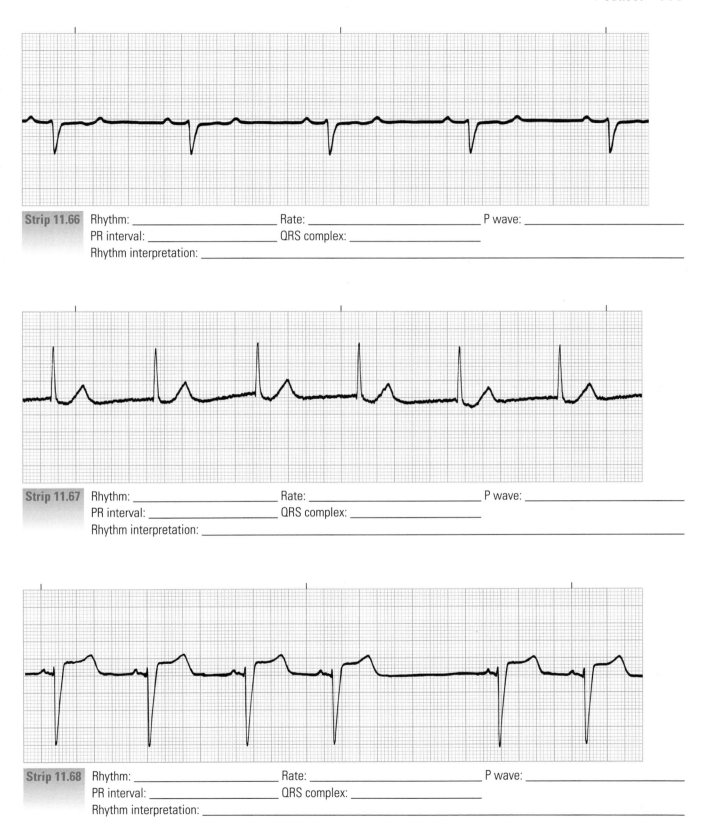

Strip 11.66 Rhythm: _____ Rate: _____ P wave: _____
PR interval: _____ QRS complex: _____
Rhythm interpretation: _____

Strip 11.67 Rhythm: _____ Rate: _____ P wave: _____
PR interval: _____ QRS complex: _____
Rhythm interpretation: _____

Strip 11.68 Rhythm: _____ Rate: _____ P wave: _____
PR interval: _____ QRS complex: _____
Rhythm interpretation: _____

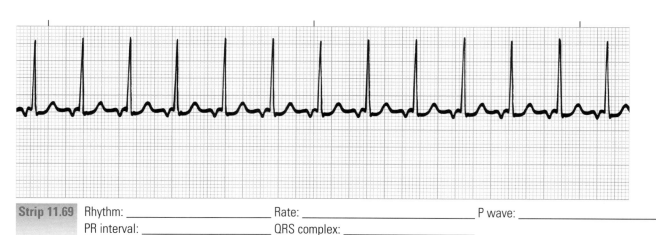

Strip 11.69 Rhythm: _____ Rate: _____ P wave: _____

PR interval: _____ QRS complex: _____

Rhythm interpretation: _____

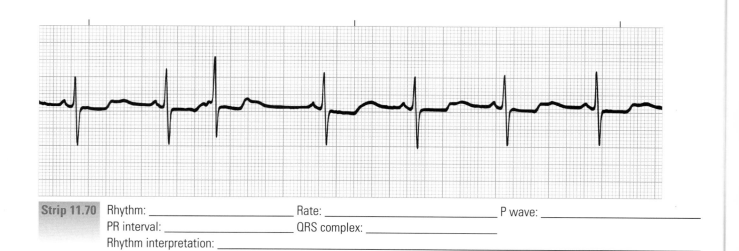

Strip 11.70 Rhythm: _____ Rate: _____ P wave: _____

PR interval: _____ QRS complex: _____

Rhythm interpretation: _____

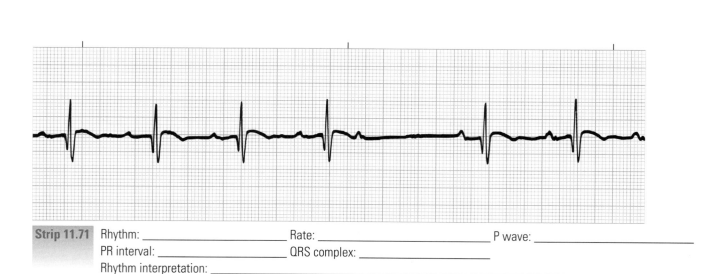

Strip 11.71 Rhythm: _____ Rate: _____ P wave: _____

PR interval: _____ QRS complex: _____

Rhythm interpretation: _____

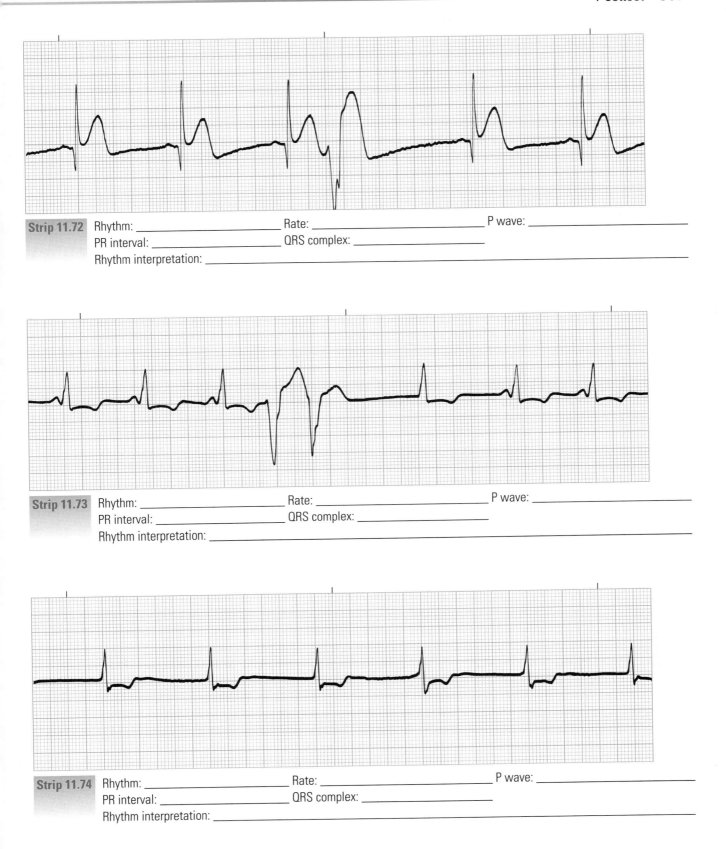

Strip 11.72 Rhythm: _____ Rate: _____ P wave: _____
PR interval: _____ QRS complex: _____
Rhythm interpretation: _____

Strip 11.73 Rhythm: _____ Rate: _____ P wave: _____
PR interval: _____ QRS complex: _____
Rhythm interpretation: _____

Strip 11.74 Rhythm: _____ Rate: _____ P wave: _____
PR interval: _____ QRS complex: _____
Rhythm interpretation: _____

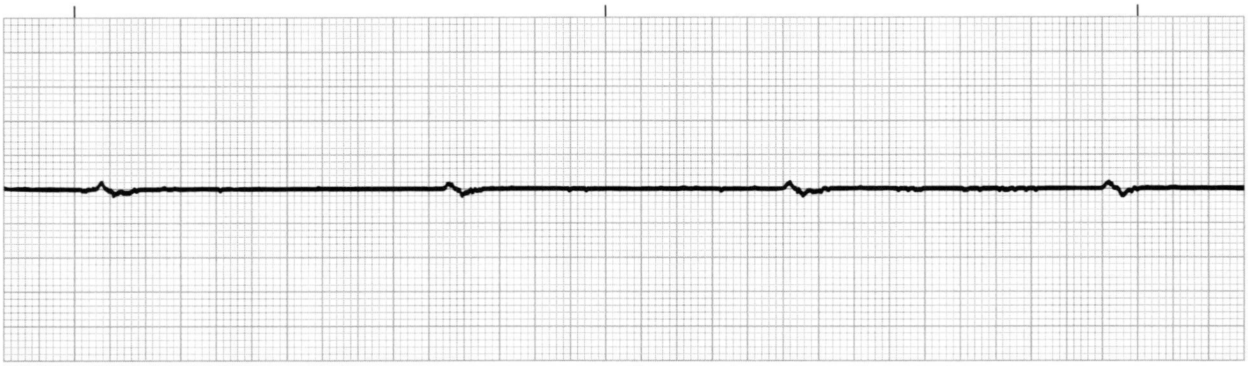

Strip 11.75 Rhythm: _____ Rate: _____ P wave: _____
PR interval: _____ QRS complex: _____
Rhythm interpretation: _____

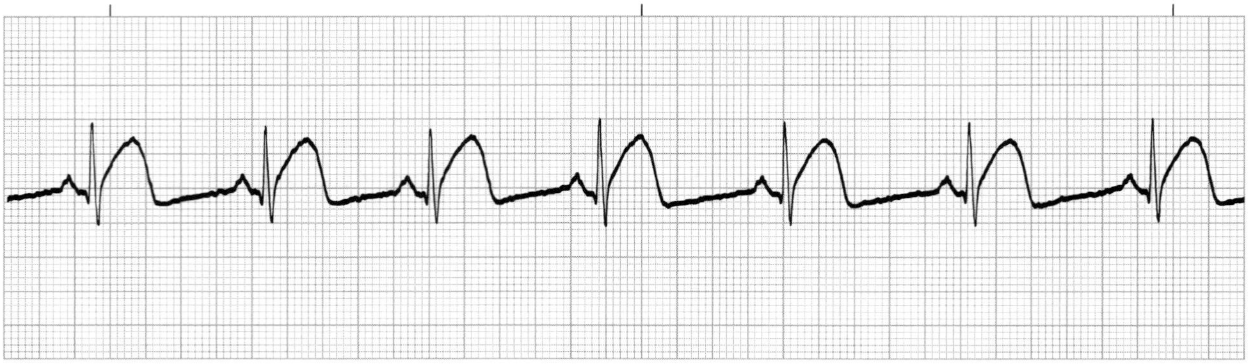

Strip 11.76 Rhythm: _____ Rate: _____ P wave: _____
PR interval: _____ QRS complex: _____
Rhythm interpretation: _____

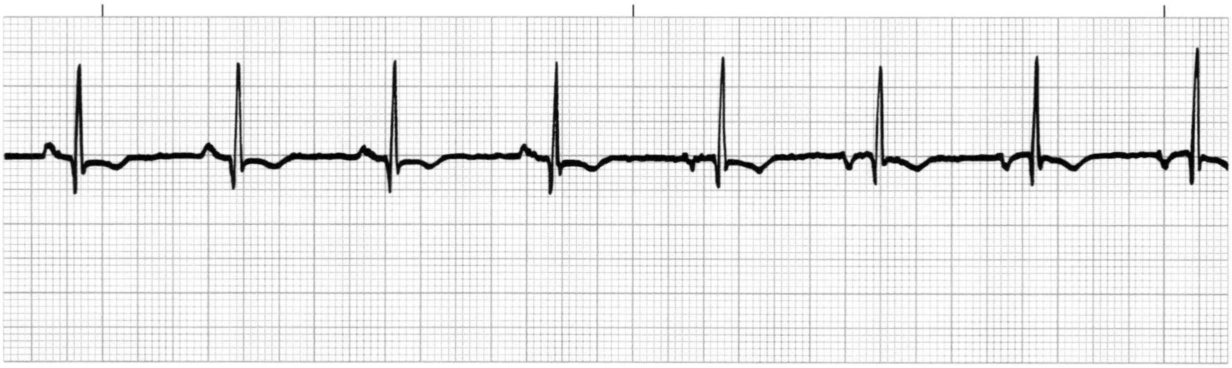

Strip 11.77 Rhythm: _____ Rate: _____ P wave: _____
PR interval: _____ QRS complex: _____
Rhythm interpretation: _____

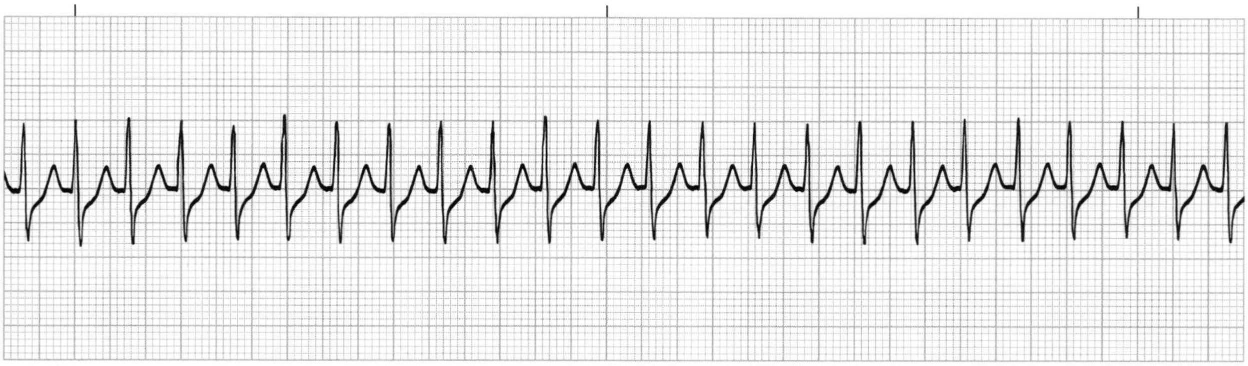

Strip 11.78 Rhythm: _____ Rate: _____ P wave: _____
PR interval: _____ QRS complex: _____
Rhythm interpretation: _____

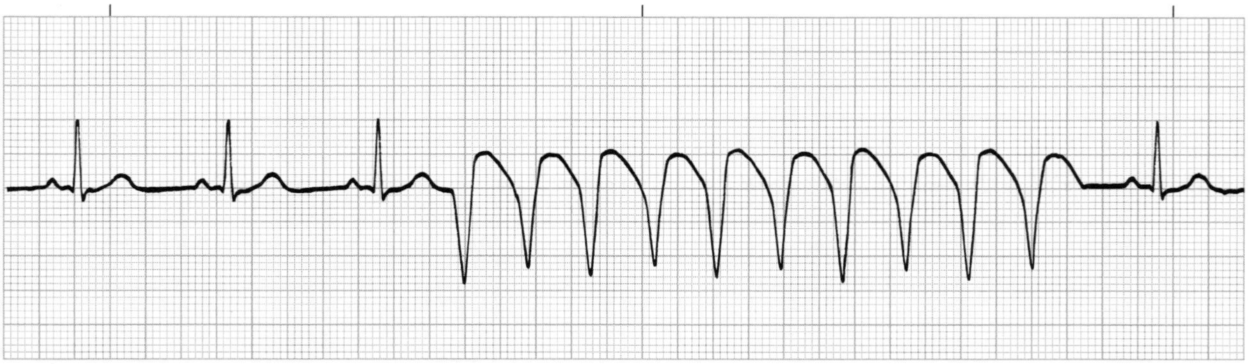

Strip 11.79 Rhythm: _____ Rate: _____ P wave: _____
PR interval: _____ QRS complex: _____
Rhythm interpretation: _____

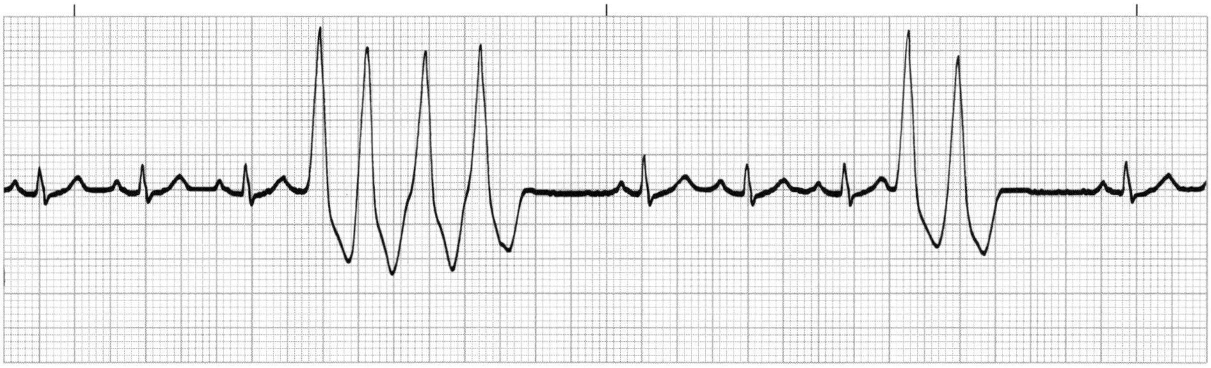

Strip 11.80 Rhythm: _____ Rate: _____ P wave: _____
PR interval: _____ QRS complex: _____
Rhythm interpretation: _____

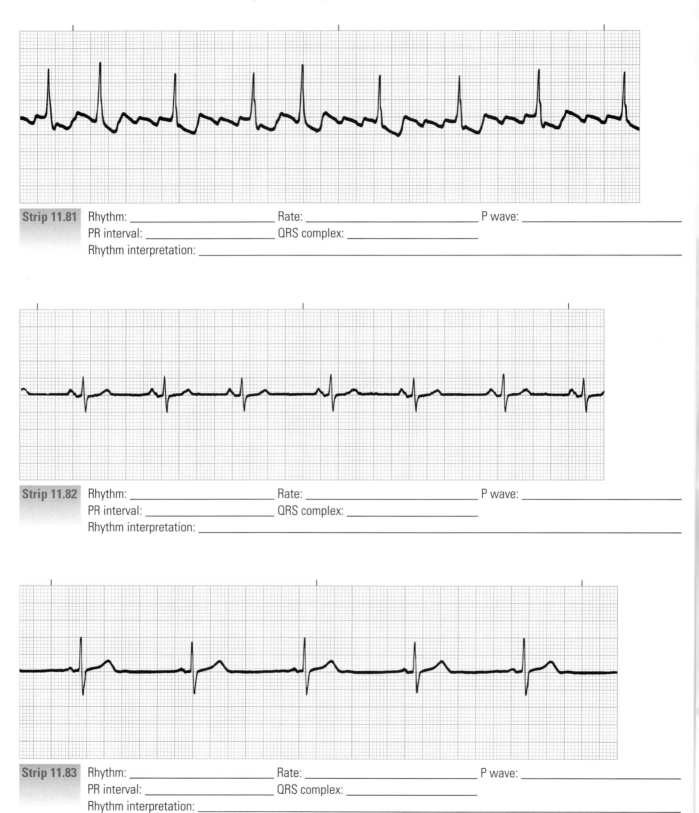

Strip 11.81 Rhythm: _____ Rate: _____ P wave: _____
PR interval: _____ QRS complex: _____
Rhythm interpretation: _____

Strip 11.82 Rhythm: _____ Rate: _____ P wave: _____
PR interval: _____ QRS complex: _____
Rhythm interpretation: _____

Strip 11.83 Rhythm: _____ Rate: _____ P wave: _____
PR interval: _____ QRS complex: _____
Rhythm interpretation: _____

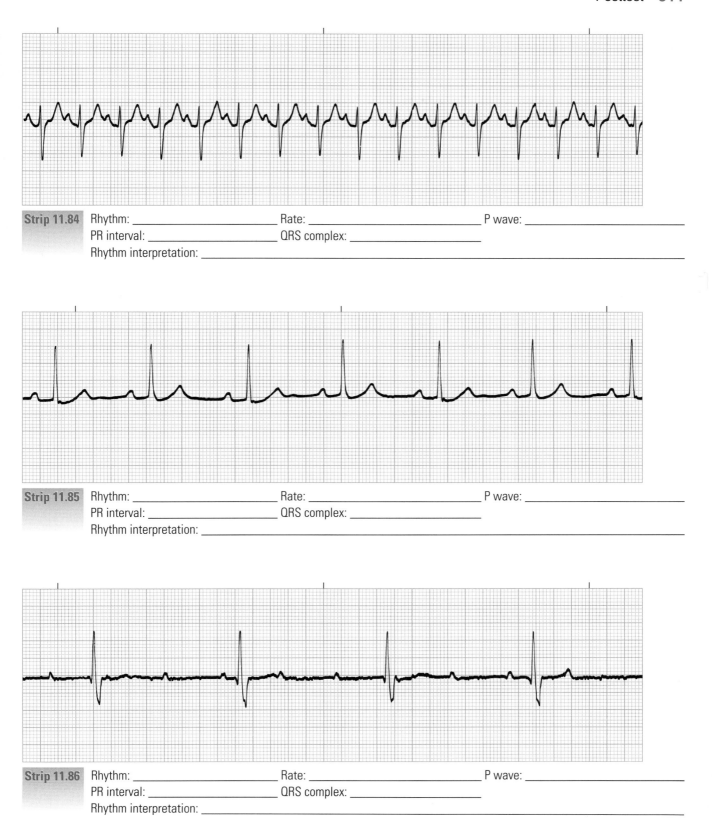

Strip 11.84   Rhythm: _____   Rate: _____   P wave: _____

PR interval: _____   QRS complex: _____

Rhythm interpretation: _____

Strip 11.85   Rhythm: _____   Rate: _____   P wave: _____

PR interval: _____   QRS complex: _____

Rhythm interpretation: _____

Strip 11.86   Rhythm: _____   Rate: _____   P wave: _____

PR interval: _____   QRS complex: _____

Rhythm interpretation: _____

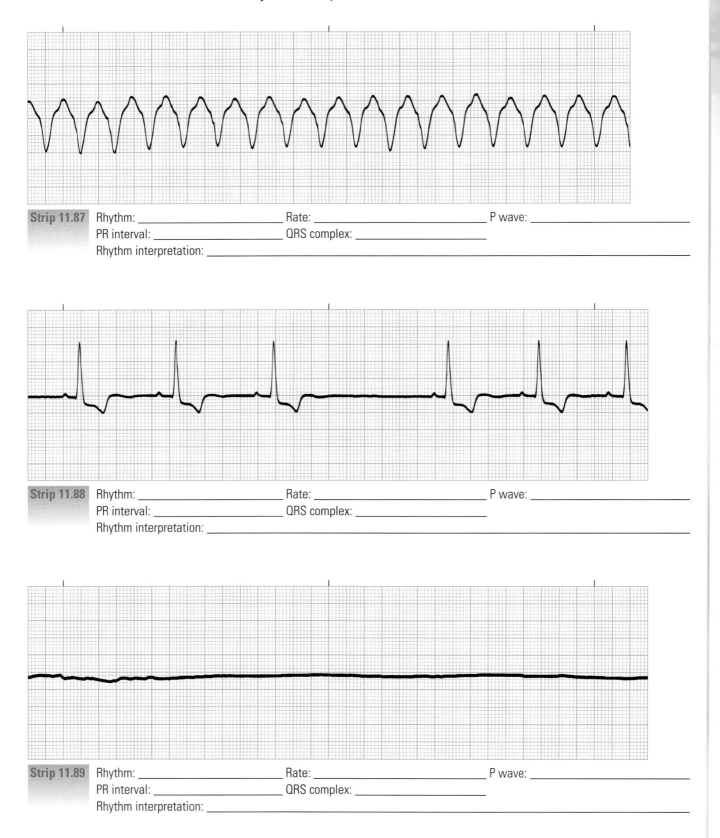

Strip 11.87 Rhythm: _____ Rate: _____ P wave: _____
PR interval: _____ QRS complex: _____
Rhythm interpretation: _____

Strip 11.88 Rhythm: _____ Rate: _____ P wave: _____
PR interval: _____ QRS complex: _____
Rhythm interpretation: _____

Strip 11.89 Rhythm: _____ Rate: _____ P wave: _____
PR interval: _____ QRS complex: _____
Rhythm interpretation: _____

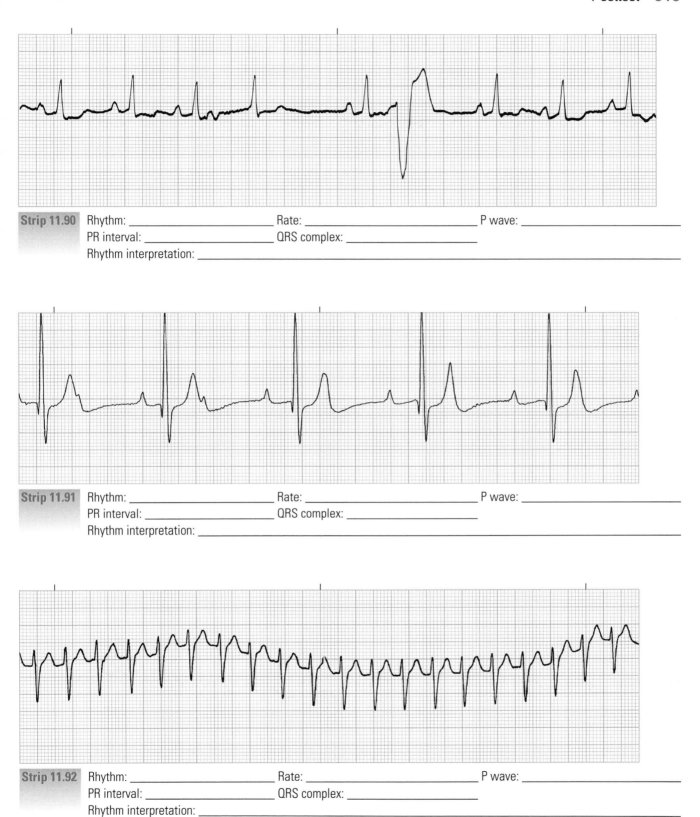

Strip 11.90 Rhythm: _____ Rate: _____ P wave: _____
PR interval: _____ QRS complex: _____
Rhythm interpretation: _____

Strip 11.91 Rhythm: _____ Rate: _____ P wave: _____
PR interval: _____ QRS complex: _____
Rhythm interpretation: _____

Strip 11.92 Rhythm: _____ Rate: _____ P wave: _____
PR interval: _____ QRS complex: _____
Rhythm interpretation: _____

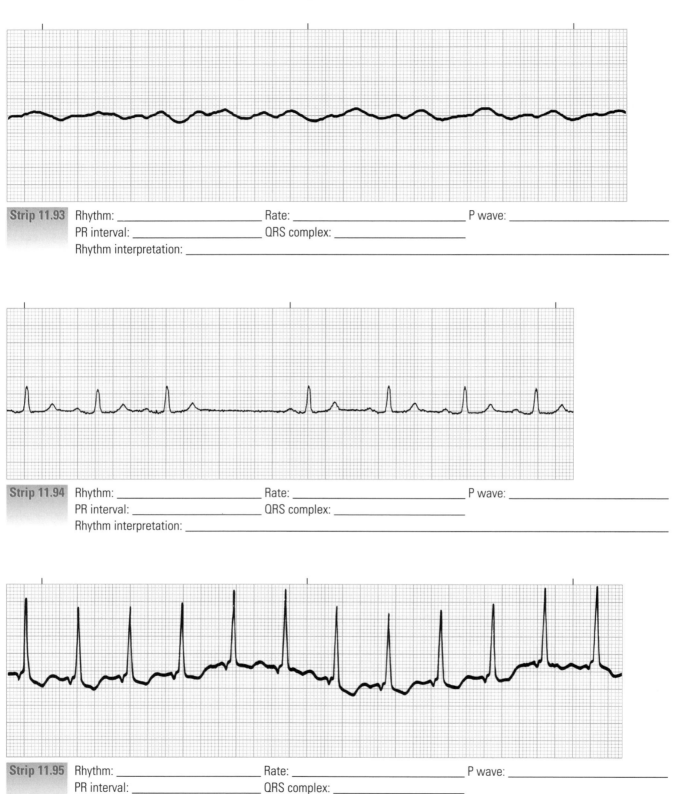

Strip 11.93   Rhythm: _____ Rate: _____ P wave: _____
PR interval: _____ QRS complex: _____
Rhythm interpretation: _____

Strip 11.94   Rhythm: _____ Rate: _____ P wave: _____
PR interval: _____ QRS complex: _____
Rhythm interpretation: _____

Strip 11.95   Rhythm: _____ Rate: _____ P wave: _____
PR interval: _____ QRS complex: _____
Rhythm interpretation: _____

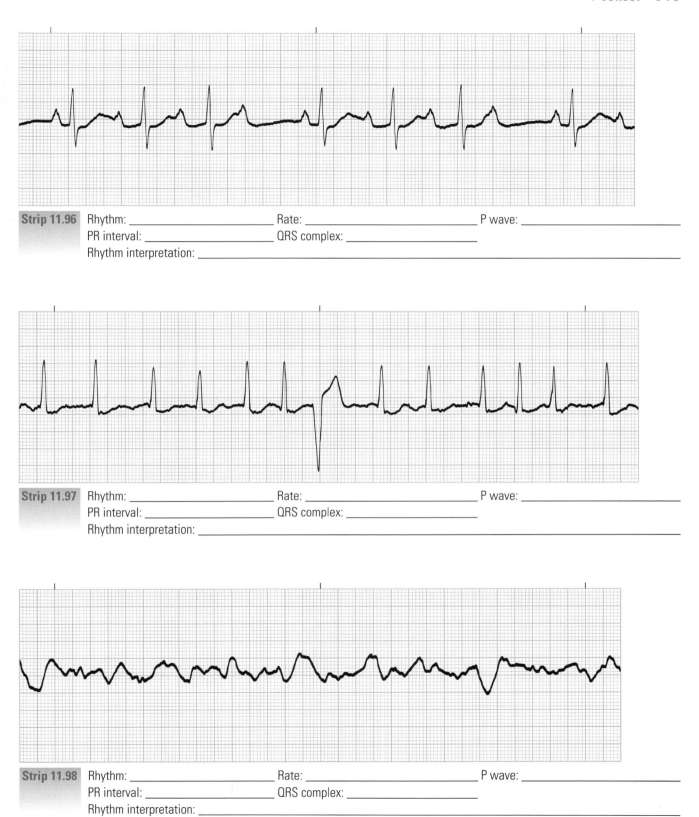

Strip 11.96 Rhythm: _____ Rate: _____ P wave: _____
PR interval: _____ QRS complex: _____
Rhythm interpretation: _____

Strip 11.97 Rhythm: _____ Rate: _____ P wave: _____
PR interval: _____ QRS complex: _____
Rhythm interpretation: _____

Strip 11.98 Rhythm: _____ Rate: _____ P wave: _____
PR interval: _____ QRS complex: _____
Rhythm interpretation: _____

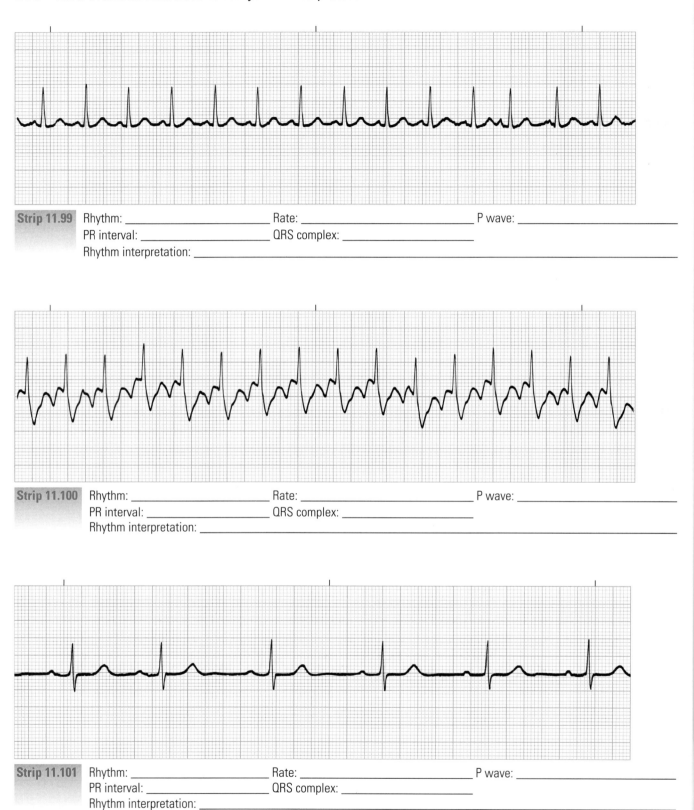

Strip 11.99   Rhythm: _____   Rate: _____   P wave: _____
PR interval: _____   QRS complex: _____
Rhythm interpretation: _____

Strip 11.100   Rhythm: _____   Rate: _____   P wave: _____
PR interval: _____   QRS complex: _____
Rhythm interpretation: _____

Strip 11.101   Rhythm: _____   Rate: _____   P wave: _____
PR interval: _____   QRS complex: _____
Rhythm interpretation: _____

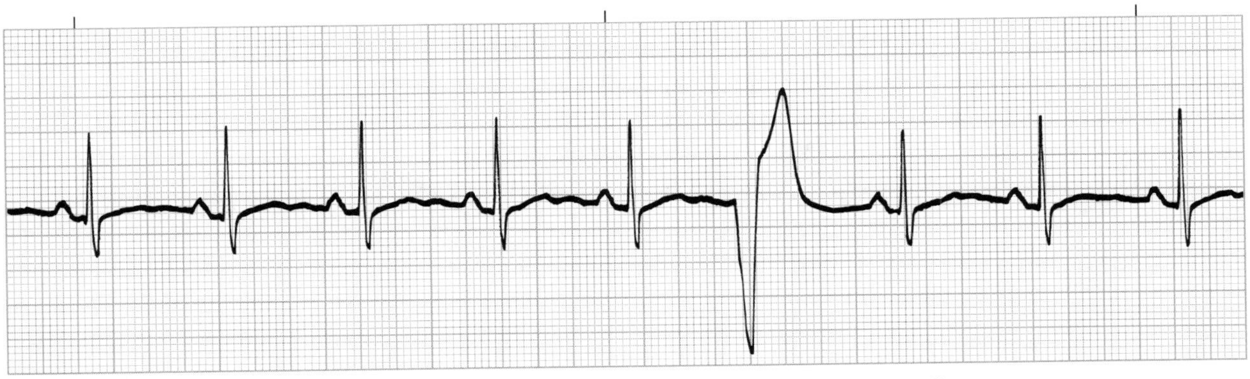

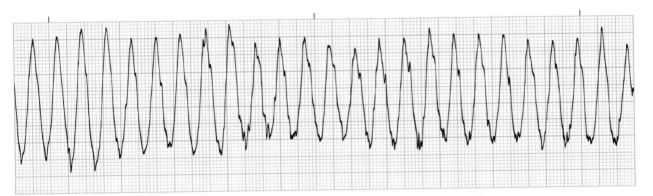

Strip 11.102　Rhythm: _____ Rate: _____ P wave: _____
PR interval: _____ QRS complex: _____
Rhythm interpretation: _____

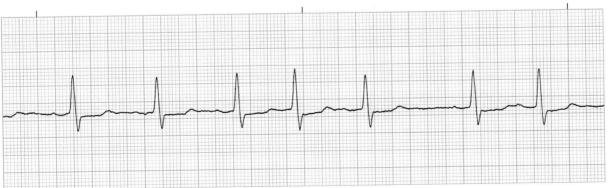

Strip 11.103　Rhythm: _____ Rate: _____ P wave: _____
PR interval: _____ QRS complex: _____
Rhythm interpretation: _____

Strip 11.104　Rhythm: _____ Rate: _____ P wave: _____
PR interval: _____ QRS complex: _____
Rhythm interpretation: _____

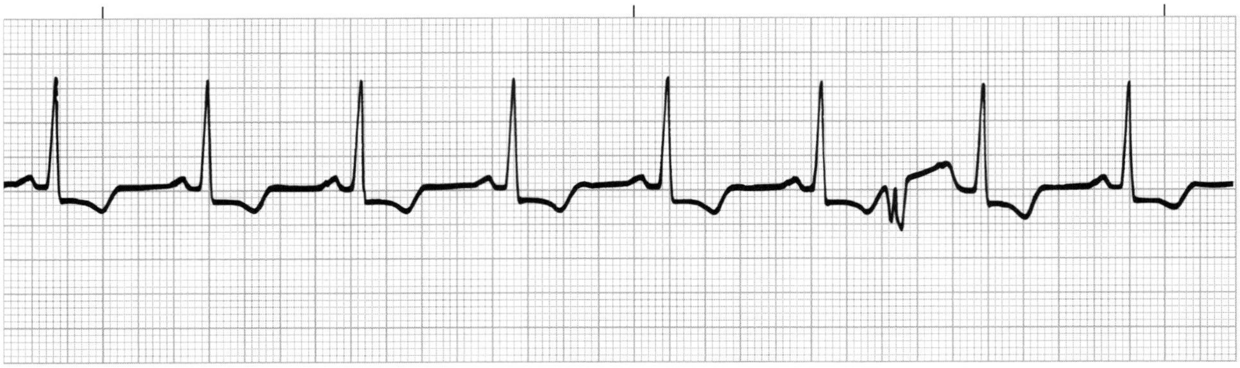

Strip 11.105   Rhythm: _____   Rate: _____   P wave: _____
PR interval: _____   QRS complex: _____
Rhythm interpretation: _____

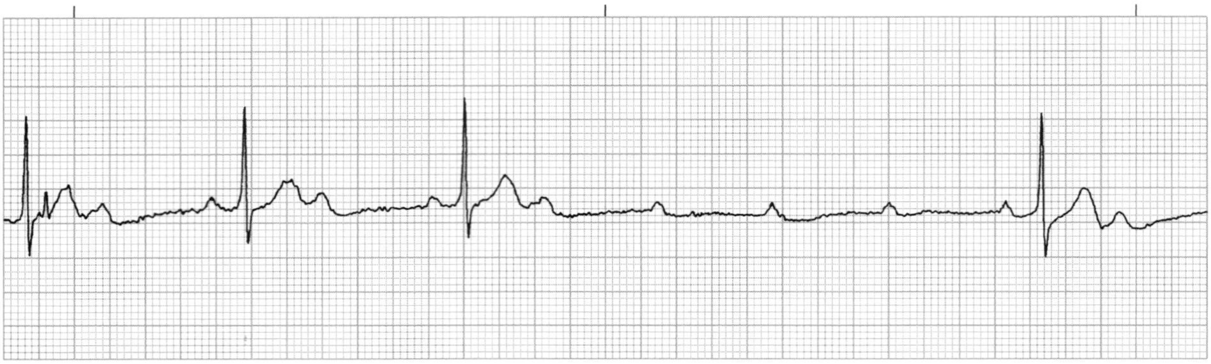

Strip 11.106   Rhythm: _____   Rate: _____   P wave: _____
PR interval: _____   QRS complex: _____
Rhythm interpretation: _____

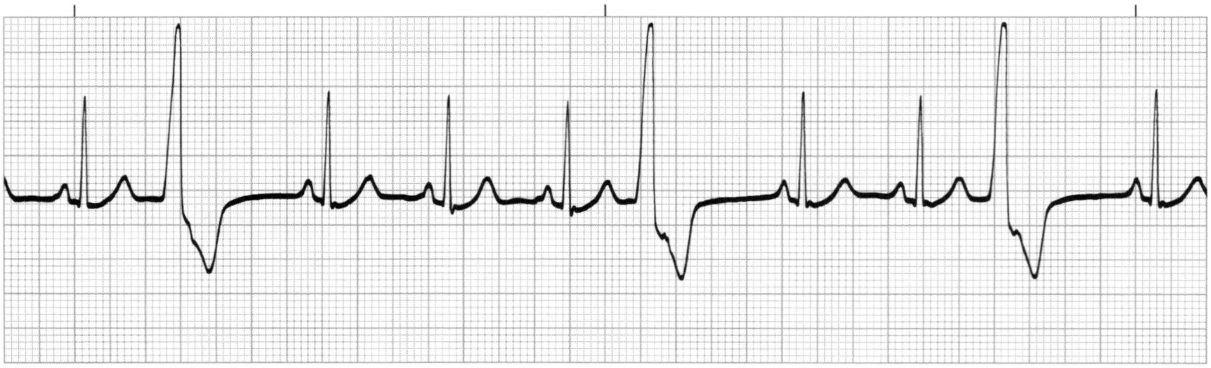

Strip 11.107   Rhythm: _____   Rate: _____   P wave: _____
PR interval: _____   QRS complex: _____
Rhythm interpretation: _____

Answer Key to Chapter 3

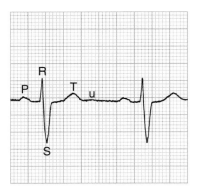

Strip 3.1

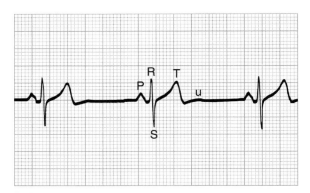

Strip 3.2

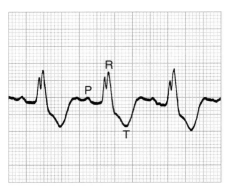

Strip 3.3

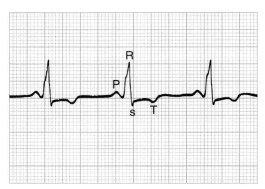

Strip 3.4

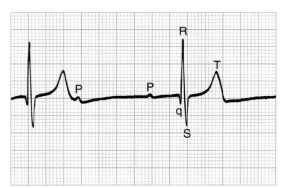

Strip 3.5

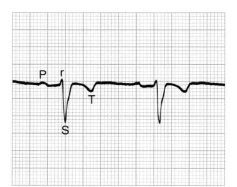

Strip 3.6

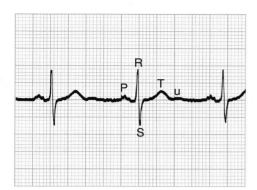

Strip 3.7

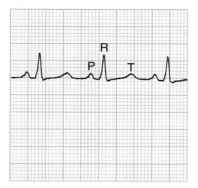

Strip 3.8

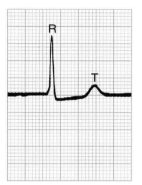

Strip 3.9

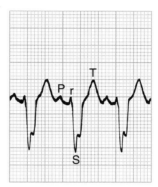

Strip 3.10

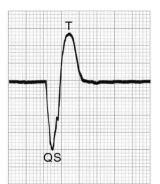

Strip 3.11

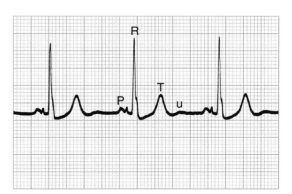

Strip 3.12

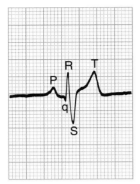

Strip 3.13

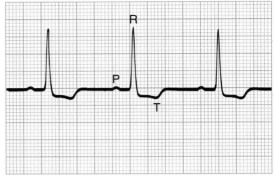

Strip 3.14

p 5.1
nterval measurement: 0.16 second
quares × 0.04 second).

ip 5.2
nterval measurement: 0.06 second
squares × 0.04 second)

ip 5.3
nterval measurement: 0.32 second
quares × 0.04 second)

ip 5.4
complex measurement: 0.04 second
quare × 0.04 second)

ip 5.5
complex measurement: 0.06 second
squares × 0.04 second)

ip 5.6
complex measurement: 0.08 second
quares × 0.04 second)

ip 5.7
QS complex measurement: 0.08 second
squares × 0.04 second)

ip 5.8
S complex measurement: 0.12 second
squares × 0.04 second)

rip 5.9
S complex measurement: 0.16 second
squares × 0.04 second)

rip 5.10
ythm: Regular
te: 72 beats/minute
waves: Sinus
interval: 0.12 to 0.16 second
RS complex: 0.04 to 0.08 second
mment. An inverted T wave is present

rip 5.11
ythm: Regular
te: 42 beats/minute
waves: Sinus
interval: 0.14 to 0.16 second
RS complex: 0.06 to 0.08 second

Strip 5.12
Rhythm: Regular
Rate: 125 beats/minute
P waves: Sinus
PR interval: 0.12 second
QRS complex: 0.08 second

Strip 5.13
Rhythm: Regular
Rate: 56 beats/minute
P waves: Sinus
PR interval: 0.16 to 0.20 second
QRS complex: 0.12 to 0.14 second

Strip 5.14
Rhythm: Regular
Rate: 88 beats/minute
P waves: Sinus
PR interval: 0.16 to 0.20 second
QRS complex: 0.06 to 0.08 second

Strip 5.15
Rhythm: Irregular
Rate: 70 beats/minute
P waves: Sinus
PR interval: 0.12 to 14 second
QRS complex: 0.08 second

Strip 5.16
Rhythm: Regular
Rate: 68 beats/minute
P waves: Sinus
PR interval: 0.16 to 0.18 second
QRS complex: 0.12 second
Comment. A U wave is present

Strip 5.17
Rhythm: Regular
Rate: 115 beats/minute
P waves: Sinus
PR interval: 0.12 to 0.14 second
QRS complex: 0.08 to 0.10 second

Strip 5.18
Rhythm: Regular
Rate: 63 beats/minute
P waves: Sinus (M-shaped)
PR interval: 0.16 second
QRS complex: 0.06 to 0.08 second
Comment. M-shaped P waves usually
indicate left atrial hypertrophy; a U wave
is present

Strip 5.19
Rhythm: Regular
Rate: 47 beats/minute
P waves: Absent
PR interval: Absent
QRS complex: 0.08 second

Strip 5.20
Rhythm: Regular
Rate: 115 beats/minute
P waves: Sinus
PR interval: 0.12 to 0.14 second
QRS complex: 0.04 to 0.06 second
Comment. ST segment depression is
present

Strip 5.21
Rhythm: Irregular
Rate: 40 beats/minute
P waves: Sinus
PR interval: 0.16 to 0.18 second
QRS complex: 0.06 to 0.08 second

Strip 6.1
Rhythm: Regular
Rate: 48 beats/minute
P waves: Sinus
PR interval: 0.16 to 0.18 second
QRS complex: 0.06 to 0.08 second
Rhythm interpretation: Sinus
bradycardia
Comment. A small U wave is present

Strip 6.2
Rhythm: Regular
Rate: 107 beats/minute
P waves: Sinus
PR interval: 0.14 to 0.16 second
QRS complex: 0.06 to 0.08 second
Rhythm interpretation: Sinus
tachycardia
Comment. An inverted T wave is present

Strip 6.3
Rhythm: Regular
Rate: 63 beats/minute
P waves: Sinus
PR interval: 0.16 to 0.18 second
QRS complex: 0.08 to 0.10 second
Rhythm interpretation: Normal sinus
rhythm

Strip 6.4
Rhythm: Regular
Rate: 107 beats/minute
P waves: Sinus
PR interval: 0.12 to 0.16 second
QRS complex: 0.04 to 0.08 second
Rhythm interpretation: Sinus
tachycardia
Comment. ST segment depression and
T-wave inversion are present

Strip 6.5
Rhythm: Regular
Rate: 54 beats/minute
P waves: Sinus
PR interval: 0.14 to 0.16 second
QRS complex: 0.06 to 0.08 second
Rhythm interpretation: Sinus
bradycardia
Comment. A U wave is present

Strip 6.6
Rhythm: Regular (basic rhythm); irregular
during pause
Rate: 100 beats/minute (basic rhythm)
P waves: Sinus (basic rhythm); absent
during pause
PR interval: 0.16 to 0.20 second
QRS complex: 0.08 to 0.10 second (basic
rhythm)
Rhythm interpretation: Normal sinus
rhythm with sinus block
Comment. ST segment depression and
T-wave inversion are present

Strip 6.7
Rhythm: Regular
Rate: 48 beats/minute
P waves: Sinus (M-shaped)
PR interval: 0.16 second
QRS complex: 0.06 to 0.08 second
Rhythm interpretation: Sinus
bradycardia
Comment. M-shaped P waves usually
indicate left atrial hypertrophy

Strip 6.8
Rhythm: Irregular
Rate: 40 beats/minute
P waves: Sinus
PR interval: 0.14 to 0.16 second
QRS complex: 0.06 to 0.08 second
Rhythm interpretation: Sinus arrhythmia
with a bradycardic rate
Comment. A U wave is present

Strip 6.9
Rhythm: Regular (basic rhythm); irregular
during pause
Rate: 58 beats/minute (basic rhythm)
P waves: Sinus (basic rhythm); absent
during pause
PR interval: 0.16 to 0.20 second (basic
rhythm); absent during pause
QRS complex: 0.08 to 0.10 second (basic
rhythm); absent during pause
Rhythm interpretation: Sinus bradycardia
with sinus arrest
Comment. ST segment depression and
T-wave inversion are present

Strip 6.10
Rhythm: Regular
Rate: 125 beats/minute
P waves: Sinus
PR interval: 0.12 to 0.14 second
QRS complex: 0.06 to 0.08 second
Rhythm interpretation: Sinus
tachycardia

Strip 6.11
Rhythm: Regular
Rate: 75 beats/minute
P waves: Sinus
PR interval: 0.16 to 0.20 second
QRS complex: 0.06 to 0.08 second
Rhythm interpretation: Normal sinus
rhythm
Comment. A depressed ST segment and
biphasic T waves are present

Strip 6.12
Rhythm: Regular
Rate: 47 beats/minute
P waves: Sinus
PR interval: 0.18 to 0.20 second
QRS complex: 0.06 to 0.08 second
Rhythm interpretation: Sinus
bradycardia
Comment. An elevated ST segment is
present

Strip 6.13
Rhythm: Irregular
Rate: 80 beats/minute
P waves: Sinus
PR interval: 0.12 to 0.14 second
QRS complex: 0.08 second
Rhythm interpretation: Sinus
arrhythmia

Strip 6.14
Rhythm: Regular
Rate: 63 beats/minute
P waves: Sinus
PR interval: 0.18 to 0.20 second
QRS complex: 0.06 to 0.08 second
Rhythm interpretation: Normal sinus
rhythm
Comment. ST segment depression and
T-wave inversion are present

Strip 6.15
Rhythm: Regular (basic rhythm); irregular
during pause
Rate: 84 beats/minute (basic rhythm);
slows to 56 beats/minute after the
pause (temporary rate suppression
may occur after a pause in the basic
rhythm)
P waves: Sinus (basic rhythm); absent
during pause
PR interval: 0.16 to 0.20 second (basic
rhythm); absent during pause
QRS complex: 0.08 to 0.10 second (basic
rhythm); absent during pause
Rhythm interpretation: Normal sinus
rhythm with sinus arrest

Strip 6.16
Rhythm: Regular
Rate: 125 beats/minute
P waves: Sinus
PR interval: 0.12 to 0.14 second
QRS complex: 0.06 to 0.08 second
Rhythm interpretation: Sinus
tachycardia

Strip 6.17
Rhythm: Regular
Rate: 54 beats/minute
P waves: Sinus
PR interval: 0.16 to 0.20 second
QRS complex: 0.08 to 0.10 second
Rhythm interpretation: Sinus
bradycardia
Comment. A U wave is present

Strip 6.18
Rhythm: Irregular
Rate: 60 beats/minute
P waves: Sinus
PR interval: 0.16 to 0.18 second
QRS complex: 0.06 to 0.08 second
Rhythm interpretation: Sinus
arrhythmia

Strip 6.19
Rhythm: Regular
Rate: 72 beats/minute
P waves: Sinus
PR interval: 0.12 second
QRS complex: 0.04 to 0.06 second
Rhythm interpretation: Normal sinus rhythm

Strip 6.20
Rhythm: Regular (basic rhythm); irregular during pause
Rate: 88 beats/minute (basic rhythm)
P waves: Sinus (basic rhythm); absent during pause
PR interval: 0.14 to 0.16 second (basic rhythm)
QRS complex: 0.08 to 0.10 second (basic rhythm)
Rhythm interpretation: Normal sinus rhythm with sinus block
Comment. A U wave is present

Strip 6.21
Rhythm: Regular
Rate: 107 beats/minute
P waves: Sinus
PR interval: 0.12 to 0.14 second
QRS complex: 0.08 to 0.10 second
Rhythm interpretation: Sinus tachycardia
Comment. ST segment elevation is present

Strip 6.22
Rhythm: Regular
Rate: 60 beats/minute
P waves: Sinus
PR interval: 0.12 second
QRS complex: 0.08 second
Rhythm interpretation: Normal sinus rhythm
Comment. T-wave inversion is present

Strip 6.23
Rhythm: Irregular
Rate: 70 beats/minute
P waves: Sinus
PR interval: 0.12 to 0.16 second
QRS complex: 0.06 to 0.08 second
Rhythm interpretation: Sinus arrhythmia

Strip 6.24
Rhythm: Regular (basic rhythm); irregular during pause
Rate: 60 beats/minute (basic rhythm); slows to 47 beats/minute after a pause (temporary rate suppression can occur after a pause in the basic rhythm)
P waves: Sinus (basic rhythm); absent during pause
PR interval: 0.16 to 0.20 second (basic rhythm); absent during pause
QRS complex: 0.04 to 0.06 second (basic rhythm); absent during pause
Rhythm interpretation: Normal sinus rhythm with sinus arrest

Strip 6.25
Rhythm: Regular
Rate: 125 beats/minute
P waves: Sinus
PR interval: 0.12 to 0.14 second
QRS complex: 0.04 to 0.06 second
Rhythm interpretation: Sinus tachycardia

Strip 6.26
Rhythm: Regular
Rate: 58 beats/minute
P waves: Sinus
PR interval: 0.12 to 0.16 second
QRS complex: 0.06 to 0.08 second
Rhythm interpretation: Sinus bradycardia
Comment. Biphasic T waves are present

Strip 6.27
Rhythm: Regular (basic rhythm); irregular during pause
Rate: 72 beats/minute (basic rhythm)
P waves: Sinus (basic rhythm); absent during pause
PR interval: 0.12 to 0.14 second (basic rhythm); absent during pause
QRS complex: 0.08 to 0.10 second (basic rhythm); absent during pause
Rhythm interpretation: Normal sinus rhythm with sinus block

Strip 6.28
Rhythm: Irregular
Rate: 60 beats/minute
P waves: Sinus
PR interval: 0.12 to 0.14 second
QRS complex: 0.08 to 0.10 second
Rhythm interpretation: Sinus arrhythmia
Comment. A U wave is present

Strip 6.29
Rhythm: Regular
Rate: 65 beats/minute
P waves: Sinus
PR interval: 0.20 second
QRS complex: 0.08 to 0.10 second
Rhythm interpretation: Normal sinus rhythm
Comment. ST segment depression and T-wave inversion are present

Strip 6.30
Rhythm: Regular (basic rhythm); irregular during pause
Rate: 68 beats/minute (basic rhythm); slows to 63 beats/minute after pause (temporary rate suppression can occur after a pause in the basic rhythm—after several cycles, the rate returns to the basic rate)
P waves: Sinus (basic rhythm); absent during pause
PR interval: 0.16 second (basic rhythm); absent during pause
QRS complex: 0.06 to 0.08 second (basic rhythm); absent during pause
Rhythm interpretation: Normal sinus rhythm with sinus arrest
Comment. A U wave is present

Strip 6.31
Rhythm: Regular
Rate: 54 beats/minute
P waves: Sinus
PR interval: 0.14 to 0.16 second
QRS complex: 0.04 to 0.08 second
Rhythm interpretation: Sinus bradycardia

Strip 6.32
Rhythm: Irregular
Rate: 60 beats/minute
P waves: Sinus
PR interval: 0.16 second
QRS complex: 0.06 to 0.08 second
Rhythm interpretation: Sinus arrhythmia

Strip 6.33
Rhythm: Regular
Rate: 115 beats/minute
P wave: Sinus
PR interval: 0.14 to 0.16 second
QRS complex: 0.06 to 0.08 second
Rhythm interpretation: Sinus tachycardia

Strip 6.34
Rhythm: Regular
Rate: 94 beats/minute
P waves: Sinus
PR interval: 0.16 to 0.20 second
QRS complex: 0.08 to 0.10 second
Rhythm interpretation: Normal sinus rhythm

Strip 6.35
Rhythm: Irregular
Rate: 50 beats/minute
P waves: Sinus
PR interval: 0.16 second
QRS complex: 0.04 to 0.06 second
Rhythm interpretation: Sinus arrhythmia with a bradycardic rate

Strip 6.36
Rhythm: Regular
Rate: 40 beats/minute
P waves: Sinus
PR interval: 0.18 to 0.20 second
QRS complex: 0.04 to 0.08 second
Rhythm interpretation: Sinus bradycardia
Comment. ST segment depression is present

Strip 6.37
Rhythm: Regular (basic rhythm); irregular during pause
Rate: 88 beats/minute (basic rhythm)
P waves: Sinus (basic rhythm); absent during pause
PR interval: 0.20 second (basic rhythm); absent during pause
QRS complex: 0.06 to 0.08 second (basic rhythm); absent during pause
Rhythm interpretation: Normal sinus rhythm with sinus arrest
Comment. ST segment depression is present

Strip 6.38
Rhythm: Regular
Rate: 107 beats/minute
P waves: Sinus
PR interval: 0.16 to 0.18 second
QRS complex: 0.06 to 0.08 second
Rhythm interpretation: Sinus tachycardia

Strip 6.39
Rhythm: Regular
Rate: 107 beats/minute
P waves: Sinus
PR interval: 0.16 second
QRS complex: 0.06 to 0.08 second
Rhythm interpretation: Sinus tachycardia
Comment. ST segment elevation is present

Strip 6.40
Rhythm: Regular
Rate: 50 beats/minute
P waves: Sinus
PR interval: 0.16 to 0.18 second
QRS complex: 0.04 to 0.06 second
Rhythm interpretation: Sinus bradycardia
Comment. A U wave is present

Strip 6.41
Rhythm: Regular
Rate: 84 beats/minute
P waves: Sinus
PR interval: 0.12 to 0.16 second
QRS complex: 0.06 to 0.08 second
Rhythm interpretation: Normal sinus rhythm

Strip 6.42
Rhythm: Irregular
Rate: 60 beats/minute
P waves: Sinus
PR interval: 0.14 to 0.16 second
QRS complex: 0.06 to 0.08 second
Rhythm interpretation: Sinus arrhythmia

Strip 6.43
Rhythm: Regular (basic rhythm); irregular during pause
Rate: 63 beats/minute (basic rhythm)
P waves: Sinus (basic rhythm); absent during pause
PR interval: 0.20 second (basic rhythm); absent during pause
QRS complex: 0.04 to 0.06 second (basic rhythm); absent during pause
Rhythm interpretation: Normal sinus rhythm with sinus arrest
Comment. ST segment depression is present

Strip 6.44
Rhythm: Irregular
Rate: 60 beats/minute
P waves: Sinus
PR interval: 0.12 to 0.16 second
QRS complex: 0.04 to 0.06 second
Rhythm interpretation: Sinus arrhythmia

Strip 6.45
Rhythm: Regular
Rate: 27 beats/minute
P waves: Sinus
PR interval: 0.12 to 0.16 second
QRS complex: 0.08 to 0.10 second
Rhythm interpretation: Sinus bradycardia with extremely slow rate
Comment. ST segment depression is present

Strip 6.46
Rhythm: Irregular
Rate: 50 beats/minute
P waves: Sinus
PR interval: 0.12 to 0.14 second
QRS complex: 0.06 to 0.08 second
Rhythm interpretation: Sinus arrhythmia with a bradycardic rate

Strip 6.47
Rhythm: Regular
Rate: 136 beats/minute
P waves: Sinus
PR interval: 0.14 to 0.16 second
QRS complex: 0.06 to 0.08 second
Rhythm interpretation: Sinus tachycardia

Strip 6.48
Rhythm: Irregular
Rate: 60 beats/minute
P waves: Sinus
PR interval: 0.16 to 0.18 second
QRS complex: 0.06 to 0.08 second
Rhythm interpretation: Sinus arrhythmia

Strip 6.49
Rhythm: Regular
Rate: 52 beats/minute
P waves: Sinus
PR interval: 0.12 second
QRS complex: 0.08 second
Rhythm interpretation: Sinus bradycardia

Strip 6.50
Rhythm: Regular
Rate: 88 beats/minute
P waves: Sinus
PR interval: 0.12 to 0.14 second
QRS complex: 0.08 to 0.10 second
Rhythm interpretation: Normal sinus rhythm

Strip 6.51
Rhythm: Regular
Rate: 107 beats/minute
P waves: Sinus
PR interval: 0.12 to 0.16 second
QRS complex: 0.08 to 0.10 second
Rhythm interpretation: Sinus
tachycardia

Strip 6.52
Rhythm: Regular (basic rhythm); irregular
during pause
Rate: 60 beats/minute (basic rhythm);
slows to 31 beats/minute during
pause (temporary rate suppression
is common after a pause in the basic
rhythm)
P waves: Sinus (basic rhythm); absent
during pause
PR interval: 0.16 to 0.20 second (basic
rhythm); absent during pause
QRS complex: 0.06 to 0.08 second (basic
rhythm); absent during pause
Rhythm interpretation: Normal sinus
rhythm with sinus arrest
Comment. ST segment depression and
T-wave inversion are present

Strip 6.53
Rhythm: Irregular
Rate: 80 beats/minute
P waves: Sinus
PR interval: 0.12 to 0.14 second
QRS complex: 0.06 to 0.08 second
Rhythm interpretation: Sinus
arrhythmia

Strip 6.54
Rhythm: Regular (basic rhythm); irregular
during pause
Rate: 88 beats/minute (basic rhythm)
rate slows to 54 beats/minute after
the pause (temporary rate suppression
can occur after a pause in the basic
rhythm)
P waves: Sinus (basic rhythm); absent
during pause
PR interval: 0.14 to 0.18 second (basic
rhythm); absent during pause
QRS complex: 0.08 to 0.10 second (basic
rhythm); absent during pause
Rhythm interpretation: Normal sinus
rhythm with sinus block

Strip 6.55
Rhythm: Regular
Rate: 79 beats/minute
P waves: Sinus
PR interval: 0.18 to 0.20 second
QRS complex: 0.06 to 0.08 second
Rhythm interpretation: Normal sinus
rhythm
Comment. Inverted T waves are
present

Strip 6.56
Rhythm: Regular
Rate: 72 beats/minute
P waves: Sinus
PR interval: 0.12 to 0.16 second
QRS complex: 0.06 to 0.08 second
Rhythm interpretation: Normal sinus
rhythm
Comment. ST segment depression and
T-wave inversion are present

Strip 6.57
Rhythm: Irregular
Rate: 40 beats/minute
P waves: Sinus
PR interval: 0.16 to 0.18 second
QRS complex: 0.08 second
Rhythm interpretation: Sinus arrhythmia
with a bradycardic rate
Comment. A U wave is present

Strip 6.58
Rhythm: Regular
Rate: 72 beats/minute
P waves: Sinus
PR interval: 0.14 to 0.16 second
QRS complex: 0.06 to 0.08 second
Rhythm interpretation: Normal sinus
rhythm

Strip 6.59
Rhythm: Regular (rhythm varies by 2 small
squares)
Rate: 52 to 54 beats/minute
P waves: Sinus
PR interval: 0.12 second
QRS complex: 0.08 to 0.10 second
Rhythm interpretation: Sinus
bradycardia
Comment. An elevated ST segment is
present

Strip 6.60
Rhythm: Regular (basic rhythm); irregular
during pause
Rate: 88 beats/minute (basic rhythm)
P waves: Sinus (basic rhythm); absent
during pause
PR interval: 0.16 to 0.20 second (basic
rhythm); absent during pause
QRS complex: 0.08 to 0.10 second (basic
rhythm); absent during pause
Rhythm interpretation: Normal sinus
rhythm with sinus block
Comment. ST segment depression is
present

Strip 6.61
Rhythm: Regular
Rate: 72 beats/minute
P waves: Sinus
PR interval: 0.12 to 0.14 second
QRS complex: 0.06 to 0.08 second
Rhythm interpretation: Normal sinus
rhythm
Comment. T-wave inversion is present

Strip 6.62
Rhythm: Regular
Rate: 107 beats/minute
P waves: Sinus
PR interval: 0.14 to 0.18 second
QRS complex: 0.06 to 0.08 second
Rhythm interpretation: Sinus
tachycardia

Strip 6.63
Rhythm: Regular
Rate: 44 beats/minute
P waves: Sinus
PR interval: 0.18 to 0.20 second
QRS complex: 0.06 to 0.08 second
Rhythm interpretation: Sinus
bradycardia
Comment. A U wave is present

Strip 6.64
Rhythm: Regular
Rate: 68 beats/minute
P waves: Sinus
PR interval: 0.14 to 0.16 second
QRS complex: 0.06 to 0.08 second
Rhythm interpretation: Normal sinus
rhythm

Strip 6.65
Rhythm: Regular
Rate: 107 beats/minute
P waves: Sinus
PR interval: 0.18 to 0.20 second
QRS complex: 0.08 to 0.10 second
Rhythm interpretation: Sinus tachycardia
Comment. ST segment elevation is present

Strip 6.66
Rhythm: Regular
Rate: 107 beats/minute
P waves: Sinus
PR interval: 0.12 to 0.16 second
QRS complex: 0.04 to 0.06 second
Rhythm interpretation: Sinus tachycardia

Strip 6.67
Rhythm: Regular
Rate: 54 beats/minute
P waves: Sinus
PR interval: 0.14 to 0.16 second
QRS complex: 0.04 second
Rhythm interpretation: Sinus bradycardia

Strip 6.68
Rhythm: Regular
Rate: 72 beats/minute
P waves: Sinus
PR interval: 0.14 to 0.18 second
QRS complex: 0.08 to 0.10 second
Rhythm interpretation: Normal sinus rhythm

Strip 6.69
Rhythm: Regular
Rate: 136 beats/minute
P waves: Sinus
PR interval: 0.14 to 0.16 second
QRS complex: 0.08 to 0.10 second
Rhythm interpretation: Sinus tachycardia
Comment. ST segment elevation is present

Strip 6.70
Rhythm: Regular (basic rhythm); irregular during pause
Rate: 56 beats/minute (basic rhythm); slows to 50 beats/minute after the pause (temporary rate suppression can occur after a pause in the basic rhythm—after several cycles the rate returns to the basic rate)
P waves: Sinus (basic rhythm); absent during pause
PR interval: 0.12 to 0.16 second (basic rhythm); absent during pause
QRS complex: 0.08 to 0.10 second (basic rhythm); absent during pause
Rhythm interpretation: Sinus bradycardia with sinus arrest

Strip 6.71
Rhythm: Regular
Rate: 115 beats/minute
P waves: Sinus
PR interval: 0.12 to 0.16 second
QRS complex: 0.08 to 0.10 second
Rhythm interpretation: Sinus tachycardia
Comment. ST segment depression is present

Strip 6.72
Rhythm: Regular
Rate: 79 beats/minute
P waves: Sinus
PR interval: 0.14 to 0.16 second
QRS complex: 0.06 to 0.08 second
Rhythm interpretation: Normal sinus rhythm
Comment. ST segment depression and biphasic T waves are present

Strip 6.73
Rhythm: Regular
Rate: 54 beats/minute
P waves: Sinus
PR interval: 0.16 second
QRS complex: 0.08 second
Rhythm interpretation: Sinus bradycardia
Comment. ST segment elevation is present

Strip 6.74
Rhythm: Regular
Rate: 94 beats/minute
P waves: Sinus
PR interval: 0.12 to 0.14 second
QRS complex: 0.06 to 0.08 second
Rhythm interpretation: Normal sinus rhythm

Strip 6.75
Rhythm: Irregular
Rate: 60 beats/minute
P waves: Sinus
PR interval: 0.14 to 0.16 second
QRS complex: 0.06 to 0.08 second
Rhythm interpretation: Sinus arrhythmia

Strip 6.76
Rhythm: Regular
Rate: 150 beats/minute
P waves: Sinus
PR interval: 0.12 to 0.14 second
QRS complex: 0.04 to 0.06 second
Rhythm interpretation: Sinus tachycardia

Strip 6.77
Rhythm: Regular
Rate: 79 beats/minute
P waves: Sinus
PR interval: 0.18 to 0.20 second
QRS complex: 0.08 to 0.10 second
Rhythm interpretation: Normal sinus rhythm
Comment. ST segment elevation is present

Strip 6.78
Rhythm: Regular
Rate: 40 beats/minute
P waves: Sinus
PR interval: 0.14 to 0.20 second
QRS complex: 0.08 second
Rhythm interpretation: Sinus bradycardia

Strip 6.79
Rhythm: Regular (basic rhythm); irregular during pause
Rate: 107 beats/minute (basic rhythm); rate slows to 94 beats/minute for one cycle after the pause (temporary rate suppression can occur after a pause in the basic rhythm).
P waves: Sinus (basic rhythm); absent during pause
PR interval: 0.16 to 0.18 second (basic rhythm); absent during pause
QRS complex: 0.10 second (basic rhythm); absent during pause
Rhythm interpretation: Sinus tachycardia with sinus block
Comment. Baseline artifact is present

Strip 6.80
Rhythm: Regular
Rate: 84 beats/minute
P waves: Sinus
PR interval: 0.16 second
QRS complex: 0.06 second
Rhythm interpretation: Normal sinus rhythm
Comment. T-wave inversion is present

Strip 6.81
Rhythm: Regular
Rate: 56 beats/minute
P waves: Sinus
PR interval: 0.16 to 0.18 second
QRS complex: 0.06 to 0.08 second
Rhythm interpretation: Sinus bradycardia
Comment. T-wave inversion is present

Strip 6.82
Rhythm: Regular
Rate: 125 beats/minute
P waves: Sinus
PR interval: 0.18 to 0.20 second
QRS complex: 0.04 to 0.06 second
Rhythm interpretation: Sinus tachycardia

Strip 6.83
Rhythm: Irregular (basic rhythm)
Rate: 60 beats/minute (basic rhythm)
P waves: Sinus (basic rhythm); absent during pause
PR interval: 0.14 to 0.16 second (basic rhythm); absent during pause
QRS complex: 0.04 second (basic rhythm); absent during pause
Rhythm interpretation: Sinus arrhythmia with sinus pause (with an irregular basic rhythm it's impossible to distinguish sinus arrest from sinus block, so the rhythm is best interpreted using the broad term sinus pause)

Strip 6.84
Rhythm: Regular
Rate: 79 beats/minute
P waves: Sinus
PR interval: 0.12 second
QRS complex: 0.04 to 0.08 second
Rhythm interpretation: Normal sinus rhythm
Comment. ST segment elevation is present

Strip 6.85
Rhythm: Regular
Rate: 136 beats/minute
P waves: Sinus
PR interval: 0.14 to 0.16 second
QRS complex: 0.06 to 0.08 second
Rhythm interpretation: Sinus tachycardia

Strip 6.86
Rhythm: Regular
Rate: 54 beats/minute
P waves: Sinus
PR interval: 0.16 to 0.18 second
QRS complex: 0.06 to 0.08 second
Rhythm interpretation: Sinus bradycardia

Strip 6.87
Rhythm: Regular (basic rhythm); irregular during pause
Rate: 84 beats/minute (basic rhythm); slows to 75 beats/minute for one cycle after the pause (temporary rate suppression is common after a pause in the basic rhythm).
P waves: Sinus (basic rhythm); absent during pause
PR interval: 0.16 to 0.18 second (basic rhythm); absent during pause
QRS complex: 0.08 to 0.10 second (basic rhythm); absent during pause
Rhythm interpretation: Normal sinus rhythm with sinus arrest

Strip 6.88
Rhythm: Regular
Rate: 100 beats/minute
P waves: Sinus
PR interval: 0.12 to 0.16 second
QRS complex: 0.08 to 0.10 second
Rhythm interpretation: Normal sinus rhythm
Comment. ST segment elevation is present

Strip 6.89
Rhythm: Regular
Rate: 54 beats/minute
P waves: Sinus
PR interval: 0.16 to 0.18 second
QRS complex: 0.06 to 0.08 second
Rhythm interpretation: Sinus bradycardia
Comment. ST segment elevation and T-wave inversion are present

Strip 6.90
Rhythm: Regular (basic rhythm); irregular during pause
Rate: 72 beats/minute (basic rhythm); slows to 68 beats/minute for two cycles after the pause (temporary rate suppression can occur after a pause in the basic rhythm).
P waves: Sinus (basic rhythm); absent during pause
PR interval: 0.12 to 0.14 second (basic rhythm); absent during pause
QRS complex: 0.06 to 0.08 second (basic rhythm); absent during pause
Rhythm interpretation: Normal sinus rhythm with sinus arrest
Comment. T-wave inversion is present

Strip 6.91
Rhythm: Regular
Rate: 63 beats/minute
P waves: Sinus
PR interval: 0.12 to 0.16 second
QRS complex: 0.06 to 0.08 second
Rhythm interpretation: Normal sinus rhythm
Comment. A U wave is present

Strip 6.92
Rhythm: Regular
Rate: 63 beats/minute
P waves: Sinus
PR interval: 0.20 second
QRS complex: 0.08 second
Rhythm interpretation: Normal sinus rhythm
Comment. ST segment depression and T-wave inversion are present

Strip 6.93
Rhythm: Regular (basic rhythm); irregular during pause
Rate: 79 beats/minute (basic rhythm); rate slows to 72 beats/minute after the pause (temporary rate suppression can occur after a pause in the basic rhythm).
P waves: Sinus (basic rhythm); absent during pause
PR interval: 0.16 to 0.20 second (basic rhythm); absent during pause
QRS complex: 0.08 to 0.10 second (basic rhythm); absent during pause
Rhythm interpretation: Normal sinus rhythm with sinus arrest
Comment. ST segment depression and T-wave inversion are present

Strip 6.94
Rhythm: Regular
Rate: 100 beats/minute
P waves: Sinus
PR interval: 0.12 to 0.16 second
QRS complex: 0.06 to 0.08 second
Rhythm interpretation: Normal sinus rhythm

Strip 6.95
Rhythm: Regular
Rate: 72 beats/minute
P waves: Sinus
PR interval: 0.16 to 0.20 second
QRS complex: 0.06 to 0.08 second
Rhythm interpretation: Normal sinus rhythm
Comment. A U wave is present

Strip 6.96
Rhythm: Irregular
Rate: 60 beats/minute
P waves: Sinus
PR interval: 0.12 to 0.14 second
QRS complex: 0.06 to 0.08 second
Rhythm interpretation: Sinus arrhythmia

Strip 6.97
Rhythm: Irregular
Rate: 40 beats/minute
P waves: Sinus (basic rhythm); absent during pause
PR interval: 0.16 to 0.20 second (basic rhythm); absent during pause
QRS complex: 0.06 to 0.08 second (basic rhythm); absent during pause
Rhythm interpretation: Sinus arrhythmia with a bradycardic rate and a sinus pause (with an irregular basic rhythm it's impossible to distinguish sinus arrest from sinus block, so the rhythm is best interpreted using the broad term sinus pause)

Strip 6.98
Rhythm: Regular
Rate: 107 beats/minute
P waves: Sinus
PR interval: 0.16 to 0.18 second
QRS complex: 0.06 to 0.08 second
Rhythm interpretation: Sinus tachycardia
Comment. ST segment elevation is present

Strip 6.99
Rhythm: Irregular
Rate: 60 beats/minute
P waves: Sinus
PR interval: 0.16 to 0.18 second
QRS complex: 0.06 to 0.08 second
Rhythm interpretation: Sinus arrhythmia

Strip 7.1
Rhythm: Irregular
Rate: Atrial: Not measurable
Ventricular: 60 beats/minute
P waves: Fibrillatory waves are present
PR interval: Not measurable
QRS complex: 0.06 to 0.08 second
Rhythm interpretation: Atrial fibrillation (controlled rate)
Comment. ST segment depression is present

Strip 7.2
Rhythm: Regular
Rate: 188 beats/minute
P waves: Hidden in T waves (TP waves)
PR interval: Not measurable
QRS complex: 0.06 to 0.08 second
Rhythm interpretation: Paroxysmal atrial tachycardia

Strip 7.3
Rhythm: Regular (basic rhythm); irregular with PACs
Rate: 94 beats/minute (basic rhythm)
P waves: Sinus (basic rhythm); premature and abnormal (PACs)
PR interval: 0.12 second (basic rhythm); 0.12 to 0.14 second (PACs)
QRS complex: 0.08 to 0.10 second (basic rhythm): 0.08 second (PACs)
Rhythm interpretation: Normal sinus rhythm with two PACs (fourth and eighth complexes)
Comment. ST segment depression is present

Strip 7.4
Rhythm: Regular (off by one square)
Rate: 65 to 68 beats/minute
P waves: Vary in size, shape, and direction
PR interval: 0.12 to 0.16 second
QRS complex: 0.06 to 0.08 second
Rhythm interpretation: Wandering atrial pacemaker

Strip 7.5
Rhythm: Regular (basic rhythm); irregular with PAC
Rate: 125 beats/minute (basic rhythm)
P waves: Sinus (basic rhythm); premature and pointed (PAC)
PR interval: 0.12 second (basic rhythm); 0.12 second (PAC)
QRS complex: 0.04 to 0.06 second (basic rhythm); 0.08 second (PAC)
Rhythm interpretation: Sinus tachycardia with one PAC (eighth complex)

Strip 7.6
Rhythm: Regular
Rate: 188 beats/minute
P waves: Hidden in T waves (TP waves)
PR interval: Not measurable
QRS complex: 0.06 to 0.08 second
Rhythm interpretation: Paroxysmal atrial tachycardia

Strip 7.7
Rhythm: Regular (basic rhythm); irregular with nonconducted PAC
Rate: 88 beats/minute (basic rhythm)
P waves: Sinus (basic rhythm); premature and abnormal with nonconducted PAC
PR interval: 0.16 to 0.18 second
QRS complex: 0.06 to 0.08 second
Rhythm interpretation: Normal sinus rhythm with nonconducted PAC (after the seventh QRS complex)
Comment. ST segment depression is present

Strip 7.8
Rhythm: Irregular
Rate: Atrial: 240 beats/minute
Ventricular: 80 beats/minute
P waves: Flutter waves present (varying ratios)
PR interval: Not measurable
QRS complex: 0.08 to 0.10 second
Rhythm interpretation: Atrial flutter with variable AV conduction

Strip 7.9
Rhythm: Irregular
Rate: 70 beats/minute
P waves: Vary in size, shape, and direction
PR interval: 0.12 to 0.14 second
QRS complex: 0.06 to 0.08 second
Rhythm interpretation: Wandering atrial pacemaker

Strip 7.10
Rhythm: Irregular
Rate: Atrial: Not measurable
Ventricular: 60 beats/minute
P waves: Fibrillatory waves are present
PR interval: Not measurable
QRS complex: 0.04 to 0.06 second
Rhythm interpretation: Atrial fibrillation (controlled rate)

Strip 7.11
Rhythm: Regular (basic rhythm); irregular with PAC
Rate: 72 beats/minute (basic rhythm)
P waves: Sinus (basic rhythm); premature and pointed with PAC
PR interval: 0.18 to 0.20 second (basic rhythm); 0.20 second (PAC)
QRS complex: 0.04 to 0.08 second (basic rhythm); 0.04 second (PAC)
Rhythm interpretation: Normal sinus rhythm with one PAC (sixth complex)

Strip 7.12
Rhythm: Regular
Rate: Atrial: 237 beats/minute
Ventricular: 79 beats/minute
P waves: Three flutter waves to each QRS complex
PR interval: Not measurable
QRS complex: 0.04 to 0.06 second
Rhythm interpretation: Atrial flutter with 3:1 AV conduction

Strip 7.13
Rhythm: Regular (basic rhythm); irregular with nonconducted PAC
Rate: 107 beats/minute (basic rhythm)
P waves: Sinus (basic rhythm); premature and abnormal with nonconducted PAC
PR interval: 0.18 to 0.20 second
QRS complex: 0.04 to 0.06 second
Rhythm interpretation: Sinus tachycardia with one nonconducted PAC (after the fifth QRS complex)

Strip 7.14
Rhythm: Irregular
Rate: Atrial: Not measurable
Ventricular: 160 beats/minute
P waves: Fibrillatory waves
PR interval: Not measurable
QRS complex: 0.04 to 0.08 second
Rhythm interpretation: Atrial fibrillation (uncontrolled rate)
Comment: ST segment depression is present

Strip 7.15
Rhythm: Both rhythms regular (off by one square in second rhythm)
Rate: First rhythm: 167 beats/minute
Second rhythm: 94 to 100 beats/minute
P waves: First rhythm: Hidden in T waves (TP waves)
Second rhythm: Sinus
PR interval: First rhythm: Not measurable
Second rhythm: 0.16 to 0.20 second
QRS complex: 0.06 to 0.08 second (both rhythms)
Rhythm interpretation: Paroxysmal atrial tachycardia converting to normal sinus rhythm

Strip 7.16
Rhythm: Regular
Rate: Atrial: 300 beats/minute
Ventricular: 100 beats/minute
P waves: Three flutter waves before each QRS complex
PR interval: Not measurable
QRS complex: 0.08 second
Rhythm interpretation: Atrial flutter with 3:1 AV conduction

Strip 7.17
Rhythm: Irregular
Rate: Atrial: Not measurable
Ventricular: 40 beats/minute
P waves: Fibrillatory waves
PR interval: Not measurable
QRS complex: 0.08 second
Rhythm interpretation: Atrial fibrillation (controlled rate)

Strip 7.18
Rhythm: Irregular
Rate: Atrial: 210 beats/minute
Ventricular: 50 beats/minute
P waves: Flutter waves (varying ratios)
PR interval: Not measurable
QRS complex: 0.08 second
Rhythm interpretation: Atrial flutter with variable AV conduction

Strip 7.19
Rhythm: Regular (basic rhythm); irregular with PACs and nonconducted PACs
Rate: 79 to 84 beats/minute (basic rhythm)
P waves: Sinus (basic rhythm); premature and abnormal (PACs and nonconducted PACs)
PR interval: 0.16 to 0.20 second (basic rhythm and PACs)
QRS complex: 0.06 to 0.08 second (basic rhythm and PACs)
Rhythm interpretation: Normal sinus rhythm with two PACs (third and ninth complexes) and two nonconducted PACs (after the fourth and fifth complexes).
Comment: ST segment depression is present

Strip 7.20
Rhythm: Regular
Rate: 188 beats/minute
P waves: Hidden in T waves (TP waves)
PR interval: Not measurable
QRS complex: 0.08 to 0.10 second
Rhythm interpretation: Paroxysmal atrial tachycardia
Comment: ST segment depression is present

Strip 7.21
Rhythm: Regular (basic rhythm); irregular with nonconducted PAC
Rate: 75 beats/minute (basic rhythm); slows to 72 beats/minute for two cycles after a pause in the rhythm (temporary rate suppression is common after a pause in the basic rhythm).
P waves: Sinus (basic rhythm); premature and pointed without QRS complex after the third QRS complex
PR interval: 0.16 to 0.18 second
QRS complex: 0.06 to 0.08 second
Rhythm interpretation: Normal sinus rhythm with one nonconducted PAC (after third QRS complex)
Comment: A U wave is present

Strip 7.22
Rhythm: Regular
Rate: Atrial: 260 beats/minute
Ventricular: 65 beats/minute
P waves: Four flutter waves to each QRS complex
PR interval: Not measurable
QRS complex: 0.08 second
Rhythm interpretation: Atrial flutter with 4:1 AV conduction

Strip 7.23
Rhythm: Regular (basic rhythm); irregular with nonconducted PAC
Rate: 79 beats/minute (basic rhythm)
P waves: Sinus (basic rhythm); premature and abnormal with nonconducted PAC
PR interval: 0.14 to 0.20 second
QRS complex: 0.06 to 0.08 second
Rhythm interpretation: Normal sinus rhythm with one nonconducted PAC (after the fourth QRS complex)
Comment: ST segment depression and T-wave inversion are present

Strip 7.24
Rhythm: Irregular
Rate: Atrial: Not measurable
Ventricular: 70 beats/minute
P waves: Fibrillatory waves are present
PR interval: Not measurable
QRS complex: 0.06 to 0.08 second
Rhythm interpretation: Atrial fibrillation (controlled rate)
Comment: ST segment depression is present

Strip 7.25
Rhythm: Irregular
Rate: 50 beats/minute
P waves: Vary in size, shape, direction
across strip
PR interval: 0.08 to 0.10 second
QRS complex: 0.06 to 0.08 second
Rhythm interpretation: Wandering atrial
pacemaker

Strip 7.26
Rhythm: Regular (basic rhythm); irregular
with PAC
Rate: 68 beats/minute (basic rhythm)
P waves: Sinus (basic rhythm); premature
and inverted (PAC)
PR interval: 0.12 to 0.14 second (basic
rhythm); 0.12 second (PAC)
QRS complex: 0.06 to 0.08 second (basic
rhythm); 0.08 second (PAC)
Rhythm interpretation: Normal
sinus rhythm with one PAC (fourth
complex)
Comment. A U wave is present

Strip 7.27
Rhythm: Regular
Rate: Atrial: 232 beats/minute
Ventricular: 58 beats/minute
P waves: Four flutter waves to each QRS
complex
PR interval: Not measurable
QRS complex: 0.06 to 0.08 second
Rhythm interpretation: Atrial flutter with
4:1 AV conduction

Strip 7.28
Rhythm: Regular (basic rhythm); irregular
with PACs
Rate: 42 beats/minute (basic rhythm)
measured between the fifth and sixth
complexes
P waves: Sinus (basic rhythm); premature
and abnormal (PACs)
PR interval: 0.12 to 0.16 second (basic
rhythm); 0.16 second (PACs)
QRS complex 0.08 to 0.10 second (basic
rhythm and PACs)
Rhythm interpretation: Sinus bradycardia
with four PACs (second, fourth, seventh,
and ninth complexes)

Strip 7.29
Rhythm: Regular
Rate: 150 beats/minute
P waves: Hidden in preceding T wave
(TP waves)
PR interval: Not measurable
QRS complex: 0.08 second
Rhythm interpretation: Paroxysmal atrial
tachycardia

Strip 7.30
Rhythm: Regular
Rate: Atrial: 272 beats/minute
Ventricular: 136 beats/minute
P waves: Two flutter waves to each QRS
complex
PR interval: Not measurable
QRS complex: 0.06 second
Rhythm interpretation: Atrial flutter with
2:1 AV conduction

Strip 7.31
Rhythm: Regular (basic rhythm); irregular
with PACs and atrial fibrillation
Rate: 68 beats/minute (basic rhythm);
140 beats/minute (atrial fibrillation)
P waves: Sinus (basic rhythm); fibrillatory
waves (atrial fibrillation)
PR interval: 0.12 to 0.14 second (basic
rhythm); 0.12 to 0.20 second (PACs)
QRS complex: 0.06 to 0.10 second (basic
rhythm, atrial fib, and PACs)
Rhythm interpretation: Normal sinus
rhythm with two PACs (second and fifth
complexes); last PAC initiates atrial
fibrillation
Comment. ST segment depression is
present

Strip 7.32
Rhythm: Regular (basic rhythm); irregular
with nonconducted PAC
Rate: 94 beats/minute (basic rhythm);
slows to 84 beats/minute for one
cycle after the pause (temporary rate
suppression can occur after a pause in the
basic rhythm)
P waves: Sinus (basic rhythm); premature,
abnormal P wave without a QRS complex
hidden in T wave after the seventh QRS
complex
PR interval: 0.12 to 0.20 second
QRS complex: 0.06 to 0.08 second
Rhythm interpretation: Normal sinus
rhythm with one nonconducted PAC (after
the seventh QRS complex

Strip 7.33
Rhythm: Regular (basic rhythm); irregular
with PAC
Rate: 45 beats/minute (basic rhythm)
P waves: Sinus (basic rhythm); premature
and pointed with PAC
PR interval: 0.18 to 0.20 second (basic
rhythm); 0.20 second (PAC)
QRS complex: 0.08 second (basic rhythm
and PAC)
Rhythm interpretation: Sinus bradycardia
with one PAC (fifth complex)
Comment. A U wave is present

Strip 7.34
Rhythm: Irregular
Rate: Atrial: Not measurable
Ventricular: 50 beats/minute
P waves: Fibrillatory waves are present
PR interval: Not measurable
QRS complex: 0.06 to 0.08 second
Rhythm interpretation: Atrial fibrillation
(controlled rate)
Comment. ST segment depression and
T-wave inversion are present

Strip 7.35
Rhythm: Regular
Rate: 188 beats/minute
P waves: Hidden in T waves (TP waves)
PR interval: Not measurable
QRS complex: 0.04 to 0.08 second
Rhythm interpretation: Paroxysmal atrial
tachycardia
Comment. ST segment depression is
present

Strip 7.36
Rhythm: Regular (basic rhythm); irregular
with PACs
Rate: 65 beats/minute (basic rhythm);
rate slows to 60 beats/minute following
pause with second PAC (temporary rate
suppression can occur following a pause
in the basic rhythm)
P waves: Sinus (basic rhythm); pointed
and abnormal with PACs
PR interval: 0.14 to 0.16 second (basic
rhythm); 0.14 to 0.16 second (PACs)
QRS complex: 0.06 to 0.08 second (basic
rhythm); 0.04 to 0.06 second (PACs)
Rhythm interpretation: Normal sinus
rhythm with two PACs (fourth and sixth
complexes)

Strip 7.37
Rhythm: Irregular
Rate: Atrial: 260 beats/minute
Ventricular: 70 beats/minute
P waves: Flutter waves present (varying ratios)
PR interval: Not measurable
QRS complex: 0.04 to 0.08 second
Rhythm interpretation: Atrial flutter with variable AV conduction

Strip 7.38
Rhythm: Regular
Rate: 150 beats/minute
P waves: Hidden in T waves (TP waves)
PR interval: Not measurable
QRS complex: 0.06 to 0.98 second
Rhythm interpretation: Paroxysmal atrial tachycardia

Strip 7.39
Rhythm: Regular (basic rhythm); irregular with PAC
Rate: 136 beats/minute (basic rhythm)
P waves: Sinus (basic rhythm); premature and pointed (PAC)
PR interval: 0.16 to 0.20 second (basic rhythm); 0.20 second (PAC)
QRS complex: 0.06 to 0.08 second (basic rhythm); 0.06 second (PAC)
Rhythm interpretation: Sinus tachycardia with one PAC (eleventh complex)

Strip 7.40
Rhythm: Irregular to regular
Rate: First rhythm: 120 beats/minute
Second rhythm: 88 beats/minute
P waves: First rhythm: Fibrillatory waves
Second rhythm: Sinus
PR interval: First rhythm: Not measurable
Second rhythm: 0.12 to 0.16 second
QRS complex: First rhythm: 0.06 to 0.08 second
Second rhythm: 0.06 second
Rhythm interpretation: Atrial fibrillation (uncontrolled rate) converting to normal sinus rhythm

Strip 7.41
Rhythm: Regular (basic rhythm); irregular with nonconducted PAC
Rate: 79 beats/minute (basic rhythm)
P waves: Sinus (basic rhythm); premature, abnormal P wave hidden in the T wave after the seventh QRS complex
PR interval: 0.20 second
QRS complex: 0.08 to 0.10 second
Rhythm interpretation: Normal sinus rhythm with one nonconducted PAC hidden in the T wave after the seventh QRS complex
Comment: A U wave is present

Strip 7.42
Rhythm: Regular (basic rhythm); irregular with PAC
Rate: 84 beats/minute (basic rhythm)
P waves: Sinus (basic rhythm); abnormal, pointed (PAC)
PR interval: 0.12 to 0.14 second (basic rhythm); 0.28 second (PAC)
QRS complex: 0.06 to 0.08 second (basic rhythm); 0.06 second (PAC)
Rhythm interpretation: Normal sinus rhythm with one PAC (conducted with long PR interval)
Comment: T-wave inversion is present

Strip 7.43
Rhythm: Regular
Rate: 68 beats/minute
P waves: Vary in size, shape, direction across strip
PR interval: 0.12 to 0.16 second
QRS complex: 0.06 to 0.08 second
Rhythm interpretation: Wandering atrial pacemaker

Strip 7.44
Rhythm: Regular (basic rhythm); irregular with PACs
Rate: 79 beats/minute (basic rhythm)
P waves: Sinus (basic rhythm); premature and pointed (PACs)
PR interval: 0.16 to 0.18 second (basic rhythm); 0.12 second (PAC)
QRS complex: 0.06 to 0.08 second (basic rhythm and PACs)
Rhythm interpretation: Normal sinus rhythm with 3 PACs (third, sixth, and ninth complexes) occurring in a trigeminal pattern

Strip 7.45
Rhythm: Regular
Rate: 214 beats/minute
P waves: Hidden in T waves (TP waves)
PR interval: Not measurable
QRS complex: 0.06 to 0.08 second
Rhythm interpretation: Paroxysmal atrial tachycardia

Strip 7.46
Rhythm: Regular (basis rhythm); irregular with PAC
Rate: 79 beats/minute (basic rhythm)
P waves: Sinus (basic rhythm); premature and pointed (PAC)
PR interval: 0.14 to 0.16 second (basic rhythm); 0.12 second (PAC)
QRS complex: 0.06 to 0.08 second (basic rhythm); 0.08 second (PAC)
Rhythm interpretation: Normal sinus rhythm with one PAC (fifth complex)

Strip 7.47
Rhythm: Regular (basic rhythm); irregular with PAC
Rate: 100 beats/minute (basic rhythm)
P waves: Sinus (basic rhythm); premature and abnormal (PAC)
PR interval: 0.12 to 0.16 second (basic rhythm); 0.12 second (PAC)
QRS complex: 0.04 to 0.08 second (basic rhythm); 0.04 second (PAC)
Rhythm interpretation: Normal sinus rhythm with one PAC
Comment: ST segment depression is present

Strip 7.48
Rhythm: Irregular
Rate: Atrial: Not measurable
Ventricular: 150 beats/minute
P waves: Fibrillatory waves present
PR interval: Not measurable
QRS complex: 0.04 to 0.08 second
Rhythm interpretation: Atrial fibrillation (uncontrolled rate)
Comment: ST segment depression is present

Strip 7.49
Rhythm: Regular
Rate: Atrial: 250 beats/minute
Ventricular: 125 beats/minute
P waves: Two flutter waves to each QRS complex
PR interval: Not measurable
QRS complex: 0.08 second
Rhythm interpretation: Atrial flutter with 2:1 AV conduction

Strip 7.50
Rhythm: Irregular
Rate: Atrial: 220 beats/minute
Ventricular: 30 beats/minute
P waves: Flutter waves are present
(varying ratios)
PR interval: Not measurable
QRS complex: 0.06 to 0.08 second
Rhythm interpretation: Atrial flutter with
variable AV conduction

Strip 7.51
Rhythm: Regular
Rate: 150 beats/minute
P waves: Hidden in T waves (TP waves)
PR interval: Not measurable
QRS complex: 0.08 to 0.10 second
Rhythm interpretation: Paroxysmal atrial
tachycardia

Strip 7.52
Rhythm: Regular (basic rhythm); irregular
with PACs
Rate: 65 beats/minute (basic rhythm)
P waves: Sinus (basic rhythm); abnormal
and inverted with PACs
PR interval: 0.20 second (basic rhythm);
0.12 second (PACs)
QRS complex: 0.06 to 0.08 second (basic
rhythm and PACs)
Rhythm interpretation: Normal sinus
rhythm with paired PACs

Strip 7.53
Rhythm: Irregular
Rate: Atrial: Not measurable
Ventricular: 70 beats/minute
P waves: Fibrillatory waves
PR interval: Not measurable
QRS complex: 0.06 to 0.08 second
Rhythm interpretation: Atrial fibrillation
(controlled rate)
Comment. ST segment depression is present

Strip 7.54
Rhythm: Regular (basic rhythm); irregular
with PAC
Rate: 94 beats/minute (basic rhythm)
P waves: Sinus (basic rhythm); premature
and pointed (PAC)
PR interval: 0.12 to 0.16 second (basic
rhythm); 0.16 second (PAC)
QRS complex: 0.06 to 0.08 second (basic
rhythm and PAC)
Rhythm interpretation: Normal sinus
rhythm with one PAC (eighth complex)
Comment. ST segment depression is present

Strip 7.55
Rhythm: First rhythm: Irregular
Second rhythm: Regular
Rate: First rhythm: 120 beats/minute
Second rhythm: 75 beats/minute
P waves: First rhythm: Fibrillatory waves
Second rhythm: Sinus
PR interval: First rhythm: Not measurable
Second rhythm: 0.12 to 0.14 second
QRS complex: 0.04 to 0.08 second (both
rhythms)
Rhythm interpretation: Atrial fibrillation
(uncontrolled rate) to normal sinus rhythm

Strip 7.56
Rhythm: Regular (basic rhythm); irregular
with PAC
Rate: 84 beats/minute (basic rhythm)
P waves: Sinus (basic rhythm); premature
and pointed with PAC
PR interval: 0.12 to 0.16 second (basic
rhythm); 0.12 second (PAC)
QRS complex: 0.06 to 0.08 second (basic
rhythm); 0.08 second (PAC)
Rhythm interpretation: Normal sinus
rhythm with one PAC (fifth complex)

Strip 7.57
Rhythm: Regular
Rate: Atrial: 300 beats/minute
Ventricular: 75 beats/minute
P waves: Four flutter waves to each QRS
complex
PR interval: Not measurable
QRS complex: 0.06 to 0.08 second
Rhythm interpretation: Atrial flutter with
4:1 AV conduction

Strip 7.58
Rhythm: Regular (basic rhythm); irregular
with nonconducted PAC
Rate: 88 beats/minute (basic rhythm);
rate slows to 72 beats/minute after the
pause following the nonconducted PAC
(temporary rate suppression is common
following a pause in the basic rhythm)
P waves: Sinus (basic rhythm); premature
abnormal P wave without a QRS complex
hidden in the T wave after the seventh
QRS complex
PR interval: 0.12 to 0.14 second
QRS complex: 0.08 to 0.10 second
Rhythm interpretation: Normal sinus
rhythm with one nonconducted PAC (after
the seventh QRS complex)

Strip 7.59
Rhythm: Irregular
Rate: 70 beats/minute
P waves: Vary in size, shape, and direction
across the strip
PR interval: 0.16 second
QRS complex: 0.06 to 0.08 second
Rhythm interpretation: Wandering atrial
pacemaker
Comment. T-wave inversion is present

Strip 7.60
Rhythm: Irregular
Rate: Atrial: Not measurable
Ventricular: 50 beats/minute
P waves: Fibrillatory waves are present
PR interval: Not measurable
QRS complex: 0.04 to 0.06 second
Rhythm interpretation: Atrial fibrillation
(controlled rate)
Comment. ST segment depression and
T-wave inversion are present

Strip 7.61
Rhythm: Irregular
Rate: Atrial: Not measurable
Ventricular: 130 beats/minute
P waves: Fibrillatory waves are present
PR interval: Not measurable
QRS complex: 0.04 to 0.08 second
Rhythm interpretation: Atrial fibrillation
(uncontrolled rate)
Comment. ST segment depression is present

Strip 7.62
Rhythm: Regular (basic rhythm); irregular
with PAC
Rate: 58 beats/minute (basic rhythm)
P waves: Sinus (basic rhythm); premature
and abnormal (PAC)
PR interval: 0.16 to 0.20 second (basic
rhythm); 0.20 second (PAC)
QRS complex: 0.06 to 0.08 second (basic
rhythm); 0.06 second (PAC)
Rhythm interpretation: Sinus bradycardia
with one PAC (fifth complex)
Comment. A U wave is present

Strip 7.63
Rhythm: Irregular
Rate: Atrial: Not measurable
Ventricular: 40 beats/minute
P waves: Fibrillatory waves are present
PR interval: Not measurable
QRS complex: 0.08 to 0.10 second
Rhythm interpretation: Atrial fibrillation
(controlled rate)

Strip 7.64
Rhythm: Regular
Rate: 214 beats/minute
P waves: Hidden in T waves (TP waves)
PR interval: Not measurable
QRS complex: 0.08 second
Rhythm interpretation: Paroxysmal atrial tachycardia

Strip 7.65
Rhythm: Regular (basic rhythm); irregular with PAC
Rate: 52 beats/minute (basic rhythm)
P waves: Sinus (basic rhythm); premature and pointed P wave associated with PAC hidden in the T wave after the fourth QRS complex
PR interval: 0.16 to 0.18 second (basic rhythm)
QRS complex: 0.06 to 0.08 second (basic rhythm); 0.06 second (PAC)
Rhythm interpretation: Sinus bradycardia with one PAC (fifth complex)
Comment. A U wave is present

Strip 7.66
Rhythm: Regular (basic rhythm); irregular with PACs and nonconducted PAC
Rate: 94 beats/minute (basic rhythm)
P waves: Sinus (basic rhythm); premature, pointed P wave hidden in T wave following third QRS complex (nonconducted PAC); premature, pointed P waves with PACs (seventh and tenth complexes)
PR interval: 0.12 second (basic rhythm)
QRS complex: 0.08 to 0.10 second (basic rhythm and PACs)
Rhythm interpretation: Normal sinus rhythm with one nonconducted PAC (following third QRS complex) and two PACs (7th and 10th complexes)

Strip 7.67
Rhythm: Irregular
Rate: 70 beats/minute
P waves: Vary in size, shape, and direction across strip
PR interval: 0.12 to 0.20 second
QRS complex: 0.08 to 0.10 second
Rhythm interpretation: Wandering atrial pacemaker

Strip 7.68
Rhythm: Regular
Rate: 150 beats/minute
P waves: Hidden in T waves (TP waves)
PR interval: Not measurable
QRS complex: 0.04 to 0.08 second
Rhythm interpretation: Paroxysmal atrial tachycardia
Comment. ST segment depression is present

Strip 7.69
Rhythm: Irregular
Rate: Atrial: 260 beats/minute
Ventricular: 70 beats/minute
P waves: Flutter waves are present (varying ratios)
PR interval: Not measurable
QRS complex: 0.06 to 0.08 second
Rhythm interpretation: Atrial flutter with variable AV conduction

Strip 7.70
Rhythm: Irregular
Rate: Atrial: Not measurable
Ventricular: 40 beats/minute
P waves: Fibrillatory waves are present
PR interval: Not measurable
QRS complex: 0.08 to 0.10 second
Rhythm interpretation: Atrial fibrillation (controlled rate)

Strip 7.71
Rhythm: Regular (basic rhythm); irregular with PACs
Rate: 88 beats/minute (basic rhythm)
P waves: Sinus (basic rhythm); premature and abnormal (PACs)
PR interval: 0.16 to 0.18 second (basic rhythm)
QRS complex: 0.06 to 0.08 second (basic rhythm); 0.08 second (PACs)
Rhythm interpretation: Normal sinus rhythm with paired PACs (third and fourth complexes)

Strip 7.72
Rhythm: Regular (basic rhythm); irregular with PACs
Rate: 60 beats/minute (basic rhythm)
P waves: Sinus (basic rhythm); premature and different from sinus P waves (PACs)
PR interval: 0.16 to 0.20 second (basic rhythm); 0.16 second (PACs)
QRS complex: 0.06 to 0.08 second (basic rhythm and PACs)
Rhythm interpretation: Normal sinus rhythm with two PACs (third and sixth complexes); PACs occur in a trigeminal pattern

Strip 7.73
Rhythm: Regular
Rate: Atrial: 272 beats/minute
Ventricular: 136 beats/minute
P waves: Two flutter waves before each QRS complex
PR interval: Not measurable
QRS complex: 0.08 second
Rhythm interpretation: Atrial flutter with 2:1 AV conduction

Strip 7.74
Rhythm: Regular (basic rhythm); irregular with PAC
Rate: 63 beats/minute (basic rhythm)
P waves: Sinus (basic rhythm); premature and abnormal with PAC
PR interval: 0.12 to 0.14 second (basic rhythm); 0.12 second (PAC)
QRS complex: 0.06 to 0.08 second (basic rhythm); 0.08 second (PAC)
Rhythm interpretation: Normal sinus rhythm with one PAC (fourth complex)
Comment. A small U wave is present

Strip 7.75
Rhythm: Regular
Rate: 188 beats/minute
P waves: Hidden in T waves (TP waves)
PR interval: Not measurable
QRS complex: 0.08 to 0.10 second
Rhythm interpretation: Paroxysmal atrial tachycardia

Strip 7.76
Rhythm: Irregular
Rate: Atrial: Not measurable
Ventricular: 130 beats/minute
P waves: Fibrillatory waves are present
PR interval: Not measurable
QRS complex: 0.04 to 0.06 second
Rhythm interpretation: Atrial fibrillation (uncontrolled rate)
Comment. ST segment depression is present

Strip 7.77
Rhythm: Regular
Rate: 88 beats/minute
P waves: Vary in size, shape, and direction across strip
PR interval: 0.14 to 0.16 second
QRS complex: 0.04 to 0.08 second
Rhythm interpretation: Wandering atrial pacemaker
Comment. T-wave inversion is present

Strip 7.78
Rhythm: Irregular
Rate: 90 beats/minute
P waves: Vary in size, shape, and direction across strip
PR interval: 0.12 to 0.20 second
QRS complex: 0.06 to 0.08 second
Rhythm interpretation: Wandering atrial pacemaker

Strip 7.79
Rhythm: Irregular
Rate: Atrial: 280 beats/minute
Ventricular: 100 beats/minute
P waves: Flutter waves are present (varying ratios)
PR interval: Not measurable
QRS complex: 0.04 to 0.06 second
Rhythm interpretation: Atrial flutter with variable AV conduction

Strip 7.80
Rhythm: Regular (basic rhythm); irregular with PAC and nonconducted PACs
Rate: 100 beats/minute (basic rhythm)
P waves: Sinus (basic rhythm); premature and abnormal (PAC and nonconducted PACs)
PR interval: 0.16 to 0.20 second (basic rhythm); 0.16 second (PAC)
QRS complex: 0.04 to 0.08 second (basic rhythm); 0.08 second (PAC)
Rhythm interpretation: Normal sinus rhythm with two nonconducted PACs (after the third and eighth)
QRS complexes) and one PAC (tenth complex)

Strip 7.81
Rhythm: Regular
Rate: 68 beats/minute
P waves: Vary in size, shape, and direction across strip
PR interval: 0.12 to 0.16 second
QRS complex: 0.08 second
Rhythm interpretation: Wandering atrial pacemaker
Comment. A U wave is present

Strip 7.82
Rhythm: Regular
Rate: Atrial: 260 beats/minute
Ventricular: 65 beats/minute
P waves: Four flutter waves to each QRS complex
PR interval: Not measurable
QRS complex: 0.08 to 0.10 second
Rhythm interpretation: Atrial flutter with 4:1 AV conduction

Strip 7.83
Rhythm: Regular
Rate: 167 beats/minute
P waves: Hidden in T waves (TP waves)
PR interval: Not measurable
QRS complex: 0.08 to 0.10 second
Rhythm interpretation: Paroxysmal atrial tachycardia

Strip 7.84
Rhythm: Irregular
Rate: 50 beats/minute
P waves: Fibrillatory waves
PR interval: Not measurable
QRS complex: 0.08 to 0.10 second
Rhythm interpretation: Atrial fibrillation (controlled rate)

Strip 7.85
Rhythm: Irregular
Rate: 40 beats/minute
P waves: Vary in size, shape, and direction across strip
PR interval: 0.14 to 0.16 second
QRS complex: 0.08 second
Rhythm interpretation: Wandering atrial pacemaker

Strip 7.86
Rhythm: Regular (basic rhythm); irregular with PAC
Rate: 115 beats/minute
P waves: Sinus (basic rhythm); small and pointed (PAC)
PR interval: 0.12 (basic rhythm); 0.08 second (PAC)
QRS complex: 0.06 to 0.08 second (basic rhythm); 0.08 second (PAC)
Rhythm interpretation: Sinus tachycardia with one PAC (10th complex)

Strip 7.87
Rhythm: Irregular
Rate: Atrial: Not measurable
Ventricular: 50 beats/minute
P waves: Fibrillatory waves
PR interval: Not measurable
QRS complex: 0.04 to 0.06 second
Rhythm interpretation: Atrial fibrillation (controlled rate)

Strip 7.88
Rhythm: First rhythm: Regular
Second rhythm: Irregular
Rate: First rhythm: 79 beats/minute
Second rhythm: 140 beats/minute
P waves: First rhythm: Sinus
Second rhythm: Fibrillatory waves
PR interval: First rhythm: 0.12 to 0.14 second
Second rhythm: Not measurable
QRS complex: 0.04 to 0.08 second (both rhythms)
Rhythm interpretation: Normal sinus rhythm changing to atrial fibrillation (uncontrolled rate)

Strip 7.89
Rhythm: Regular (basic rhythm); irregular with nonconducted PAC
Rate: 84 beats/minute (basic rhythm)
P waves: Sinus (basic rhythm); premature and pointed (nonconducted PAC)
PR interval: 0.16 to 0.20 second
QRS complex: 0.04 to 0.08 second
Rhythm interpretation: Normal sinus rhythm with one nonconducted PAC (after fifth QRS complex)
Comment. ST segment depression is present

Strip 7.90
Rhythm: Regular (basic rhythm) measured between first and second QRS complexes; irregular with (PACs)
Rate: 75 beats/minute (basic rhythm)
P waves: Sinus (basic rhythm); premature and pointed (PACs)
PR interval: 0.16 to 0.18 second (basic rhythm); 0.12 to 0.16 second (PACs)
QRS complex: 0.04 to 0.08 second (basic rhythm); 0.06 to 0.08 second (PACs)
Rhythm interpretation: Normal sinus rhythm with paired PACs (third and fourth complexes) and single PACs (sixth and eighth complexes)

Strip 7.91
Rhythm: Regular (basic rhythm); irregular with PAC
Rate: 63 beats/minute (basic rhythm)
P waves: Sinus (basic rhythm); premature and abnormal (PAC)
PR interval: 0.16 to 0.18 second (basic rhythm); 0.16 second (PAC)
QRS complex: 0.04 to 0.06 second (basic rhythm); 0.06 second (PAC)
Rhythm interpretation: Normal sinus rhythm with one PAC (fifth complex)
Comment. A U wave is present

Strip 7.92
Rhythm: Regular
Rate: Atrial: 235 beats/minute
Ventricular: 47 beats/minute
P waves: Five flutter waves before each QRS complex
PR interval: Not measurable
QRS complex: 0.08 second
Rhythm interpretation: Atrial flutter with 5:1 AV conduction
Comment: T-wave inversion is present

Strip 7.93
Rhythm: Regular
Rate: 150 beats/minute
P waves: Hidden in T waves (TP waves)
PR interval: Not measurable
QRS complex: 0.04 to 0.08 second
Rhythm interpretation: Paroxysmal atrial tachycardia

Strip 7.94
Rhythm: Irregular
Rate: Atrial: Not measurable
Ventricular: 50 beats/minute
P waves: Fibrillatory waves are present
PR interval: Not measurable
QRS complex: 0.04 to 0.06 second
Rhythm interpretation: Atrial fibrillation (controlled rate)
Comment: ST segment depression is present

Strip 7.95
Rhythm: Regular (basic rhythm); irregular after a burst of PAT
Rate: 84 beats/minute (basic rhythm); 188 beats/minute (PAT)
P waves: Sinus (basic rhythm); premature and abnormal (PAT)
PR interval: 0.16 to 0.20 second (basic rhythm); not measurable in PAT
QRS complex: 0.04 to 0.06 second (basic rhythm and PAT)
Rhythm interpretation: Normal sinus rhythm with three-beat run of PAT (three consecutive PACs after the fourth QRS complex)

Strip 7.96
Rhythm: Regular
Rate: 75 beats/minute
P waves: Sinus
PR interval: 0.16 to 0.20 second
QRS complex: 0.06 to 0.08 second
Rhythm interpretation: Normal sinus rhythm
Comment: A U wave is present

Strip 7.97
Rhythm: Regular (basic rhythm)—off by one square; irregular with PACs
Rate: 84 to 88 beats/minute (basic rhythm)
P waves: Sinus (basic rhythm); premature and abnormal (PACs)
PR interval: 0.14 to 0.16 second (basic rhythm); 0.16 second (PACs)
QRS complex: 0.06 to 0.08 second (basic rhythm and PACs)
Rhythm interpretation: Normal sinus rhythm with PACs every fourth beat (quadrigeminal pattern)

Strip 7.98
Rhythm: Regular
Rate: 107 beats/minute
P waves: Sinus
PR interval: 0.12 to 0.16 second
QRS complex: 0.04 to 0.06 second
Rhythm interpretation: Sinus tachycardia

Strip 7.99
Rhythm: Regular
Rate: Atrial: 250 beats/minute
Ventricular: 125 beats/minute
P waves: Two flutter waves before each QRS complex
PR interval: Not measurable
QRS complex: 0.08 second
Rhythm interpretation: Atrial flutter with 2:1 AV conduction

Strip 7.100
Rhythm: Regular (basic rhythm); irregular during pause
Rate: 48 beats/minute (basic rhythm)
P waves: Sinus (basic rhythm); absent during pause
PR interval: 0.20 second (basic rhythm); absent during pause
QRS complex: 0.06 to 0.08 second (basic rhythm); absent during pause
Rhythm interpretation: Sinus bradycardia with sinus arrest

Strip 7.101
Rhythm: Irregular
Rate: 90 beats/minute
P waves: Vary in size, shape, and direction across strip
PR interval: 0.12 to 0.20 second
QRS complex: 0.06 to 0.08 second
Rhythm interpretation: Wandering atrial pacemaker

Strip 7.102
Rhythm: Regular (off by one square)
Rate: 45 to 47 beats/minute
P waves: Sinus
PR interval: 0.16 to 0.20 second
QRS complex: 0.04 to 0.08 second
Rhythm interpretation: Sinus bradycardia
Comment: T-wave inversion is present

Strip 7.103
Rhythm: Regular (first and second rhythms)
Rate: 88 beats/minute (basic rhythm); 188 beats/minute (PAT)
P waves: Sinus (basic rhythm); hidden in T waves (PAT)
PR interval: 0.16 to 0.18 second (basic rhythm)
QRS complex: 0.06 to 0.08 second (basic rhythm); 0.04 to 0.08 second (PAT)
Rhythm interpretation: Normal sinus rhythm with PAC (fourth complex) initiating an eight-beat run of PAT followed by a return to NSR

Strip 7.104
Rhythm: Irregular
Rate: Atrial: Not measurable
Ventricular: 100 beats/minute
P waves: Fibrillatory waves
PR interval: Not measurable
QRS complex: 0.08 to 0.10 second
Rhythm interpretation: Atrial fibrillation (controlled rate)

Strip 7.105
Rhythm: Irregular
Rate: 60 beats/minute
P waves: Sinus
PR interval: 0.14 to 0.16 second
QRS complex: 0.06 to 0.08 second
Rhythm interpretation: Sinus arrhythmia

Strip 7.106
Rhythm: First rhythm: Regular
Second rhythm: Irregular
Rate: First rhythm: 75 beats/minute
Second rhythm: 140 beats/minute
P waves: First rhythm: Sinus
Second rhythm: Fibrillatory and flutter waves
PR interval: First rhythm: 0.12 second
Second rhythm: Not measurable
QRS complex: 0.08 to 0.10 second (first and second rhythms)
Rhythm interpretation: Normal sinus rhythm with PAC (fifth complex) changing to atrial fib/flutter

Strip 7.107
Rhythm: Regular
Rate: 84 beats/minute
P waves: Sinus
PR interval: 0.12 to 0.14 second
QRS complex: 0.06 to 0.08 second
Rhythm interpretation: Normal sinus rhythm

Strip 8.1
Rhythm: Regular (basic rhythm); irregular with PJC
Rate: 79 beats/minute (basic rhythm)
P waves: Sinus (basic rhythm); inverted with PJC
PR interval: 0.12 to 0.14 second (basic rhythm); 0.08 second (PJC)
QRS complex: 0.06 to 0.08 second (basic rhythm); 0.08 second (PJC)
Rhythm interpretation: Normal sinus rhythm with one PJC (seventh complex)

Strip 8.2
Rhythm: Regular
Rate: 65 beats/minute
P waves: Sinus
PR interval: 0.32 to 0.36 second (PR consistent)
QRS complex: 0.06 to 0.08 second
Rhythm interpretation: Normal sinus rhythm with first-degree AV block
Comment: An inverted T wave is present

Strip 8.3
Rhythm: Regular (atrial and ventricular)
Rate: Atrial: 94 beats/minute
Ventricular: 32 beats/minute
P waves: Three sinus P waves before each QRS complex
PR interval: 0.14 to 0.16 second (PR consistent)
QRS complex: 0.12 second
Rhythm interpretation: Mobitz II with 3:1 AV conduction (third P wave is hidden in T waves)

Strip 8.4
Rhythm: Regular (basic rhythm); irregular with junctional escape beat
Rate: 58 beats/minute (basic rhythm)
P waves: Sinus (basic rhythm); hidden P wave with junctional escape beat
PR interval: 0.16 to 0.18 second (basic rhythm)
QRS complex: 0.08 to 0.10 second (basic rhythm); 0.10 second (junctional escape beat)
Rhythm interpretation: Sinus bradycardia with junctional escape beat (fourth complex) after pause in basic rhythm

Strip 8.5
Rhythm: Regular (first and second rhythms)
Rate: First rhythm: 84 beats/minute
Second rhythm: 94 beats/minute
P waves: First rhythm: Sinus
Second rhythm: Inverted
PR interval: First rhythm: 0.12 second
Second rhythm: 0.06 to 0.08 second
QRS complex: 0.06 to 0.08 second (first and second rhythms)
Rhythm interpretation: Normal sinus rhythm changing to accelerated junctional rhythm

Strip 8.6
Rhythm: Regular
Rate: 84 beats/minute
P waves: Sinus
PR interval: 0.22 to 0.24 second (PR consistent)
QRS complex: 0.08 to 0.10 second
Rhythm interpretation: Normal sinus rhythm with first-degree AV block

Strip 8.7
Rhythm: Regular
Rate: 65 beats/minute
P waves: Inverted before each QRS complex
PR interval: 0.08 second
QRS complex: 0.08 to 0.10 second
Rhythm interpretation: Accelerated junctional rhythm
Comment: ST segment elevation and T-wave inversion are present

Strip 8.8
Rhythm: Atrial (regular); Ventricular (irregular)
Rate: Atrial: 75 beats/minute
Ventricular: 70 beats/minute
P waves: Sinus
PR interval: Lengthens from 0.28 to 0.32 second (PR varies)
QRS complex: 0.06 to 0.08 second
Rhythm interpretation: Second-degree AV block, Mobitz I
Comment: ST segment depression and T-wave inversion are present

Strip 8.9
Rhythm: Regular
Rate: 47 beats/minute
P waves: Hidden in QRS complex
PR interval: Not measurable
QRS complex: 0.08 second
Rhythm interpretation: Junctional rhythm
Comment: ST segment depression is present

Strip 8.10
Rhythm: Atrial: Regular
Ventricular: Irregular
Rate: Atrial: 75 beats/minute
Ventricular: 30 beats/minute
P waves: Two sinus P waves before each QRS complex
PR interval: 0.20 to 0.22 second (PR consistent)
QRS complex: 0.10 second
Rhythm interpretation: Second-degree AV block, Mobitz II
Comment: Clinical correlation is suggested to diagnose Mobitz II when 2:1 AV conduction is present with a narrow QRS complex

Strip 8.11
Rhythm: Regular (Atrial and ventricular)
Rate: Atrial: 60 beats/minute
Ventricular: 33 beats/minute
P waves: Sinus (bear no relationship to QRS complex)
PR interval: PR varies
QRS complex: 0.12 second
Rhythm interpretation: Third-degree AV block
Comment: ST segment depression and T-wave inversion are present

Strip 8.12
Rhythm: First rhythm (unable to measure). Second rhythm: Regular
Rate: 75 beats/minute (second rhythm)
P waves: Sinus (sinus beat); squiggle (PAC); inverted before QRS (second rhythm)
PR interval: 0.16 second (sinus beat); 0.16 second (PAC); 0.08 second (second rhythm)
QRS complex: 0.06 to 0.08 second
Rhythm interpretation: Sinus beat followed by a PAC changing to accelerated junctional rhythm

Strip 8.13
Rhythm: Regular
Rate: 65 beats/minute
P waves: Sinus
PR interval: 0.44 to 0.48 second (PR consistent)
QRS complex: 0.08 to 0.10 second
Rhythm interpretation: Normal sinus rhythm with first-degree AV block
Comment: ST segment elevation is present

Strip 8.14
Rhythm: Regular (basic rhythm); irregular with PJC
Rate: 136 beats/minute (basic rhythm)
P waves: Sinus (basic rhythm); hidden P wave with PJC
PR interval: 0.12 to 0.14 second
QRS complex: 0.04 to 0.06 second; 0.06 (PJC)
Rhythm interpretation: Sinus tachycardia with one PJC (13th complex)

Strip 8.15
Rhythm: Regular
Rate: 84 beats/minute
P waves: Sinus
PR interval: 0.24 to 0.28 second (PR consistent)
QRS complex: 0.06 to 0.08 second
Rhythm interpretation: Normal sinus rhythm with first-degree AV block
Comment: ST segment depression is present

Strip 8.16
Rhythm: Regular (basic rhythm); irregular with premature beat
Rate: 58 beats/minute (basic rhythm)
P waves: Sinus (basic rhythm); inverted (premature beat)
PR interval: 0.16 to 0.18 second (basic rhythm); 0.08 second (PJC)
QRS complex: 0.06 to 0.08 second (basic rhythm); 0.08 second (PJC)
Rhythm interpretation: Sinus bradycardia with one PJC (fourth complex)
Comment: ST segment depression is present

Strip 8.17
Rhythm: Regular (atrial and ventricular rhythms)
Rate: Atrial: 80 beats/minute
Ventricular: 40 beats/minute
P waves: Sinus
PR interval: 0.16 to 0.18 second (PR consistent)
QRS complex: 0.14 to 0.16 second
Rhythm interpretation: Second-degree AV block, Mobitz II
Comment: ST segment depression is present

Strip 8.18
Rhythm: Atrial (regular); Ventricular (irregular)
Rate: Atrial: 65 beats/minute
Ventricular: 50 beats/minute
P waves: Sinus
PR interval: PR lengthens from 0.20 to 0.48 second (PR varies)
QRS complex: 0.04 to 0.06 second
Rhythm interpretation: Second-degree AV block, Mobitz I

Strip 8.19
Rhythm: Regular
Rate: 125 beats/minute
P waves: Inverted before each QRS complex
PR interval: 0.08 to 0.10 second
QRS complex: 0.06 to 0.08 second
Rhythm interpretation: Junctional tachycardia

Strip 8.20
Rhythm: Regular (atrial and ventricular)
Rate: Atrial: 100 beats/minute
Ventricular: 38 beats/minute
P waves: Sinus (bear no relationship to QRS complex)
PR interval: PR varies
QRS complex: 0.06 to 0.08 second
Rhythm interpretation: Third-degree AV block
Comment: ST segment depression is present

Strip 8.21
Rhythm: Regular (basic rhythm); irregular with PJC
Rate: 60 beats/minute (basic rhythm)
P waves: Sinus (basic rhythm); premature and inverted (PJC)
PR interval: 0.12 to 0.14 second (basic rhythm); 0.08 second (PJC)
QRS complex: 0.08 second (basic rhythm and PJC)
Rhythm interpretation: Normal sinus rhythm with one PJC (fourth complex)

Strip 8.22
Rhythm: Regular (basic rhythm); off by two squares
Rate: 54 to 58 beats/minute
P waves: Sinus (basic rhythm); hidden in QRS complex (junctional escape beats)
PR interval: 0.16 to 0.18 second (basic rhythm)
QRS complex: 0.08 to 10 second (basic rhythm and junctional escape beats)
Rhythm interpretation: Sinus bradycardia with a pause followed by two junctional escape beats
Comment: Specific pause (sinus arrest or sinus block) cannot be identified due to the presence of the escape beats).

Strip 8.23
Rhythm: Regular
Rate: 72 beats/minute
P waves: Sinus
PR interval; 0.32 to 0.34 second (PR consistent)
QRS complex: 0.04 to 0.06 second
Rhythm interpretation: Normal sinus rhythm with first-degree AV block

Strip 8.24
Rhythm: Atrial (regular); Ventricular (irregular)
Rate: Atrial: 68 beats/minute
Ventricular: 60 beats/minute
P waves: Sinus
PR interval: Lengthens from 0.30 to 0.36 second (PR varies)
QRS complex: 0.08 second
Rhythm interpretation: Second-degree AV block, Mobitz I
Comment: A U wave is present

Strip 8.25
Rhythm: Regular
Rate: 75 beats/minute
P waves: Sinus
PR interval: 0.28 to 0.32 second (PR consistent)
QRS complex: 0.06 to 0.08 second
Rhythm interpretation: Normal sinus rhythm with first-degree AV block

Strip 8.26
Rhythm: Regular (basic rhythm); irregular with premature beats
Rate: 100 beats/minute (basic rhythm)
P waves: Sinus (basic rhythm); pointed P wave (PAC); inverted P wave (PJCs)
PR interval: 0.20 second (basic rhythm); 0.16 second (PAC); 0.06 second (PJCs)
QRS complex: 0.06 to 0.08 second (basic rhythm and premature beats)
Rhythm interpretation: Normal sinus rhythm with one PAC (seventh complex) and paired PJCs (eighth and ninth complexes)
Comment. ST segment depression is present

Strip 8.27
Rhythm: Regular
Rate: 65 beats/minute
P waves: Inverted before each QRS complex
PR interval: 0.08 second
QRS complex: 0.06 to 0.08 second
Rhythm interpretation: Accelerated junctional rhythm
Comment. ST segment elevation is present

Strip 8.28
Rhythm: Regular (basic rhythm); irregular with nonconducted PAC
Rate: 60 beats/minute (basic rhythm)
P waves: Sinus (basic rhythm)
PR interval: 0.28 to 0.30 second (PR consistent)
QRS complex: 0.08 second
Rhythm interpretation: Normal sinus rhythm with first-degree AV block and one nonconducted PAC

Strip 8.29
Rhythm: Regular (atrial); Irregular (ventricular)
Rate: Atrial: 72 beats/minute
Ventricular: 50 beats/minute
P waves: Sinus
PR interval: Lengthens from 0.26 to 0.36 second (PR varies)
QRS complex: 0.08 to 0.10 second
Rhythm interpretation: Second-degree AV block, Mobitz I
Comment. T-wave inversion is present

Strip 8.30
Rhythm: Regular (atrial and ventricular)
Rate: Atrial: 136 beats/minute
Ventricular: 23 beats/minute
P waves: Sinus (bear no relationship to QRS complexes)
PR interval: PR varies
QRS complex: 0.12 second
Rhythm interpretation: Third-degree AV block

Strip 8.31
Rhythm: Regular (atrial and ventricular); both off by two squares
Rate: Atrial: 80 beats/minute
Ventricular: 30 beats/minute
P waves: Three sinus P waves to each QRS complex
PR interval: 0.20 to 0.22 second (PR consistent)
QRS complex: 0.14 to 0.16 second
Rhythm interpretation: Second-degree AV block, Mobitz II with 3:1 AV conduction
Comment. ST segment depression and T-wave inversion are present

Strip 8.32
Rhythm: Regular (atrial and ventricular)
Rate: Atrial: 75 beats/minute
Ventricular: 34 beats/minute
P waves: Sinus (bear no relationship to QRS complexes)
PR interval: PR varies
QRS complex: 0.12 to 0.14 second
Rhythm interpretation: Third-degree AV block
Comment. ST segment elevation is present

Strip 8.33
Rhythm: Regular (basic rhythm); irregular with PAC
Rate: 100 beats/minute (basic rhythm)
P waves: Inverted before the QRS complex (basic rhythm); upright and pointed (PAC)
PR interval: 0.08 second (basic rhythm); 0.12 second (PAC)
QRS complex: 0.06 to 0.08 second (basic rhythm); 0.08 second (PAC)
Rhythm interpretation: Accelerated junctional rhythm with one PAC (sixth complex)
Comment. ST segment depression is present

Strip 8.34
Rhythm: Regular (atrial); Irregular (ventricular)
Rate: Atrial: 70 beats/minute
Ventricular: 50 beats/minute
P waves: Sinus
PR interval: Lengthens from 0.28 to 0.36 second (PR varies)
QRS complex: 0.08 to 0.10 second
Rhythm interpretation: Second-degree AV block, Mobitz I

Strip 8.35
Rhythm: Regular
Rate; 60 beats/minute
P waves: Sinus
PR interval: 0.24 to 0.26 second (PR consistent)
QRS complex: 0.06 to 0.08 second
Rhythm interpretation: Normal sinus rhythm with first-degree AV block

Strip 8.36
Rhythm: Regular
Rate: 41 beats/minute
P waves: Inverted after the QRS complex
PR interval: 0.04 to 0.06 second
QRS complex: 0.06 to 0.08 second
Rhythm interpretation: Junctional rhythm

Strip 8.37
Rhythm: Regular (basic rhythm); irregular with PJCs
Rate: 58 beats/minute (basic rhythm)
P waves: Sinus (basic rhythm); inverted with PJCs
PR interval: 0.16 second (basic rhythm); 0.08 to 0.10 second (PJCs)
QRS complex: 0.04 to 0.08 second (basic rhythm); 0.06 to 0.08 second (PJCs)
Rhythm interpretation: Sinus bradycardia with two PJCs (fourth and sixth complexes)
Comment. A U wave is present

Strip 8.38
Rhythm: Regular
Rate: 60 beats/minute
P waves: Inverted
PR interval: 0.08 to 0.10 second
QRS complex: 0.06 to 0.08 second
Rhythm interpretation: Junctional rhythm

Strip 8.39
Rhythm: Regular (atrial and ventricular)
Rate: Atrial: 70 beats/minute
Ventricular: 36 beats/minute
P waves: Sinus (bear no relationship to
QRS complexes)
PR interval: PR varies
QRS complex: 0.12 to 0.14 second
Rhythm interpretation: Third-degree AV block
Comment. ST segment depression is present

Strip 8.40
Rhythm: Regular (atrial and ventricular)
Rate: Atrial: 68 beats/minute
Ventricular: 28 beats/minute
P waves: Sinus (bear no relationship to
QRS complexes)
PR interval: PR varies
QRS complex: 0.12 to 0.14 second
Rhythm interpretation: Third-degree AV block
Comment. T-wave inversion is present

Strip 8.41
Rhythm: Regular
Rate: 84 beats/minute
P waves: Hidden in QRS complexes
PR interval: Not measurable
QRS complex: 0.06 to 0.08 second
Rhythm interpretation: Accelerated
junctional rhythm

Strip 8.42
Rhythm: Regular (atrial and ventricular)
Rate: Atrial: 115 beats/minute
Ventricular: 40 beats/minute
P waves: Three sinus P waves before each
QRS complex
PR interval: 0.22 to 0.24 second
(PR consistent)
QRS complex: 0.12 second
Rhythm interpretation: Second-degree AV
block, Mobitz II

Strip 8.43
Rhythm: Regular (first and second rhythms)
Rate: First rhythm: 48 beats/minute
Second rhythm: 56 beats/minute
P waves: First rhythm (sinus); Second
rhythm (hidden in QRS)
PR interval: First rhythm (0.16 to
0.18 second)
QRS complex: First rhythm (0.06 second);
Second rhythm (0.04 to 0.06 second)
Rhythm interpretation: Sinus bradycardia
changing to junctional rhythm and
returning to a sinus beat

Strip 8.44
Rhythm: Regular (basic rhythm); irregular
with premature beats
Rate: 60 beats/minute (basic rhythm)
P waves: Sinus (basic rhythm); premature
and abnormal (premature beats)
PR interval: 0.12 to 0.16 second (basic
rhythm); 0.16 (PAC); 0.08 second (PJC)
QRS complex: 0.06 to 0.08 second (basic
rhythm and premature beats)
Rhythm interpretation: Normal sinus
rhythm with one PAC (fourth complex) and
one PJC (fifth complex)
Comment. ST segment depression and
T-wave inversion are present

Strip 8.45
Rhythm: Regular (atrial and ventricular)
Rate: Atrial: 70 beats/minute
Ventricular: 32 beats/minute
P waves: Sinus (bear no relationship to
QRS complexes)
PR interval: PR varies
QRS complex: 0.12 second
Rhythm interpretation: Third-degree AV
block
Comment. ST segment elevation is
present

Strip 8.46
Rhythm: Irregular
Rate: 40 beats/minute
P waves: Sinus
PR interval: 0.28 second (PR consistent)
QRS complex: 0.08 to 0.10 second
Rhythm interpretation: Sinus arrhythmia
with a bradycardic rate and first-degree
AV block
Comment. A U wave is present

Strip 8.47
Rhythm: Regular (atrial); Irregular
(ventricular)
Rate: Atrial: 80 beats/minute
Ventricular: 50 beats/minute
P waves: Sinus
PR interval: Lengthens from 0.20 to
0.40 second (PR varies)
QRS complex: 0.08 to 0.10 second
Rhythm interpretation: Second-degree AV
block, Mobitz I

Strip 8.48
Rhythm: Regular (atrial and ventricular)
Rate: Atrial: 107 beats/minute
Ventricular: 35 beats/minute
P waves: Three sinus P waves before each
QRS complex
PR interval: 0.12 to 0.14 second
(PR consistent)
QRS complex: 0.08 to 0.10 second
Rhythm interpretation: Second-degree AV
block, Mobitz II with 3:1 AV conduction

Strip 8.49
Rhythm: Irregular
Rate: 40 beats/minute
P waves: Inverted before each QRS complex
PR interval: 0.06 to 0.08 second
QRS complex: 0.08 to 0.10 second
Rhythm interpretation: Junctional rhythm
Comment. ST segment depression is present

Strip 8.50
Rhythm: Regular (basic rhythm); irregular
with PJCs and junctional escape beat)
Rate: 94 beats/minute (basic rhythm)
P waves: Sinus (basic rhythm); inverted
(PJCs and junctional escape beat)
PR interval: 0.14 to 0.16 second (basic
rhythm); 0.10 second (PJCs and junctional
escape beat)
QRS complex: 0.08 second (basic rhythm,
PJCs, and junctional escape beat)
Rhythm interpretation: Normal sinus
rhythm with two PJCs (fourth and eighth
complexes) and one junctional escape
beat (ninth complex)

Strip 8.51
Rhythm: Regular (atrial—off by two
squares); Irregular (ventricular)
Rate: Atrial: 60 to 65 beats/minute
Ventricular: 50 beats/minute
P waves: Sinus
PR interval: Lengthens from 0.28 to
0.40 second (PR varies)
QRS complex: 0.08 second
Rhythm interpretation: Second-degree AV
block, Mobitz I

Strip 8.52
Rhythm: Regular
Rate 63 beats/minute
P waves: Hidden in QRS complex
PR interval: Not measurable
QRS complex: 0.08 second
Rhythm interpretation: Accelerated
junctional rhythm

Strip 8.53
Rhythm: Regular (atrial—off by two squares); Irregular (ventricular)
Rate: Atrial: 90 beats/minute
Ventricular: 40 beats/minute
P waves: Sinus (two or three P waves before each QRS complex)
PR interval: 0.12 second (PR consistent)
QRS complex: 0.12 second
Rhythm interpretation: Second-degree AV block, Mobitz II with 2:1 and 3:1 AV conduction

Strip 8.54
Rhythm: Regular
Rate: 94 beats/minute
P waves: Inverted before each QRS complex
PR interval: 0.08 second
QRS complex: 0.06 to 0.08 second
Rhythm interpretation: Accelerated junctional rhythm

Strip 8.55
Rhythm: Regular (basic rhythm)
Rate: 55 beats/minute (basic rhythm)
P waves: Sinus (basic rhythm); no P wave seen with fourth QRS complex; fifth QRS complex has P wave on top of the preceding T wave
PR interval: 0.20 second (basic rhythm)
QRS complex: 0.06 to 0.08 second (basic rhythm); 0.06 second (junctional beat); 0.08 second (PAC)
Rhythm interpretation: Sinus bradycardia with a pause followed by a junctional escape beat (fourth complex) and a PAC (fifth complex)

Strip 8.56
Rhythm: Regular (first and second rhythms)
Rate: First rhythm (72 beats/minute); Second rhythm (140 beats/minute)
P waves: First rhythm (sinus); Second rhythm (inverted)
PR interval: First rhythm (0.12 second); Second rhythm (0.08 to 0.10 second)
QRS complex: 0.06 to 0.08 second (both rhythms)
Rhythm interpretation: Normal sinus rhythm changing to junctional tachycardia
Comment: ST segment depression is present

Strip 8.57
Rhythm: Regular
Rate: 50 beats/minute
P waves: Sinus
PR interval: 0.24 second (PR consistent)
QRS complex: 0.08 to 0.10 second
Rhythm interpretation: Sinus bradycardia with first-degree AV block
Comment: ST segment depression is present

Strip 8.58
Rhythm: Regular (atrial and ventricular)
Rate: Atrial: 94 beats/minute
Ventricular: 54 beats/minute
P waves: Sinus (bear no relationship to QRS complexes)
PR interval: PR varies
QRS complex: 0.16 second
Rhythm interpretation: Third-degree AV block

Strip 8.59
Rhythm: Regular (atrial); Irregular (ventricular)
Rate: Atrial: 80 beats/minute
Ventricular: 60 beats/minute
P waves: Sinus
PR interval: Lengthens from 0.24 to 0.40 second (PR varies)
QRS complex: 0.08 second
Rhythm interpretation: Second-degree AV block, Mobitz I

Strip 8.60
Rhythm: Regular (basic rhythm); irregular with premature beats
Rate: 60 beats/minute (basic rhythm)
P waves: Sinus (basic rhythm); abnormal with premature beats
PR interval: 0.12 second (basic rhythm); 0.16 second (PAC); 0.08 to 0.10 second (PJCs)
QRS complex: 0.08 second (basic rhythm and premature beats)
Rhythm interpretation: Normal sinus rhythm with one PAC (third complex) and paired PJCs (sixth and seventh complexes)

Strip 8.61
Rhythm: Regular
Rate: 47 beats/minute
P waves: Hidden in the QRS complex
PR interval: Not measurable
QRS complex: 0.08 to 0.10 second
Rhythm interpretation: Junctional rhythm
Comment: Tall peaked T wave is present

Strip 8.62
Rhythm: Regular (basic rhythm); irregular with nonconducted PAC
Rate: 84 beats/minute (basic rhythm); slows to 63 beats/minute after the pause (temporary rate suppression is common after a pause in the basic rhythm)
P waves: Sinus (basic rhythm); premature, pointed P wave distorting T wave after the sixth QRS complex
PR interval: 0.24 to 0.28 second (PR consistent)
QRS complex: 0.08 to 0.10 second
Rhythm interpretation: Normal sinus rhythm with first-degree AV block and a nonconducted PAC after the sixth QRS complex

Strip 8.63
Rhythm: Cannot be determined for sure (only one basic R-R interval in strip)
Rate: 56 beats/minute (basic rhythm); measured from sixth to seventh complexes
P waves: Sinus (basic rhythm); inverted P wave with PJC; squiggle before PAC
PR interval: 0.16 to 0.18 second (basic rhythm); 0.08 second (PJC); 0.20 second (PAC)
QRS complex: 0.06 to 0.08 second (basic rhythm); 0.08 second (PJC and PAC); 0.04 second (junctional escape beat)
Rhythm interpretation: Sinus bradycardia with PJC (second complex), PAC (fourth complex), and a junctional escape beat (fifth complex)

Strip 8.64
Rhythm: Regular (atrial and ventricular)
Rate: Atrial: 72 beats/minute
Ventricular: 31 beats/minute
P waves: Sinus (bear no relationship to QRS complexes)
PR interval: PR varies
QRS complex: 0.12 second
Rhythm interpretation: Third-degree AV block
Comment: ST segment elevation is present

Strip 8.65
Rhythm: Regular (atrial and ventricular)
Rate: Atrial: 90 beats/minute
Ventricular: 45 beats/minute
P waves: Two sinus P waves to each QRS complex
PR interval: 0.24 to 0.28 second (PR consistent)
QRS complex: 0.12 second
Rhythm interpretation: Second-degree AV block, Mobitz II with 2:1 AV conduction
Comment: ST segment elevation is present

Strip 8.66
Rhythm: Regular
Rate: 79 beats/minute
P waves: Inverted before each QRS complex
PR interval: 0.08 to 0.10 second
QRS complex: 0.04 to 0.08 second
Rhythm interpretation: Accelerated junctional rhythm

Strip 8.67
Rhythm: Regular
Rate: 94 beats/minute
P waves: Sinus
PR interval: 0.24 second (PR consistent)
QRS complex: 0.08 second
Rhythm interpretation: Normal sinus rhythm with first-degree AV block

Strip 8.68
Rhythm: Regular (basic rhythm); irregular with premature beats
Rate: 72 beats/minute (basic rhythm)
P waves: Sinus (basic rhythm); abnormal with premature beats
PR interval: 0.12 to 0.16 second (basic rhythm); 0.12 second (PACs); 0.10 second (PJC)
QRS complex: 0.06 to 0.08 second (basic rhythm and premature beats)
Rhythm interpretation: Normal sinus rhythm with two PACs (third and eighth complexes) and one PJC (fifth complex)
Comment. A U wave is present

Strip 8.69
Rhythm: Regular (basic rhythm); irregular with premature beats
Rate: 54 beats/minute (basic rhythm)
P waves: Hidden (basic rhythm); abnormal with premature beats
PR interval: Not measurable (basic rhythm); 0.12 to 0.16 second (PACs)
QRS complex: 0.06 to 0.08 second (basic rhythm and premature beats)
Rhythm interpretation: Junctional rhythm with two PACs (second and fifth complexes)
Comment. ST segment depression is present

Strip 8.70
Rhythm: Regular (atrial); Irregular (ventricular)
Rate: Atrial: 79 beats/minute
Ventricular: 70 beats/minute
P waves: Sinus
PR interval: Lengthens from 0.24 to 0.28 second (PR varies)
QRS complex: 0.08 second
Rhythm interpretation: Second-degree AV block, Mobitz I

Strip 8.71
Rhythm: Regular (atrial); Irregular (ventricular)
Rate: Atrial: 84 beats/minute
Ventricular: 30 beats/minute
P waves: Two to three sinus P waves before each QRS complex
PR interval: 0.12 second (PR consistent)
QRS complex: 0.12 second
Rhythm interpretation: Second-degree AV block, Mobitz II with 2:1 and 3:1 AV conduction

Strip 8.72
Rhythm: Regular (atrial and ventricular)
Rate: Atrial: 94 beats/minute
Ventricular: 40 beats/minute
P waves: Sinus (bear no relationship to QRS complexes)
PR interval: PR varies
QRS complex: 0.10 second
Rhythm interpretation: Third-degree AV block

Strip 8.73
Rhythm: Regular
Rate: 84 beats/minute
P waves: Hidden in QRS complexes
PR interval: Not measurable
QRS complex: 0.06 to 0.08 second
Rhythm interpretation: Accelerated junctional rhythm
Comment. ST segment depression and T-wave inversion are present

Strip 8.74
Rhythm: Regular (atrial); Irregular (ventricular)
Rate: Atrial: 54 beats/minute
Ventricular: 50 beats/minute
P waves: Sinus
PR interval: Lengthens from 0.32 to 0.44 second (PR varies)
QRS complex: 0.08 second
Rhythm interpretation: Second-degree AV block, Mobitz I

Strip 8.75
Rhythm: Regular (basic rhythm); irregular with escape beat
Rate: 58 beats/minute (basic rhythm)
P waves: Sinus (basic rhythm); hidden P wave (escape beat)
PR interval: 0.16 to 0.20 second (basic rhythm)
QRS complex: 0.08 to 0.10 second (basic rhythm); 0.08 second (escape beat)
Rhythm interpretation: Sinus bradycardia with junctional escape beat (fourth complex) after a pause in the basic rhythm

Strip 8.76
Rhythm: Regular
Rate: 47 beats/minute
P waves: Hidden in the QRS complex
PR interval: Not measurable
QRS complex: 0.06 to 0.08 second
Rhythm interpretation: Junctional rhythm
Comment. ST segment depression is present

Strip 8.77
Rhythm: Regular (atrial and ventricular)
Rate: Atrial: 94 beats/minute
Ventricular: 44 beats/minute
P waves: Sinus (bear no relationship to QRS complexes)
PR interval: PR varies
QRS complex: 0.14 to 0.16 second
Rhythm interpretation: Third-degree AV block
Comment. ST segment elevation is present

Strip 8.78
Rhythm: Regular (basic rhythm); irregular with premature beats
Rate: 68 beats/minute (basic rhythm)
P waves: Sinus (basic rhythm); abnormal P waves with premature beats
PR interval: 0.12 to 0.14 second (basic rhythm); 0.12 second (PAC); 0.10 second (PJC)
QRS complex: 0.06 to 0.08 second (basic rhythm and premature beats)
Rhythm interpretation: Normal sinus rhythm with one PAC (third complex) and one PJC (seventh complex)
Comment. A U wave is present

Strip 8.79
Rhythm: Regular (basic rhythm); irregular with premature beats
Rate: 75 beats/minute (basic rhythm)
P waves: Sinus (basic rhythm); inverted (PJC); squiggle (PAC)
PR interval: 0.14 to 0.16 second (basic rhythm); 0.08 second (PJC); 0.16 second (PAC)
QRS complex: 0.04 to 0.08 second (basic rhythm); 0.08 second (PJC); 0.06 second (PAC)
Rhythm interpretation: Normal sinus rhythm with one PJC (third complex) and one PAC (sixth complex)

Strip 8.80
Rhythm: Regular (basic rhythm); irregular with nonconducted PAC
Rate: 72 beats/minute (basic rhythm)
P waves: Sinus (basic rhythm); premature, pointed P wave without a QRS complex after the sixth QRS complex
PR interval: 0.22 to 0.24 second (PR consistent)
QRS complex: 0.04 to 0.06 second
Rhythm interpretation: Normal sinus rhythm with first-degree AV block and one nonconducted PAC (after the sixth QRS complex)
Comment. ST segment depression and T-wave inversion are present

Strip 8.81
Rhythm: Regular
Rate: 94 beats/minute
P waves: Inverted before each QRS complex
PR interval: 0.08 second
QRS complex: 0.08 second
Rhythm interpretation: Accelerated junctional rhythm

Strip 8.82
Rhythm: Regular (atrial); Irregular (ventricular)
Rate: Atrial: 68 beats/minute
Ventricular: 50 beats/minute
P waves: Sinus
PR interval: Lengthens from 0.26 to 0.40 second (PR varies)
QRS complex: 0.06 to 0.08 second
Rhythm interpretation: Second-degree AV block, Mobitz I
Comment. ST depression is present

Strip 8.83
Rhythm: Regular
Rate: 107 beats/minute
P waves: Inverted before each QRS complex
PR interval: 0.08 second
QRS complex: 0.08 to 0.10 second
Rhythm interpretation: Junctional tachycardia

Strip 8.84
Rhythm: Regular (both rhythms)
Rate: First rhythm: 79 beats/minute
Second rhythm: 84 beats/minute
P waves: First rhythm (sinus); Second rhythm (inverted)
PR interval: First rhythm (0.14 to 0.16 second); Second rhythm (0.08 second)
QRS complex: 0.06 to 0.08 second (both rhythms)
Rhythm interpretation: Normal sinus rhythm changing to accelerated junctional rhythm

Strip 8.85
Rhythm: Regular (atrial and ventricular)
Rate: Atrial: 75 beats/minute
Ventricular: 38 beats/minute
P waves: Two sinus P waves before each QRS complex
PR interval: 0.16 second (PR consistent)
QRS complex: 0.16 second
Rhythm interpretation: Second-degree AV block, Mobitz II with 2:1 AV conduction

Strip 8.86
Rhythm: Regular
Rate: 60 beats/minute
P waves: Sinus
PR interval: 0.24 second (PR consistent)
QRS complex: 0.08 second
Rhythm interpretation: Normal sinus rhythm with first-degree AV block
Comment. ST segment depression and T-wave inversion are present

Strip 8.87
Rhythm: Regular (atrial and ventricular)
Rate: Atrial: 88 beats/minute
Ventricular: 33 beats/minute
P waves: Sinus (bear no relationship to QRS complexes)
PR interval: PR varies
QRS complex: 0.12 to 0.14 second
Rhythm interpretation: Third-degree AV block

Strip 8.88
Rhythm: Regular (basic rhythm); irregular with premature and escape beats)
Rate: 60 beats/minute (basic rhythm)
P waves: Sinus (basic rhythm); pointed (atrial beat); inverted (junctional beats)
PR interval: 0.12 to 0.14 second (basic rhythm); 0.12 second (atrial beat); 0.08 second (junctional beats)
QRS complex: 0.06 to 0.08 second (basic rhythm, atrial and junctional beats)
Rhythm interpretation: Normal sinus rhythm with one PJC (third complex), one atrial escape beat (fourth complex), and one junctional escape beat (fifth complex)

Strip 8.89
Rhythm: Regular (atrial); Irregular (ventricular)
Rate: Atrial: 68 beats/minute
Ventricular: 50 beats/minute
P waves: Sinus
PR interval: Lengthens from 0.32 to 0.40 second (PR varies)
QRS complex: 0.08 to 0.10 second
Rhythm interpretation: Second-degree AV block, Mobitz I

Strip 8.90
Rhythm: Regular
Rate: 107 beats/minute
P waves: Inverted before each QRS complex
PR interval: 0.08 to 0.10 second
QRS complex: 0.06 to 0.08 second
Rhythm interpretation: Junctional tachycardia

Strip 8.91
Rhythm: Regular (basic rhythm); irregular with nonconducted PAC
Rate: 88 beats/minute (basic rhythm)
P waves: Sinus (basic rhythm); premature, pointed P wave deforming T wave after the sixth QRS complex; pointed, abnormal P wave with the seventh QRS complex
PR interval 0.20 to 0.24 second (basic rhythm) PR consistent; 0.14 second (atrial escape beat)
QRS complex: 0.06 to 0.08 second (basic rhythm); 0.08 second (atrial escape beat)
Rhythm interpretation: Normal sinus rhythm with first-degree AV block, a nonconducted PAC (after sixth complex), and an atrial escape beat (seventh complex)

Strip 8.92
Rhythm: Regular (atrial); Irregular (ventricular)
Rate: Atrial: 75 beats/minute
Ventricular: 30 beats/minute
P waves: Two to three sinus P waves before each QRS complex
PR interval: 0.16 second (PR consistent)
QRS complex: 0.12 second
Rhythm interpretation: Second-degree AV block, Mobitz II with 2:1 and 3:1 AV conduction
Comment: ST segment depression is present

Strip 8.93
Rhythm: Regular
Rate: 65 beats/minute
P waves: Inverted before each QRS complex
PR interval: 0.08 to 0.10 second
QRS complex: 0.04 to 0.06 second
Rhythm interpretation: Accelerated junctional rhythm
Comment: ST segment elevation is present

Strip 8.94
Rhythm: Regular (basic rhythm); irregular with PJC
Rate: 75 beats/minute (basic rhythm)
P waves: Sinus (basic rhythm); inverted with PJC
PR interval: 0.12 to 0.16 second (basic rhythm); 0.10 second (PJC)
QRS complex: 0.08 second (basic rhythm); 0.08 second (PJC)
Rhythm interpretation: Normal sinus rhythm with one PJC (fifth complex)
Comment: ST segment depression is present

Strip 8.95
Rhythm: Regular (atrial) off by two squares; Regular (ventricular) off by one square
Rate: Atrial: 80 beats/minute
Ventricular: 40 beats/minute
P waves: Two sinus P waves before each QRS complex
PR interval: 0.12 second (PR consistent)
QRS complex: 0.12 to 0.14 second
Rhythm interpretation: Second-degree AV block, Mobitz II with 2:1 AV conduction
Comment: ST segment elevation is present

Strip 8.96
Rhythm: Regular (atrial); Irregular (ventricular)
Rate: Atrial: 75 beats/minute
Ventricular: 70 beats/minute
P waves: Sinus
PR interval: Lengthens from 0.36 to 0.40 second (PR varies)
QRS complex: 0.04 to 0.06 second
Rhythm interpretation: Second-degree AV block, Mobitz I

Strip 8.97
Rhythm: Regular
Rate: 40 beats/minute
P waves: Hidden in the QRS complex
PR interval: Not measurable
QRS complex: 0.08 to 0.10 second
Rhythm interpretation: Junctional rhythm
Comment: ST segment elevation is present

Strip 8.98
Rhythm: Regular (atrial and ventricular)
Rate: Atrial: 80 beats/minute
Ventricular: 40 beats/minute
P waves: Two sinus P waves to each QRS complex
PR interval: 0.22 to 0.24 second (PR consistent)
QRS complex: 0.08 to 0.10 second
Rhythm interpretation: Second-degree AV block, Mobitz II
Comment: ST segment elevation is present; clinical correlation is suggested to diagnose Mobitz II when 2:1 conduction is present with a narrow QRS complex

Strip 8.99
Rhythm: Regular (basic rhythm); irregular with PJCs
Rate: 94 beats/minute (basic rhythm)
P waves: Sinus (basic rhythm); inverted with PJCs
PR interval: 0.14 to 0.16 second (basic rhythm); 0.10 second (PJCs)
QRS complex: 0.08 to 0.10 second (basic rhythm); 0.06 to 0.08 second (PJCs)
Rhythm interpretation: Normal sinus rhythm with two PJCs (fourth and eighth complexes)

Strip 8.100
Rhythm: Regular (basic rhythm); irregular after PJC and run of PJT
Rate: 100 beats/minute (basic rhythm); 136 beats/minute (PJT)
P waves: Sinus (basic rhythm); inverted with PJC and run of PJT
PR interval: 0.12 to 0.14 second (basic rhythm); 0.08 second (PJC and PJT)
QRS complex: 0.04 to 0.08 second (basic rhythm); 0.06 to 0.08 second (PJC and PJT)
Rhythm interpretation: Normal sinus rhythm with one PJC (fifth complex) and a three-beat run of PJT (8th, 9th, and 10th complexes)

Strip 8.101
Rhythm: Regular
Rate: 42 beats/minute
P waves: Hidden in QRS complexes
PR interval: Not measurable
QRS complex: 0.08 to 0.10 second
Rhythm interpretation: Junctional rhythm
Comment: ST segment depression is present

Strip 8.102
Rhythm: Regular
Rate: 79 beats/minute
P waves: Sinus
PR interval: 0.12 to 0.14 second
QRS complex: 0.06 to 0.08 second
Rhythm interpretation: Normal sinus rhythm

Strip 8.103
Rhythm: Irregular
Rate: Atrial: 240 beats/minute
Ventricular: 90 beats/minute
P waves: Flutter waves
PR interval: Not measurable
QRS complex: 0.04 to 0.06 second
Rhythm interpretation: Atrial flutter with variable AV conduction

Strip 8.104
Rhythm: Regular (basic rhythm); irregular with PJC
Rate: 58 beats/minute (basic rhythm)
P waves: Sinus (basic rhythm); inverted following PJC
PR interval: 0.12 to 0.14 second (basic rhythm); 0.06 second (PJC)
QRS complex: 0.06 to 0.08 second (basic rhythm); 0.10 second (PJC)
Rhythm interpretation: Sinus bradycardia with one PJC (fifth complex)

Strip 8.105
Rhythm: Regular (basic rhythm); irregular with PAC
Rate: 58 beats/minute (basic rhythm)
P waves: Sinus (basic rhythm); pointed (PAC)
PR interval: 0.28 to 0.30 second (basic rhythm) PR consistent; 0.30 second (PAC)
QRS complex: 0.08 to 0.10 second (basic rhythm); 0.08 second (PAC)
Rhythm interpretation: Sinus bradycardia with first-degree AV block and one PAC (fourth complex)

Strip 8.106
Rhythm: Irregular
Rate: 90 beats/minute
P waves: Vary in size, shape, and direction across strip
PR interval: 0.12 to 0.18 second
QRS complex: 0.06 to 0.08 second
Rhythm interpretation: Wandering atrial pacemaker

Strip 8.107
Rhythm: Regular (basic rhythm); irregular during pause
Rate: 72 beats/minute (basic rhythm); rate slows to 60 beats/minute following pause (temporary rate suppression is common following a pause in the basic rhythm)
P waves: Sinus (basic rhythm); absent during pause
PR interval: 0.22 to 0.24 second (basic rhythm) PR consistent; absent during pause
QRS complex: 0.08 to 0.10 second (basic rhythm); absent during pause
Rhythm interpretation: Normal sinus rhythm with first-degree AV block and sinus arrest

Strip 8.108
Rhythm: Regular (atrial and ventricular)
Rate: Atrial: 84 beats/minute
Ventricular: 41 beats/minute
P waves: Two sinus P waves before each QRS complex
PR interval: 0.16 to 0.18 second (PR consistent)
QRS complex: 0.12 to 0.14 second
Rhythm interpretation: Second-degree AV block, Mobitz II

Strip 8.109
Rhythm: Regular
Rate: 115 beats/minute
P waves: Inverted before each QRS complex
PR interval: 0.10 second
QRS complex: 0.06 to 0.08 second
Rhythm interpretation: Junctional tachycardia

Strip 8.110
Rhythm: Regular (basic rhythm)
Rate: 40 beats/minute
P waves: Sinus (basic rhythm); one premature, pointed P wave without QRS complex following second QRS complex
PR interval: 0.24 to 0.26 second (PR consistent)
QRS complex: 0.08 to 0.10 second
Rhythm interpretation: Sinus bradycardia with first-degree AV block and one nonconducted PAC (following second QRS complex)

Strip 8.111
Rhythm: Irregular
Rate: 80 beats/minute
P waves: Sinus
PR interval: 0.12 to 0.16 second
QRS complex: 0.04 to 0.06 second
Rhythm interpretation: Sinus arrhythmia

Strip 8.112
Rhythm: Regular (atrial and ventricular)
Rate: Atrial: 72 beats/minute
Ventricular: 35 beats/minute
P waves: Sinus (bear no relationship to QRS complexes)
PR interval: PR varies
QRS complex: 0.12 second
Rhythm interpretation: Third-degree AV block
Comment: ST segment depression is present

Strip 8.113
Rhythm: Irregular
Rate: 60 beats/minute
P waves: Fibrillatory waves
PR interval: Not measurable
QRS complex: 0.04 to 0.06 second
Rhythm interpretation: Atrial fibrillation (controlled rate)

Strip 8.114
Rhythm: Regular (off by one square)
Rate: 48 to 50 beats/minute
P waves: Sinus
PR interval: 0.16 to 0.20 second
QRS complex: 0.06 to 0.08 second
Rhythm interpretation: Sinus bradycardia

Strip 8.115
Rhythm: Regular
Rate: 167 beats/minute
P waves: Hidden in T waves (TP waves)
PR interval: Not measurable
QRS complex: 0.04 to 0.08 second
Rhythm interpretation: Paroxysmal atrial tachycardia

Strip 8.116
Rhythm: Regular
Rate: 58 beats/minute
P waves: Hidden in QRS complex
PR interval: Not measurable
QRS complex: 0.08 to 0.10 second
Rhythm interpretation: Junctional rhythm
Comment: ST segment elevation is present

Strip 8.117
Rhythm: Regular (atrial); Irregular (ventricular)
Rate: Atrial: 88 beats/minute
Ventricular: 60 beats/minute
P waves: Sinus
PR interval: Lengthens from 0.20 to 0.28 second (PR varies)
QRS complex: 0.04 to 0.08 second
Rhythm interpretation: Second-degree AV block, Mobitz I

Strip 8.118
Rhythm: Regular
Rate: 107 beats/minute
P waves: Sinus
PR interval: 0.14 to 0.16 second
QRS complex: 0.04 to 0.06 second
Rhythm interpretation: Sinus tachycardia

Strip 8.119
Rhythm: Regular (basic rhythm); irregular with premature beat
Rate: 88 beats/minute (basic rhythm)
P waves: Sinus (basic rhythm); small, pointed P wave with premature beat
PR interval: 0.12 to 0.14 second (basic rhythm); 0.12 second (premature beat)
QRS complex: 0.08 second (basic rhythm and premature beat)
Rhythm interpretation: Normal sinus rhythm with one PAC
Comment: ST segment depression is present

Strip 8.120
Rhythm: Regular
Rate: 65 beats/minute
P waves: Inverted before each QRS complex
PR interval: 0.08 to 0.10 second
QRS complex: 0.06 to 0.08 second
Rhythm interpretation: Accelerated junctional rhythm

Strip 9.1
Rhythm: Regular
Rate: 167 beats/minute
P waves: None identified
PR interval: Not measurable
QRS complex: 0.12 to 0.14 second
Rhythm interpretation: Ventricular tachycardia

Strip 9.2
Rhythm: Regular
Rate: 84 beats/minute
P waves: Sinus
PR interval: 0.18 to 0.20 second
QR complex: 0.12 to 0.16 second
Rhythm interpretation: Normal sinus rhythm with bundle branch block

Strip 9.3
Rhythm: Regular (basic rhythm); irregular with PVCs
Rate: 75 beats/minute (basic rhythm)
P waves: Sinus (basic rhythm)
PR interval: 0.16 to 0.20 second (basic rhythm)
QRS complex: 0.06 to 0.08 second (basic rhythm); 0.12 second (PVCs)
Rhythm interpretation: Normal sinus rhythm with two unifocal PVCs

Strip 9.4
Rhythm: Irregular
Rate: 30 beats/minute
P waves: Absent
PR interval: Not measurable
QRS complex: 0.16 second
Rhythm interpretation: Idioventricular rhythm

Strip 9.5
Rhythm: Irregular and chaotic
Rate: Not measurable
P waves: Recognizable P waves are absent; wavy, irregular deflections are seen that vary in size, shape, and height
PR interval: Not measurable
QRS complex: Absent
Rhythm interpretation: Ventricular fibrillation (coarse waveforms)

Strip 9.6
Rhythm: Regular (basic rhythm); irregular with PVCs
Rate: 100 beats/minute (basic rhythm)
P waves: Sinus (basic rhythm)
PR interval: 0.12 to 0.16 second
QRS complex: 0.08 second (basic rhythm); 0.12 second (PVCs)
Rhythm interpretation: Normal sinus rhythm with univocal PVCs in a bigeminal pattern (second, fourth, sixth, and eighth complexes)

Strip 9.7
Rhythm: Not measurable (basic rhythm); Irregular (AIVR)
Rate: 54 beats/minute (basic rhythm); 80 beats/minute (AIVR)
P waves: Sinus (basic rhythm)
PR interval: 0.16 second (basic rhythm)
QRS complex: 0.08 second (basic rhythm); 0.12 second (AIVR
Rhythm interpretation: Sinus bradycardia changing to accelerated idioventricular rhythm
Comment. ST segment depression is present in basic rhythm

Strip 9.8
Rhythm: Irregular (basic rhythm and VT)
Rate: 60 beats/minute (basic rhythm); about 190 beats/minute (VT)
P waves: Fibrillatory waves (basic rhythm)
PR interval: Not measurable
QRS complex: 0.04 to 0.08 second (basic rhythm); 0.12 to 0.14 second (VT)
Rhythm interpretation: Atrial fibrillation with five-beat run of ventricular tachycardia
Comment. ST segment depression with first rhythm

Strip 9.9
Rhythm: Regular
Rate: 250 beats/minute
P waves: None identified
PR interval: Not measurable
QRS complex: 0.16 to 0.20 second
Rhythm interpretation: Ventricular tachycardia (torsade de pointes)

Strip 9.10
Rhythm: Regular (basic rhythm); irregular with PVCs
Rate: 100 beats/minute (basic rhythm)
P waves: Sinus (basic rhythm)
PR interval: 0.16 second
QRS complex: 0.08 second (basic rhythm); 0.12 second (PVCs)
Rhythm interpretation: Normal sinus rhythm with a single unifocal PVC (fourth complex) and paired unifocal PVCs (eighth and ninth complexes)

Strip 9.11
Rhythm: Regular
Rate: 42 beats/minute
P waves: Absent
PR interval: Not measurable
QRS complex: 0.12 second
Rhythm interpretation: Idioventricular rhythm

Strip 9.12
Rhythm: Regular
Rate: 125 beats/minute
P waves: Sinus
PR interval: 0.12 second
QRS complex: 0.12 second
Rhythm interpretation: Sinus tachycardia with bundle branch block
Comment. ST segment elevation is present

Strip 9.13
Rhythm: Not measurable
Rhythm: 10 beats/minute (ventricular)
P waves: Absent
PR interval: Not measurable
QRS complex: 0.16 second
Rhythm interpretation: One ventricular complex changing to ventricular standstill (asystole)

Strip 9.14
Rhythm: Regular
Rate: 250 beats/minute
P waves: None identified
PR interval: Not measurable
QRS complex: 0.12 to 0.16 or more
Rhythm interpretation: Ventricular tachycardia

Strip 9.15
Rhythm: Regular (basic rhythm)
Rate: 50 beats/minute (basic rhythm)
P waves: Sinus (basic rhythm)
PR interval: 0.16 to 0.18 second
QRS complex: 0.08 second (basic rhythm);
0.12 second (PVC)
Rhythm interpretation: Sinus bradycardia
with one PVC (third complex)
Comment. ST segment depression is present

Strip 9.16
Rhythm: Irregular and chaotic
Rate: Not measurable
P wave: Recognizable P waves are absent;
wavy, irregular deflections are seen that
vary in size, shape, and height
PR interval: Not measurable
QRS complex: Absent
Rhythm interpretation: Ventricular
fibrillation (coarse waveforms)

Strip 9.17
Rhythm: Regular (basic rhythm)—off by
two squares
Rate: 60 beats/minute
P waves: Sinus (basic rhythm)
PR interval: 0.20 second (basic rhythm)
QRS complex: 0.08 second (basic rhythm);
0.12 second (PVC)
Rhythm interpretation: Normal sinus
rhythm with R-on-T PVC (PVC falls on
downslope of T wave)
Comment. ST segment depression is present

Strip 9.18
Rhythm: Regular
Rate: 107 beats/minute
P waves: Sinus
PR interval: 0.16 to 0.20 second
QRS complex: 0.12 second
Rhythm interpretation: Sinus tachycardia
with bundle branch block
Comment. ST segment elevation is present

Strip 9.19
Rhythm: Irregular
Rate: Atrial: 300 beats/minute
Ventricular: 50 beats/minute
P waves: Flutter waves are present
PR interval: Not measurable
QRS complex: 0.04 to 0.08 second (basic
rhythm); 0.12 second (PVC)
Rhythm interpretation: Atrial flutter with
variable AV conduction and one PVC (fifth
complex)

Strip 9.20
Rhythm: Regular (atrial rhythm)
Rate: 34 beats/minute (atrial)
P waves: Sinus
PR interval: Not measurable
QRS complex: Absent
Rhythm interpretation: Ventricular
standstill (asystole)

Strip 9.21
Rhythm: Irregular
Rate: 40 beats/minute
P waves: Absent
PR interval: Not measurable
QRS complex: 0.16 second
Rhythm interpretation: Idioventricular
rhythm

Strip 9.22
Rhythm: Irregular and chaotic
Rate: Not measurable
P waves: Recognizable P wave are absent;
wavy, irregular deflections are seen that
vary in size, shape, and height
PR interval: Not measurable
QRS complex: Absent
Rhythm interpretation: Ventricular
fibrillation (fine waveforms)

Strip 9.23
Rhythm: Regular
Rate: 88 beats/minute
P waves: Absent
PR interval: Not measurable
QRS complex: 0.12 second
Rhythm interpretation: Accelerated
idioventricular rhythm

Strip 9.24
Rhythm: Irregular (basic rhythm)
Rate: 60 beats/minute (basic rhythm)
P waves: Fibrillatory waves are present
PR interval: Not measurable
QRS complex: 0.04 to 0.08 second (basic
rhythm); 0.12 second (PVCs)
Rhythm interpretation: Atrial fibrillation
with paired PVCs

Strip 9.25
Rhythm: Regular (basic rhythm and VT)
Rate: 100 beats/minute (basic rhythm);
188 beats/minute (VT
P waves: Sinus (basic rhythm)
PR interval: 0.14 to 0.16 second (basic
rhythm)
QRS complex: 0.06 to 0.08 second (basic
rhythm); 0.12 second (VT and paired PVCs)
Rhythm interpretation: Normal sinus
rhythm with four-beat run of ventricular
tachycardia and paired PVCs

Strip 9.26
Rhythm: Regular (basic rhythm); irregular
with PVC
Rate: 107 beats/minute (basic rhythm)
P waves: Sinus (basic rhythm)
PR interval: 0.18 to 0.20 second
QRS complex: 0.08 to 0.10 second (basic
rhythm); 0.16 second (PVC)
Rhythm interpretation: Sinus tachycardia
with one R-on-T PVC
Comment. ST segment elevation is
present

Strip 9.27
Rhythm: Difficult to measure due to
changing polarity of QRS complexes
Rate: 250 beats/minute or greater
P waves: None identified
PR interval: Not measurable
QRS complex: 0.12 to 0.16 second or
greater
Rhythm interpretation: Ventricular
tachycardia (torsades de pointes)

Strip 9.28
Rhythm: Regular
Rate: 250 beats/minute or greater
P waves: None identified
PR interval: Not measurable
QRS complex: 0.12 to 0.16 second or
greater
Rhythm interpretation: Ventricular
tachycardia (torsades de pointes)

Strip 9.29
Rhythm: Regular
Rate: 84 beats/minute
P waves: Absent
PR interval: Not measurable
QRS complex: 0.12 to 0.14 second
Rhythm interpretation: Accelerated
idioventricular rhythm

Strip 9.30
Rhythm: Irregular and chaotic
Rate: Not measurable
P waves: Recognizable P waves are absent; wavy, irregular deflections are seen that vary in size, shape, and height
PR interval: Not measurable
QRS: Absent
Rhythm interpretation: Ventricular fibrillation (fine waveforms)

Strip 9.31
Rhythm: Regular (basic rhythm); irregular with atrial fibrillation and PVC
Rate: 107 beats/minute (basic rhythm); 160 beats/minute (atrial fibrillation)
P waves: Sinus (basic rhythm); fibrillatory waves (atrial fibrillation)
PR interval: 0.14 to 0.16 second (basic rhythm)
QRS complex: 0.04 to 0.08 second (basic rhythm); 0.04 to 0.08 second (atrial fib); 0.12 second (PVC)
Rhythm interpretation: Sinus tachycardia with one PVC changing to atrial fibrillation (atrial fibrillation was initiated by a PAC)

Strip 9.32
Rhythm: Regular (basic rhythm); irregular with PVCs)
Rate: 125 beats/minute (basic rhythm)
P waves: Sinus (basic rhythm)
PR interval: 0.14 to 0.16 second (basic rhythm)
QRS complex: 0.06 to 0.08 second (basic rhythm); 0.12 second (PVCs)
Rhythm interpretation: Sinus tachycardia with multifocal paired PVCs (eighth and ninth complexes)

Strip 9.33
Rhythm: Regular (basic rhythm)
Rate: 37 beats/minute (basic rhythm)
P waves: Sinus (basic rhythm)
PR interval: 0.12 to 0.16 second
QRS complex: 0.06 to 0.08 second (basic rhythm); 0.12 second (escape beat)
Rhythm interpretation: Sinus bradycardia with one ventricular escape beat (third complex)

Strip 9.34
Rhythm: Regular (basic rhythm and VT)
Rate: 72 beats/minute (basic rhythm); 150 beats/minute (VT)
P waves: Sinus (basic rhythm)
PR interval: 0.16 to 0.18 second
QRS complex: 0.08 second (basic rhythm); 0.12 second (VT)
Rhythm interpretation: Normal sinus rhythm with a seven-beat run of ventricular tachycardia

Strip 9.35
Rhythm: Irregular and chaotic
Rate: Not measurable
P waves: Recognizable P waves are absent; wavy, irregular deflections are seen that vary in size, shape, and height
PR interval: Not measurable
QRS complex: Absent
Rhythm interpretation: Ventricular fibrillation

Strip 9.36
Rhythm: Regular
Rate: 43 beats/minute
P waves: Absent
PR interval: Not measurable
QRS complex: 0.32 second
Rhythm interpretation: Idioventricular rhythm

Strip 9.37
Rhythm: Not measurable
Rate: 10 beats/minute (ventricular)
P waves: Absent
PR interval: Not measurable
QRS complex: 0.28 second or wider
Rhythm interpretation: One ventricular complex followed by ventricular standstill (asystole)

Strip 9.38
Rhythm: Regular
Rate: 84 beats/minute
P waves: Absent
PR interval: Not measurable
QRS complex: 0.12 to 0.16 second
Rhythm interpretation: Accelerated idioventricular rhythm

Strip 9.39
Rhythm: Regular (basic rhythm); irregular with PVC
Rate: 115 beats/minute (basic rhythm)
P waves: Inverted before each QRS complex (basic rhythm)
PR interval; 0.08 second (basic rhythm)
QRS complex: 0.06 to 0.08 second (basic rhythm); 0.12 second (PVC)
Rhythm interpretation: Junctional tachycardia with one PVC (10th complex)

Strip 9.40
Rhythm: Irregular (atrial); not measurable (ventricular)
Rate: 70 beats/minute (atrial); 10 beats/minute (ventricular)
P waves: Sinus
PR interval: 0.16 second
QRS complex: 0.10 second
Rhythm interpretation: One QRS complex changing to ventricular standstill (asystole)

Strip 9.41
Rhythm: Regular (basic rhythm); irregular with PVCs
Rate: 79 beats/minute (basic rhythm)
P waves: Sinus (basic rhythm)
PR interval: 0.16 second (basic rhythm)
QRS complex: 0.16 second (basic rhythm); 0.12 to 0.16 second (PVCs)
Rhythm interpretation: Normal sinus rhythm with bundle branch block and paired multifocal PVCs
Comment: ST segment depression is present

Strip 9.42
Rhythm: Regular (basic rhythm)
Rate: 100 beats/minute (basic rhythm)
P waves: Sinus (basic rhythm)
PR interval: 0.16 to 0.18 second (basic rhythm)
QRS complex: 0.08 second (basic rhythm); 0.12 to 0.14 second (PVCs)
Rhythm interpretation: Normal sinus rhythm with one PVC (second complex) and paired unifocal PVCs (fifth and sixth complexes and ninth and tenth complexes)

Strip 9.43
Rhythm: Regular (basic rhythm); Regular (AIVR)—off by two squares
Rate: 100 beats/minute (basic rhythm); 94 to 100 beats/minute (AIVR)
P waves: Sinus (basic rhythm)
PR interval; 0.12 second
QRS complex: 0.12 to 0.14 second (basic rhythm); 0.12 second (AIVR)
Rhythm interpretation: Normal sinus rhythm with bundle branch block with a seven-beat run of accelerated idioventricular rhythm

Strip 9.44
Rhythm: Not measurable (only one cardiac cycle)
Rate: 50 beats/minute (basic rhythm); 41 beats/minute (IVR)
P waves: Sinus (basic rhythm)
PR interval: 0.12 to 0.14 second (basic rhythm)
QRS complex: 0.06 to 0.08 second (basic rhythm); 0.12 second (IVR)
Rhythm interpretation: Sinus bradycardia changing to idioventricular rhythm
Comment. A U wave is present

Strip 9.45
Rhythm: Regular
Rate: 214 beats/minute
P waves: Not identified
PR interval: Not measurable
QRS complex: 0.16 second or wider
Rhythm interpretation: Ventricular tachycardia

Strip 9.46
Rhythm: Regular (basic rhythm); irregular with ventricular beats
Rate: 58 beats/minute (basic rhythm)
P waves: Sinus (basic rhythm)
PR interval: 0.20 second
QRS complex: 0.06 to 0.08 second (basic rhythm); 0.16 second (PVC); 0.12 second (ventricular escape beat)
Rhythm interpretation: Sinus bradycardia with one PVC (fourth complex) and one ventricular escape beat (fifth complex)
Comment. ST segment depression is present

Strip 9.47
Rhythm: Regular (basic rhythm)
Rate: 68 beats/minute (basic rhythm)
P waves: Sinus (basic rhythm)
PR interval; 0.12 to 0.14 second
QRS complex: 0.08 to 0.10 second (basic rhythm); 0.16 second (PVC)
Rhythm interpretation: Normal sinus rhythm with one R-on-T PVC

Strip 9.48
Rhythm: Not measurable
Rate: 10 beats/minute (ventricular)
P waves: Absent
PR interval: Not measurable
QRS complex: 0.12 second
Rhythm interpretation: One ventricular complex changing to ventricular standstill (asystole)

Strip 9.49
Rhythm: Regular
Rate: 75 beats/minute
P waves: Sinus
PR interval: 0.16 to 0.18 second
QRS: 0.12 second
Rhythm interpretation: Normal sinus rhythm with bundle branch block
Comment. ST segment depression is present

Strip 9.50
Rhythm: Regular
Rate: 188 beats/minute
P waves: Not identified
PR interval: Not measurable
QRS complex: 0.16 second or greater
Rhythm interpretation: Ventricular tachycardia

Strip 9.51
Rhythm: Regular (basic rhythm)
Rate: 84 beats/minute (basic rhythm)
P waves: Sinus (basic rhythm)
PR interval: 0.14 to 0.16 second (basic rhythm)
QRS complex: 0.04 to 0.08 second (basic rhythm); 0.12 second (PVCs)
Rhythm interpretation: Normal sinus rhythm with paired multifocal PVCs
Comment. ST segment depression is present

Strip 9.52
Rhythm: Regular (basic rhythm and AIVR)
Rate: 72 beats/minute (basic rhythm); 72 beats/minute (AIVR)
P waves: Sinus (basic rhythm)
PR interval: 0.12 to 0.14 second (basic rhythm)
QRS complex: 0.08 second (basic rhythm); 0.12 to 0.14 second (AIVR)
Rhythm interpretation: Normal sinus rhythm with a three-beat run of accelerated idioventricular rhythm

Strip 9.53
Rhythm: Regular
Rate: 40 beats/minute (atrial)
P waves: Sinus
PR interval: Not measurable
QRS complex: Absent
Rhythm interpretation: Ventricular standstill (asystole)

Strip 9.54
Rhythm: Regular
Rate: 50 beats/minute
P waves: Sinus
PR interval: 0.16 second
QRS complex: 0.12 second
Rhythm interpretation: Sinus bradycardia with bundle branch block

Strip 9.55
Rhythm: Regular
Rate: 41 beats/minute
P waves: Absent
PR interval: Not measurable
QRS complex: 0.16 second
Rhythm interpretation: Idioventricular rhythm

Strip 9.56
Rhythm: Regular (basic rhythm); irregular with PVCs
Rate: 84 beats/minute
P waves: Sinus (basic rhythm)
PR interval: 0.16 to 0.20 second
QRS complex: 0.16 to 0.18 second (basic rhythm); 0.16 second (PVC)
Rhythm interpretation: Normal sinus rhythm with bundle branch block and one PVC (sixth complex)
Comment. ST segment depression is present

Strip 9.57
Rhythm: Regular (basic rhythm); irregular with PVCs
Rate: 72 beats/minute (basic rhythm)
P waves: Sinus (basic rhythm)
PR interval: 0.12 to 0.14 second
QRS complex: 0.08 second (basic rhythm); 0.12 second (PVCs)
Rhythm interpretation: Normal sinus rhythm with unifocal PVCs (fourth and eighth complexes) in a quadrigeminal pattern

Strip 9.58
Rhythm: Irregular (atrial)
Rate: 50 beats/minute (atrial)
P waves: Sinus
PR interval: Not measurable
QRS complex: Absent
Rhythm interpretation: Ventricular standstill (asystole)

Strip 9.59
Rhythm: Irregular and chaotic
Rate: Not measurable
P waves: Recognizable P waves are absent; wavy, irregular deflections are seen that vary in size, shape, and height
PR interval: Not measurable
QRS complex: Absent
Rhythm interpretation: Ventricular fibrillation (coarse waveforms)

Strip 9.60
Rhythm: Not measurable
Rate: 10 beats/minute (ventricular)
P waves: Absent
PR interval: Not measurable
QRS complex: 0.24 second or greater
Rhythm interpretation: One ventricular complex changing to ventricular standstill (asystole)

Strip 9.61
Rhythm: Regular (basic rhythm and AIVR)
Rate: 100 beats/minute (basic rhythm); 100 beats/minute (AIVR)
P waves: Sinus (basic rhythm)
PR interval: 0.12 to 0.16 second
QRS complex: 0.06 to 0.08 second (basic rhythm); 0.12 second (AIVR)
Rhythm interpretation: Normal sinus rhythm changing to accelerated idioventricular rhythm

Strip 9.62
Rhythm: Regular
Rate: 40 beats/minute
P waves: Absent
PR interval: Not measurable
QRS complex: 0.16 second
Rhythm interpretation: Idioventricular rhythm

Strip 9.63
Rhythm: Regular
Rate: 167 beats/minute
P waves: Not identified
PR interval: Not measurable
QRS complex: 0.12 to 0.16 second or more
Rhythm interpretation: Ventricular tachycardia

Strip 9.64
Rhythm: Regular
Rate: 72 beats/minute
P waves: Sinus
PR interval: 0.16 to 0.18 second
QRS complex: 0.12 second
Rhythm interpretation: Normal sinus rhythm with bundle branch block

Strip 9.65
Rhythm: Irregular
Rate: 60 beats/minute
P waves: Fibrillatory waves
PR interval: Not measurable
QRS complex: 0.12 second (basic rhythm); 0.12 second (PVC)
Rhythm interpretation: Atrial fibrillation with bundle branch block and one PVC (fifth complex)

Strip 9.66
Rhythm: Difficult to measure due to changing polarity of QRS complex
Rate: 280 beats/minute or more
P waves: None identified
PR interval: Not measurable
QRS complex: 0.12 to 0.16 second
Rhythm interpretation: Ventricular tachycardia (torsades de pointes)

Strip 9.67
Rhythm: Irregular and chaotic
Rate: Not measurable
P waves: Recognizable P waves are absent; wavy, irregular deflections are seen that vary in size, shape, and height
PR interval: Not measurable
QRS complex: Absent
Rhythm interpretation: Ventricular fibrillation

Strip 9.68
Rhythm: Regular
Rate: 150 beats/minute
P waves: None identified
PR interval: Not measurable
QRS complex: 0.12 to 0.16 second
Rhythm interpretation: Ventricular tachycardia

Strip 9.69
Rhythm: Regular (basic rhythm); irregular (VT)
Rate: 115 beats/minute (basic rhythm); 188 to 214 beats/minute (VT)
P waves: Sinus (basic rhythm)
PR interval: 0.12 second (basic rhythm)
QRS complex: 0.10 second (basic rhythm); 0.12 to 0.16 second or more (VT)
Rhythm interpretation: Sinus tachycardia with 10-beat run of ventricular tachycardia
Comment: T-wave inversion is present (basic rhythm)

Strip 9.70
Rhythm: Regular
Rate: 29 beats/minute
P waves: Absent
PR interval: Not measurable
QRS complex: 0.16 second
Rhythm interpretation: Idioventricular rhythm

Strip 9.71
Rhythm: Regular
Rate: 100 beats/minute
P waves: Absent
PR interval: Not measurable
QRS complex: 0.12 second
Rhythm interpretation: Accelerated idioventricular rhythm

Strip 9.72
Rhythm: Not measurable
Rate: 10 beats/minute (ventricular)
P waves: Absent
PR interval: Not measurable
QRS complex: 0.24 second
Rhythm interpretation: One ventricular complex changing to ventricular standstill (asystole)

Strip 9.73
Rhythm: Regular
Rate: 214 beats/minute
P waves: None identified
PR interval: Not measurable
QRS complex: 0.16 to 0.20 second
Rhythm interpretation: Ventricular tachycardia followed by electric shock and return to ventricular tachycardia

Strip 9.74
Rhythm: Regular (basic rhythm); irregular with PVC
Rate: 88 beats/minute (basic rhythm)
P waves: Sinus (basic rhythm)
PR interval: 0.16 to 0.20 second
QRS complex: 0.06 to 0.08 second (basic rhythm); 0.12 to 0.14 second (PVC)
Rhythm interpretation: Normal sinus rhythm with one PVC (fourth complex)
Comment: ST segment depression is present

Strip 9.75
Rhythm: Regular
Rate: 50 beats/minute
P waves: Sinus
PR interval: 0.16 to 0.18 second
QRS complex: 0.12 to 0.14 second
Rhythm interpretation: Sinus bradycardia with bundle branch block

Strip 9.76
Rhythm: Regular (atrial)—off by two squares
Rate: 63 to 68 beats/minute (atrial)
P waves: Sinus
PR interval: Not measurable
QRS complex: Absent
Rhythm interpretation: Ventricular standstill (asystole)

Strip 9.77
Rhythm: Regular
Rate: 41 beats/minute
P waves: Absent
PR interval: Not measurable
QRS complex: 0.12 second
Rhythm interpretation: Idioventricular rhythm

Strip 9.78
Rhythm: Not measurable
Rate: 10 beats/minute (ventricular)
P waves: Absent
PR interval: Not measurable
QRS complex: 0.12 second or greater
Rhythm interpretation: One ventricular complex changing to ventricular standstill (asystole)

Strip 9.79
Rhythm: Irregular and chaotic
Rate: Not measurable
P waves: Recognizable P waves are absent; wavy, irregular deflections are seen that vary in size, shape, and height
PR interval: Not measurable
QRS complex: Absent
Rhythm interpretation: Coarse ventricular fibrillation changing to fine ventricular fibrillation

Strip 9.80
Rhythm: Regular (basic rhythm) and AIVR
Rate: 94 beats/minute (basic rhythm); 75 beats/minute (AIVR)
P waves: Sinus (basic rhythm)
PR interval: 0.16 second (basic rhythm)
QRS complex: 0.12 second (basic rhythm); 0.12 second (AIVR)
Rhythm interpretation: Normal sinus rhythm with bundle branch block and a five-beat run of accelerated idioventricular rhythm

Strip 9.81
Rhythm: Regular (atrial); not measurable (ventricular)
Rate: 94 beats/minute (atrial); 40 beats/minute (ventricular)
P waves: Sinus (bear no relationship to QRS complexes)
PR interval: PR varies
QRS complex: 0.14 to 0.16 second
Rhythm interpretation: Third-degree AV block changing to ventricular standstill (asystole)

Strip 9.82
Rhythm: Regular
Rate: 72 beats/minute
P waves: Sinus
PR interval: 0.16 to 0.18 second
QRS complex: 0.12 to 0.14 second
Rhythm interpretation: Normal sinus rhythm with bundle branch block
Comment: ST segment elevation is present

Strip 9.83
Rhythm: Regular (basic rhythm); irregular and chaotic (VF)
Rate: 214 beats/minute (basic rhythm)
P waves: None identified
PR interval: Not measurable
QRS complex: 0.12 to 0.16 second (basic rhythm)
Rhythm interpretation: Ventricular tachycardia changing to ventricular fibrillation (coarse)

Strip 9.84
Rhythm: Not measurable
Rate: 20 beats/minute (ventricular)
P waves: Absent
PR interval: Not measurable
QRS complex: 0.24 second or greater
Rhythm interpretation: Idioventricular rhythm

Strip 9.85
Rhythm: Regular (basic rhythm); irregular with PVCs
Rate: 125 beats/minute (basic rhythm)
P waves: Sinus (basic rhythm)
PR interval: 0.12 second
QRS complex: 0.04 to 0.08 second (basic rhythm); 0.12 second (PVCs)
Rhythm interpretation: Sinus tachycardia with multifocal paired PVCs (eighth and ninth complexes)

Strip 9.86
Rhythm: Regular (atrial)
Rate: 52 beats/minute (atrial)
P waves: Sinus
PR interval: Not measurable
QRS complex: Absent
Rhythm interpretation: Ventricular standstill (asystole)

Strip 9.87
Rhythm: Regular (basic rhythm); irregular (AIVR)
Rate: 68 beats/minute (basic rhythm); 80 beats/minute (AIVR)
P waves: Sinus (basic rhythm)
PR interval: 0.12 to 0.14 second (basic rhythm)
QRS complex: 0.08 second (basic rhythm); 0.12 to 0.16 second (AIVR)
Rhythm interpretation: Normal sinus rhythm with four-beat run of accelerated idioventricular rhythm

Strip 9.88
Rhythm: Regular
Rate: 167 beats/minute
P waves: None identified
PR interval: Not measurable
QRS complex: 0.12 to 0.16 second or greater
Rhythm interpretation: Ventricular tachycardia (torsades de pointes)

Strip 9.89
Rhythm: Regular (basic rhythm); irregular with PVCs
Rate: 125 beats/minute (basic rhythm)
P waves: Sinus (basic rhythm)
PR interval: 0.12 to 0.14 second
QRS complex: 0.04 to 0.08 second (basic rhythm); 0.12 second (PVCs)
Rhythm interpretation: Sinus tachycardia with paired univocal PVCs (seventh and eighth complexes)

Strip 9.90
Rhythm: Regular (atrial)
Rate: 72 beats/minute (atrial)
P waves: Sinus
PR interval: Not measurable
QRS complex: Absent
Rhythm interpretation: Ventricular standstill (asystole)

Strip 9.91
Rhythm: Regular
Rate: 188 beats/minute
P waves: None identified
PR interval: Not measurable
QRS complex: 0.16 to 0.20 second or greater
Rhythm interpretation: Ventricular tachycardia

Strip 9.92
Rhythm: Irregular and chaotic
Rate: Not measurable
P waves: Recognizable P waves are absent; wavy, irregular deflections are seen that vary in size, shape, and height
PR interval: Not measurable
QRS complex: Absent
Rhythm interpretation: Ventricular fibrillation (coarse)

Strip 9.93
Rhythm: Regular
Rate: 28 beats/minute
P waves: Absent
PR interval: Not measurable
QRS complex: 0.20 second or greater
Rhythm interpretation: Idioventricular rhythm

Strip 9.94
Rhythm: Regular
Rate: 79 beats/minute
P waves: Sinus
PR interval: 0.18 to 0.20 second
QRS complex: 0.12 to 0.16 second
Rhythm interpretation: Normal sinus rhythm with bundle branch block

Strip 9.95
Rhythm: Regular (basic rhythm)
Rate: 68 beats/minute (basic rhythm)
P waves: Sinus (basic rhythm)
PR interval: 0.16 to 0.20 second
QRS complex: 0.06 to 0.08 second (basic rhythm); 0.12 second (PVC)
Rhythm interpretation: Normal sinus rhythm with one interpolated PVC (seventh complex)
Comment: Interpolated PVCs are sandwiched between two sinus beats and have no compensatory pause. ST segment depression and T-wave inversion are present

Strip 9.96
Rhythm: Regular (basic rhythm); irregular with PVCs
Rate: 72 beats/minute (basic rhythm)
P waves: Sinus (basic rhythm)
PR interval: 0.12 to 0.16 second
QRS complex: 0.08 second (basic rhythm); 0.12 to 0.14 second (PVCs)
Rhythm interpretation: Normal sinus rhythm with PVCs in a trigeminal pattern

Strip 9.97
Rhythm: Regular
Rate: 72 beats/minute
P waves: Absent
PR interval: Not measurable
QRS complex: 0.12 to 0.14 second
Rhythm interpretation: Accelerated idioventricular rhythm

Strip 9.98
Rhythm: Regular (basic rhythm)
Rate: 68 beats/minute (basic rhythm); 150 beats/minute (VT)
P waves: Sinus (basic rhythm)
PR interval: 0.12 to 0.16 second (basic rhythm)
QRS complex: 0.06 to 0.08 second (basic rhythm); 0.12 or greater (VT)
Rhythm interpretation: Normal sinus rhythm with a three-beat run of ventricular tachycardia
Comment: T-wave inversion is present

Strip 9.99
Rhythm: Regular
Rate: 68 beats/minute
P waves: Sinus
PR interval: 0.20 second
QRS complex: 0.12 second
Rhythm interpretation: Normal sinus rhythm with bundle branch block
Comment: ST segment depression is present

Strip 9.100
Rhythm: Not measurable
Rate: 10 beats/minute (ventricular)
P waves: Absent
PR interval: Not measurable
QRS complex: 0.20 second
Rhythm interpretation: One ventricular complex changing to ventricular standstill (asystole)

Strip 9.101
Rhythm: Irregular
Rate: 60 beats/minute
P waves: Sinus
PR interval: 0.16 to 0.18 second
QRS complex: 0.06 to 0.08 second
Rhythm interpretation: Sinus arrhythmia

Strip 9.102
Rhythm: Regular
Rate: 167 beats/minute
P waves: Hidden in T waves
PR interval: Not measurable
QRS complex: 0.08 to 0.10 second
Rhythm interpretation: Paroxysmal atrial tachycardia

Strip 9.103
Rhythm: Regular
Rate: 45 beats/minute
P waves: Hidden within QRS complex
PR interval: Not measurable
QRS complex: 0.06 to 0.08 second
Rhythm interpretation: Junctional rhythm
Comment: ST segment depression is present

Strip 9.104
Rhythm: Regular
Rate: 63 beats/minute
P waves: Sinus
PR interval: 0.12 to 0.14 second
QRS complex: 0.14 to 0.16 second
Rhythm interpretation: Normal sinus rhythm with bundle branch block

Strip 9.105
Rhythm: Regular (atrial); irregular (ventricular)
Rate: 84 beats/minute (atrial); 70 beats/minute (ventricular)
P waves: Sinus
PR interval: Lengthens from 0.20 to 0.32 second (PR varies)
QRS complex: 0.08 to 0.10 second
Rhythm interpretation: Second-degree AV block, Mobitz I

Strip 9.106
Rhythm: Regular (basic rhythm); irregular with pause
Rate: 72 beats/minute (basic rhythm); rate decreases to 68 beats/minute following pause due to temporary rate suppression
P waves: Sinus (basic rhythm); absent during pause
PR interval: 0.24 second (basic rhythm); absent during pause
QRS complex: 0.04 to 0.08 second (basic rhythm); absent during pause
Rhythm interpretation: Normal sinus rhythm with first-degree AV block and sinus arrest
Comment: T-wave inversion is present

Strip 9.107
Rhythm: Regular (basic rhythm); irregular with PAC
Rate: 52 beats/minute (basic rhythm)
P waves: Sinus (basic rhythm); small, pointed P wave with PAC
PR interval: 0.14 to 0.16 second (basic rhythm); 0.12 second (PAC)
QRS complex: 0.08 to 0.10 second (basic rhythm); 0.08 second (PAC)
Rhythm interpretation: Sinus bradycardia with one PAC (fourth complex)

Strip 9.108
Rhythm: Regular (basic rhythm)
Rate: 48 beats/minute (basic rhythm)
P waves: Absent
PR interval: Not measurable
QRS complex: 0.12 to 0.16 second
Rhythm interpretation: Idioventricular rhythm changing to ventricular standstill (asystole)

Strip 9.109
Rhythm: Regular
Rate: 88 beats/minute
P waves: Sinus
PR interval: 0.28 to 0.32 second (PR consistent)
QRS complex: 0.06 to 0.10 second
Rhythm interpretation: Normal sinus rhythm with first-degree AV block
Comment: ST segment depression is present

Strip 9.110
Rhythm: Regular (basic rhythm); irregular with PVC
Rate: 75 beats/minute (basic rhythm)
P waves: Sinus
PR interval: 0.16 to 0.18 second
QRS complex: 0.06 to 0.08 second (basic rhythm); 0.12 second (PVC)
Rhythm interpretation: Normal sinus rhythm with one PVC (third complex)

Strip 9.111
Rhythm: Regular
Rate: 232 beats/minute (atrial); 58 beats/minute (ventricular)
P waves: Flutter waves are present
PR interval: Not measurable
QRS complex: 0.06 to 0.08 second
Rhythm interpretation: Atrial flutter with 4:1 AV conduction

Strip 9.112
Rhythm: Regular
Rate: 115 beats/minute
P wave: Sinus
PR interval: 0.12 to 0.16 second
QRS complex: 0.04 to 0.06 second
Rhythm interpretation: Sinus tachycardia
Comment: ST segment depression is present

Strip 9.113
Rhythm: Not measurable
Rate: 10 beats/minute (ventricular)
P waves: Absent
PR interval: Not measurable
QRS complex: 0.20 to 0.24 second
Rhythm interpretation: One ventricular complex changing to ventricular standstill (asystole)

Strip 9.114
Rhythm: Regular (basic rhythm)—off by two squares
Rate: 72 to 75 beats/minute
P waves: Vary in size, shape, and direction across strip
PR interval: 0.10 to 0.16 second
QRS complex; 0.04 to 0.08 second (basic rhythm); 0.12 second or greater (PVC)
Rhythm interpretation: Wandering atrial pacemaker with PVC (eighth complex)

Strip 9.115
Rhythm: Not measurable (basic rhythm); Regular (AIVR)—off by two squares
Rate: 75 beats/minute (basic rhythm); 72 to 79 beats/minute (AIVR)
P waves: Sinus (basic rhythm)
PR interval: 0.20 second (basic rhythm)
QRS complex: 0.04 to 0.08 second (basic rhythm); 0.12 to 0.16 second (AIVR)
Rhythm interpretation: Normal sinus rhythm with a six-beat run of accelerated idioventricular rhythm

Strip 9.116
Rhythm: Regular—off by one square
Rate: 54 to 56 beats/minute
P waves: Sinus
PR interval: 0.14 to 0.16 second
QRS complex: 0.04 second
Rhythm interpretation: Sinus bradycardia

Strip 9.117
Rhythm: Irregular
Rate: Not measurable (atrial); 70 beats/minute (ventricular)
P waves: Fibrillatory waves present
PR interval: Not measurable
QRS complex: 0.04 second
Rhythm interpretation: Atrial fibrillation, controlled rate

Strip 9.118
Rhythm: Regular
Rate: 150 beats/minute
P waves: None identified
PR interval: Not measurable
QRS complex: 0.12 second
Rhythm interpretation: Ventricular tachycardia

Strip 9.119
Rhythm: Regular
Rate: 100 beats/minute
P waves: Inverted before each QRS complex
PR interval: 0.08 to 0.10 second
QRS complex: 0.04 to 0.08 second
Rhythm interpretation: Accelerated junctional rhythm

Strip 9.120

Rhythm: Regular (atrial)—off by one
square; Regular (ventricular)
Rate: 88 to 94 beats/minute (atrial);
44 beats/minute (ventricular)
P waves: Sinus (bear no relationship to
QRS complexes)
PR interval: PR varies
QRS complex: 0.06 to 0.08 second
Rhythm interpretation: Third-degree AV block

Strip 9.121

Rhythm: Irregular and chaotic
Rate: Not measurable
P waves: Recognizable P waves are
absent; wavy, irregular deflections are
seen that vary in size, shape, and height
PR interval: Not measurable
QRS complex: Absent
Rhythm interpretation: Ventricular
fibrillation (coarse)

Strip 9.122

Rhythm: Regular
Rate: 63 beats/minute
P waves: Sinus
PR interval: 0.16 to 0.18 second
QRS complex: 0.08 to 0.10 second
Rhythm interpretation: Normal sinus rhythm
Comment: A U wave is present

Strip 9.123

Rhythm: Regular (basic rhythm); irregular
with PJCs
Rate: 72 beats/minute (basic rhythm)
P waves: Sinus (basic rhythm); inverted
with PJCs
PR interval: 0.12 to 0.16 (basic rhythm);
0.08 second (PJCs)
QRS complex: 0.08 second (basic rhythm
and PJCs)
Rhythm interpretation: Normal sinus rhythm
with two PJCs (fourth and sixth complexes)

Strip 9.124

Rhythm: Regular (atrial)—off by two
squares; Regular (ventricular)
Rate: 68 to 72 beats/minute (atrial); 34
beats/minute (ventricular)
P waves: Two sinus P waves before each
QRS complex
PR interval: 0.12 to 0.14 second (PR
consistent)
QRS complex: 0.12 second
Rhythm interpretation: Second-degree AV
block, Mobitz II

Strip 10.1

Analysis: The first three beats are
ventricular paced beats followed by one
intrinsic beat, two ventricular paced
beats, one intrinsic beat, and two
ventricular paced beats.
Interpretation: Ventricular paced
rhythm with two intrinsic beats (normal
pacemaker function)

Strip 10.2

Analysis: The first three beats are intrinsic
beats followed by a ventricular paced
beat that occurs too early, one ventricular
paced beat, two intrinsic beats, one
ventricular paced beat that occurs too
early, and one intrinsic beat.
Interpretation: Normal sinus rhythm
with one ventricular paced beat and two
episodes of undersensing (both occur with
capture). This is abnormal pacemaker
function.

Strip 10.3

Analysis: The first complex is an intrinsic
beat followed by two ventricular
paced beats, an intrinsic beat, and two
ventricular paced beats.
Interpretation: Ventricular paced
rhythm with two intrinsic beats (normal
pacemaker function).

Strip 10.4

Analysis: The first two complexes are
ventricular paced followed by a pacing
spike with failure to capture, a ventricular
paced beat, a pacing spike with failure
to capture, an intrinsic beat, a ventricular
paced beat, a pacing spike with failure to
capture, and an intrinsic beat.
Interpretation: Ventricular paced rhythm
with two intrinsic beats and three
episodes of failure to capture (abnormal
pacemaker function).

Strip 10.5

Analysis: No patient beats are seen;
pacing spikes are present that fail to
capture the ventricles.
Interpretation: Failure to capture in
the presence of ventricular standstill
(abnormal pacemaker function)

Strip 10.6

Analysis: The first five complexes are
intrinsic beats followed by two ventricular
paced beats, two intrinsic beats, and one
ventricular paced beat.
Interpretation: Ventricular paced rhythm
with seven intrinsic beats (normal
pacemaker function).

Strip 10.7

Analysis: The first complex is an
intrinsic beat followed by a ventricular
paced beat that occurs too early, two
ventricular paced beats, a fusion beat,
an intrinsic beat, a pacing spike that
occurs too early, and three intrinsic
beats.
Interpretation: Ventricular paced rhythm
with five intrinsic beats, one fusion
beat, and two episodes of undersensing
(one with capture and one without
capture). This is abnormal pacemaker
function.

Strip 10.8

Analysis: The first five complexes are
ventricular paced followed by a pause
in pacing, a ventricular paced beat
that occurs later than expected, and a
ventricular paced beat.
Interpretation: Ventricular paced rhythm
with one episode of oversensing
(pacemaker sensed the small waveform
artifact seen during the pause). This is
abnormal pacemaker function.

Strip 10.9

Analysis: The first two complexes are
ventricular paced beats followed by a
pacing spike that fails to capture, an
intrinsic beat, three ventricular paced
beats, and an intrinsic beat.
Interpretation: Ventricular paced rhythm
with two intrinsic beats and one episode
of failure to capture (abnormal pacemaker
function).

Strip 10.10

Analysis: All complexes are pacemaker
induced.
Interpretation: Ventricular paced rhythm
(normal pacemaker function).

Strip 10.11
Analysis: The first three complexes are ventricular paced beats followed by an intrinsic beat, a pacing spike that occurs too early, an intrinsic beat, a pacing spike with capture that occurs too early, and three ventricular paced beats.
Interpretation: Ventricular paced rhythm with two intrinsic beats and two episodes of undersensing (one with capture and one without capture). This represents abnormal pacemaker function.

Strip 10.12
Analysis: The first six complexes are intrinsic beats followed by two ventricular paced beats and two intrinsic beats.
Interpretation: Atrial fibrillation with two ventricular paced beats (normal pacemaker function)

Strip 10.13
Analysis: All complexes are pacemaker induced.
Interpretation: Ventricular paced rhythm (normal pacemaker function)

Strip 10.14
Analysis: The first two complexes are intrinsic beats followed by a fusion beat (note pacing spike at onset of QRS), another fusion beat, and three ventricular paced beats.
Interpretation: Ventricular paced rhythm with two intrinsic beats and two fusion beats (normal pacemaker function).

Strip 10.15
Analysis: The first three complexes are ventricular paced beats followed by a pseudofusion beat, an intrinsic beat, a ventricular paced beat, and an intrinsic beat.
Interpretation: Ventricular paced rhythm with two intrinsic beats and one pseudofusion beat (normal pacemaker function).

Strip 10.16
Analysis: The first two beats are ventricular paced beats followed by an intrinsic beat, a pacing spike that fails to capture, two ventricular paced beats, two intrinsic beats, and a ventricular paced beat.
Interpretation: Ventricular paced rhythm with three intrinsic beats and one episode of failure to capture (abnormal pacemaker function).

Strip 10.17
Analysis: The first two complexes are ventricular paced beats followed by a fusion beat, two intrinsic beats, a pacing spike that occurs too early, an intrinsic beat, a pacing spike that occurs too early, an intrinsic beat, a pacing spike with capture that occurs too early, and a ventricular paced beat.
Interpretation: Ventricular paced rhythm with four intrinsic beats, one fusion beat, and three episodes of undersensing (two episodes without capture and one episode with capture). This represents abnormal pacemaker function.

Strip 10.18
Analysis: The first two complexes are ventricular paced beats followed by a fusion beat and four intrinsic beats.
Interpretation: Ventricular paced rhythm with one fusion beat and four intrinsic beats (normal pacemaker function).

Strip 10.19
Analysis: The first four complexes are ventricular paced beats followed by an intrinsic beat and three ventricular paced beats.
Interpretation: Ventricular paced rhythm with one intrinsic beat (normal pacemaker function).

Strip 10.20
Analysis: The first complex is a ventricular paced beat followed by two pacing spikes with failure to capture, a ventricular paced beat, a pacing spike with failure to capture, a ventricular paced beat, a pacing spike with failure to capture, two ventricular paced beats, and a pacing spike with failure to capture.
Interpretation: Ventricular paced rhythm with five episodes of failure to capture (abnormal pacemaker function).

Strip 10.21
Analysis: All complexes are pacemaker induced.
Interpretation: Ventricular paced rhythm (normal pacemaker function).

Strip 10.22
Analysis: One ventricular paced beat changing to ventricular tachycardia (torsade de pointes).
Interpretation: Ventricular paced beat changing to torsade de pointes VT (normal pacemaker function).

Strip 10.23
Analysis: The first four complexes are ventricular paced beats followed by an intrinsic beat, a pacing spike that occurs too early, a fusion beat, and a ventricular paced beat.
Interpretation: Ventricular paced rhythm with one intrinsic beat, one fusion beat, and one episode of undersensing (abnormal pacemaker function).

Strip 10.24
Analysis: The first complex is a ventricular paced beat followed by a pacing spike with failure to capture, an intrinsic beat, a pacing spike with failure to capture, an intrinsic beat, a ventricular paced beat, a pacing spike with failure to capture, an intrinsic beat, a pacing spike with failure to capture, and an intrinsic beat.
Interpretation: Ventricular paced rhythm with four intrinsic beats and four episodes of failure to capture (abnormal pacemaker function).

Strip 10.25
Analysis: All complexes are pacemaker induced.
Interpretation: Ventricular paced rhythm (normal pacemaker function).

Strip 10.26
Analysis: The first complex is an intrinsic beat followed by a fusion beat, an intrinsic beat, two ventricular paced beats, four intrinsic beats, and one ventricular paced beat.
Interpretation: Ventricular paced rhythm with one fusion beat and six intrinsic beats (normal pacemaker function).

Strip 10.27
Analysis: The first four complexes are ventricular paced beats followed by ventricular standstill (asystole).
Interpretation: Ventricular paced rhythm with failure to fire resulting in ventricular standstill (abnormal pacemaker function).

Strip 10.28
Analysis: The first four complexes are ventricular paced beats followed by two pacing spikes with failure to capture, an intrinsic beat, two pacing spikes with failure to capture, and an intrinsic beat.
Interpretation: Ventricular paced rhythm with two intrinsic beats and four episodes of failure to capture (abnormal pacemaker function).

Strip 10.29
Analysis: The first two complexes are intrinsic beats followed by three ventricular paced beats and one intrinsic beat.
Interpretation: Ventricular paced rhythm with an underlying basic rhythm of atrial fibrillation (normal pacemaker function).

Strip 10.30
Analysis: The first two complexes are ventricular paced followed by an intrinsic beat, two ventricular paced beats, an intrinsic beat, a fusion beat, and a ventricular paced beat.
Interpretation: Ventricular paced rhythm with two intrinsic beats and one fusion beat (normal pacemaker function).

Strip 10.31
Analysis: The first three complexes are ventricular paced beats followed by two intrinsic beats (paired PVCs) and four ventricular paced beats.
Interpretation: Ventricular paced rhythm with two intrinsic beats (normal pacemaker function).

Strip 10.32
Analysis: The first four complexes are ventricular paced beats followed by one intrinsic beat (PVC), a pacing spike occurring too early, and three ventricular paced beats.
Interpretation: Ventricular paced rhythm with one intrinsic beat and one episode of undersensing (abnormal pacemaker function).

Strip 10.33
Analysis: The first two complexes are ventricular paced beats followed by two intrinsic beats, a fusion beat, and two ventricular paced beats.
Interpretation: Ventricular paced rhythm with two intrinsic beats and one fusion beat (normal pacemaker function).

Strip 10.34
Analysis: The first four complexes are ventricular paced beats followed by a pacing spike with failure to capture, an intrinsic beat, a pacing spike that occurs too early, and two ventricular paced beats.
Interpretation: Ventricular paced rhythm with one intrinsic beat, one episode of failure to capture, and one episode of undersensing (abnormal pacemaker function).

Strip 10.35
Analysis: The first two complexes are ventricular paced beats followed by an intrinsic beat, a fusion beat, an intrinsic beat, one ventricular paced beat that occurs too early, two ventricular paced beats, and an intrinsic beat.
Interpretation: Ventricular paced rhythm with three intrinsic beats, one fusion beat, and one episode of undersensing with capture (abnormal pacemaker function).

Strip 10.36
Analysis: The first two complexes are ventricular paced beats followed by an intrinsic beat, a pacing spike that occurs too early, three intrinsic beats, and three ventricular paced beats.
Interpretation: Ventricular paced rhythm with four intrinsic beats and one episode of undersensing (abnormal pacemaker function).

Strip 10.37
Analysis: The first five complexes are ventricular paced beats followed by an intrinsic beat and two ventricular paced beats.
Interpretation: Ventricular paced rhythm with one intrinsic beat (normal pacemaker function).

Strip 10.38
Analysis: The first four complexes are ventricular paced beats followed by a pause in pacing, a ventricular paced beat that occurs later than expected, a ventricular paced beat, and an intrinsic beat.
Interpretation: Ventricular paced rhythm with one intrinsic beat and one episode of oversensing (the pacemaker sensed the large T wave at the start of the pause). This is abnormal pacemaker function.

Strip 10.39
Analysis: The first complex is ventricular paced followed by three intrinsic beats and four ventricular paced beats.
Interpretation: Ventricular paced rhythm with three intrinsic beats (normal pacemaker function.

Strip 10.40
Analysis: The first complex is ventricular paced followed by ventricular standstill (asystole).
Interpretation: Ventricular paced beat with failure to fire resulting in ventricular standstill (abnormal pacemaker function).

Strip 10.41
Analysis: The first four beats are intrinsic beats followed by two ventricular paced beats, an intrinsic beat with a pacer spike, and two ventricular paced beats.
Interpretation: Ventricular paced rhythm with an underlying rhythm of atrial fibrillation and one pseudofusion beat (seventh complex). This is normal pacemaker function.

Strip 10.42
Analysis: The first five beats are intrinsic beats followed by one ventricular paced beat.
Interpretation: Atrial fibrillation with one ventricular paced beat.

Strip 11.1
Rhythm: Regular
Rate: 136 beats/minute
P waves: Sinus
PR interval: 0.12 second
QRS complex: 0.06 to 0.08 second
Rhythm interpretation: Sinus tachycardia

Strip 11.2
Rhythm: Regular
Rate: 72 beats/minute
P waves: Sinus
PR interval: 0.16 to 0.18 second
QRS complex: 0.12 second
Rhythm interpretation: Normal sinus rhythm with bundle branch block
Comment. A U wave is present

Strip 11.3
Rhythm: Regular (atrial); irregular (ventricular)
Rate: 79 beats/minute (atrial); 30 beats/minute (ventricular)
P waves: Sinus (two or four P waves before each QRS complex)
PR interval: 0.24 to 0.28 second (PR consistent)
QRS complex: 0.06 to 0.08 second
Rhythm interpretation: Second-degree AV block, Mobitz II with 2:1 and 4:1 AV conduction

Strip 11.4
Rhythm: Irregular
Rate: 60 beats/minute (basic rhythm)
P waves: Fibrillatory and flutter waves are present
PR interval: Not measurable
QRS complex: 0.06 to 0.08 second
Rhythm interpretation: Atrial Fib-Flutter followed by synchronized shock returning to atrial fib-flutter

Strip 11.5
Rhythm: Regular
Rate: 48 beats/minute
P waves: Hidden in QRS complexes
PR interval: Not measurable
QRS complex: 0.04 to 0.08 second
Rhythm interpretation: Junctional rhythm
Comment: ST segment depression is present

Strip 11.6
Rhythm: Regular
Rate: 188 beats/minute
P waves: Hidden in T waves
PR interval: Not measurable
QRS complex: 0.10 second
Rhythm interpretation: Paroxysmal atrial tachycardia

Strip 11.7
Rhythm: Regular
Rate: 115 beats/minute
P waves: Inverted before each QRS complex
PR interval: 0.08 to 0.10 second
QRS complex: 0.06 to 0.08 second
Rhythm interpretation: Junctional tachycardia

Strip 11.8
Rhythm: Regular (atrial and ventricular)
Rate: 75 beats/minute (atrial); 26 beats/minute (ventricular)
P waves: Sinus (bear no relationship to QRS complexes)
PR interval: PR varies
QRS complex: 0.14 to 0.16 second
Rhythm interpretation: Third-degree AV block
Comment: ST segment elevation is present

Strip 11.9
Rhythm: Regular
Rate: 188 beats/minute
P waves: None identified
PR interval: Not measurable
QRS complex: 0.16 to 0.20 second
Rhythm interpretation: Ventricular tachycardia

Strip 11.10
Rhythm: Regular
Rate: 40 beats/minute
P waves: None identified
PR interval: Not measurable
QRS complex: 0.16 second or greater
Rhythm interpretation: Idioventricular rhythm

Strip 11.11
Rhythm: Regular (basic rhythm)
Rate: 56 beats/minute (basic rhythm)
P waves: Sinus (notched)
PR interval: 0.16 to 0.20 second
QRS complex: 0.04 to 0.08 second (basic rhythm); 0.12 to 0.14 second (PVC)
Rhythm interpretation: Sinus bradycardia with one interpolated PVC
Comment: ST segment depression is present; notched P waves may indicate atrial hypertrophy

Strip 11.12
Rhythm: Regular
Rate: 84 beats/minute
P waves: Inverted before each QRS complex
PR interval: 0.08 to 0.10 second
QRS complex: 0.04 to 0.08 second
Rhythm interpretation: Accelerated junctional rhythm

Strip 11.13
Rhythm: Regular
Rate: 232 beats/minute (atrial); 58 beats/minute (ventricular)
P waves: Four flutter waves before each QRS complex
PR interval: Not measurable
QRS complex: 0.04 to 0.08 second
Rhythm interpretation: Atrial flutter with 4:1 AV conduction

Strip 11.14
Rhythm: Regular
Rate: 79 beats/minute
P waves: Sinus
PR interval: 0.16 second
QRS complex: 0.12 second
Rhythm interpretation: Normal sinus rhythm with bundle branch block
Comment: ST segment elevation is present

Strip 11.15
Rhythm: Regular
Rate: 84 beats/minute
P waves: Absent
PR interval: Not measurable
QRS complex: 0.14 to 0.16 second
Rhythm interpretation: Accelerated idioventricular rhythm

Strip 11.16
Rhythm: Regular (basic rhythm); irregular with pause
Rate: 75 beats/minute (basic rhythm)
P waves: Sinus (basic rhythm); one premature, abnormal P wave without a QRS complex (after fifth QRS complex)
PR interval: 0.24 to 0.28 second (PR consistent)
QRS complex: 0.08 second
Rhythm interpretation: Normal sinus rhythm with first-degree AV block and one nonconducted PAC (after fifth QRS complex)

Strip 11.17
Rhythm: Regular
Rate: 115 beats/minute
P waves: Sinus
PR interval: 0.14 to 0.16 second
QRS complex: 0.04 to 0.06 second
Rhythm interpretation: Sinus tachycardia

Strip 11.18
Rhythm: Regular
Rate: 48 beats/minute
P waves: Sinus
PR interval: 0.12 to 0.16 second
QRS complex: 0.08 second
Rhythm interpretation: Sinus bradycardia
Comment: ST segment elevation is present

Strip 11.19
Rhythm: Regular (basic rhythm); irregular with premature beats
Rate: 72 beats/minute (basic rhythm)
P waves: Sinus (basic rhythm); inverted with premature beats
PR interval: 0.12 to 0.14 second (basic rhythm); 0.08 second (premature beats)
QRS complex: 0.08 second (basic rhythm); 0.06 second PJCs
Rhythm interpretation: Normal sinus rhythm with two premature junctional contractions (fourth and sixth complexes)

Strip 11.20
Rhythm: Regular
Rate: 63 beats/minute
P waves: Vary in size, shape, and direction across strip
PR interval: 0.12 second
QRS complex: 0.04 to 0.08 second
Rhythm interpretation: Wandering atrial pacemaker
Comment: ST segment depression is present

Strip 11.21
Rhythm: Irregular and chaotic
Rate: Not measurable
P waves: Recognizable P waves are absent: wavy, irregular deflections are seen that vary in size, shape, and height
PR interval: Not measurable
QRS complex: Absent
Rhythm interpretation: Ventricular fibrillation (coarse)

Strip 11.22
Rhythm: Regular
Rate: 107 beats/minute
P waves: Inverted before each QRS complex
PR interval: 0.08 second
QRS complex: 0.04 second
Rhythm interpretation: Junctional tachycardia

Strip 11.23
Rhythm: Regular (atrial)
Rate: 34 beats/minute (atrial)
P waves: Sinus
PR interval: Not measurable
QRS complex: Absent
Rhythm interpretation: Ventricular standstill (asystole)

Strip 11.24
Rhythm: Irregular
Rate: 70 beats/minute
P waves: Sinus
PR interval: 0.44 to 0.48 second (PR consistent)
QRS complex: 0.08 to 0.10 second
Rhythm interpretation: Sinus arrhythmia with first-degree AV block
Comment: ST segment elevation is present

Strip 11.25
Rhythm: Regular (basic rhythm); irregular with pause
Rate: 48 beats/minute (basic rhythm)
P waves: Sinus
PR interval: 0.32 to 0.36 second (PR consistent)
QRS complex: 0.12 to 0.14 second (basic rhythm)
Rhythm interpretation: Sinus bradycardia with first-degree AV block and sinus arrest

Strip 11.26
Rhythm: Regular (atrial); irregular (ventricular)
Rate: 72 beats/minute (atrial); 40 beats/minute (ventricular)
P waves: Sinus
PR interval: Lengthens from 0.20 to 0.28 second (PR varies)
QRS complex: 0.04 to 0.06 second
Rhythm interpretation: Second-degree AV block, Mobitz I
Comment: ST segment depression is present

Strip 11.27
Rhythm: Regular
Rate: 72 beats/minute
P waves: Sinus
PR interval: 0.20 second
QRS complex: 0.08 to 0.10 second
Rhythm interpretation: Normal sinus rhythm
Comment: ST segment depression and T-wave inversion are present

Strip 11.28
Rhythm: Regular (basic rhythm); irregular with pause
Rate: 72 beats/minute (basic rhythm); rate slows to 63 beats/minute after pause (temporary rate suppression can occur after a pause in the basic rhythm)
P waves: Sinus (basic rhythm)
PR interval: 0.16 to 0.20 second (basic rhythm)
QRS complex: 0.04 to 0.08 second
Rhythm interpretation: Normal sinus rhythm with sinus arrest

Strip 11.29
Rhythm: Regular (basic rhythm); irregular with premature beats
Rate: 63 beats/minute (basic rhythm)
P waves: Sinus (basic rhythm); premature and pointed (PAC)
PR interval: 0.14 to 0.16 second (basic rhythm); 0.12 second (PAC)
QRS complex: 0.08 second (basic rhythm and PAC)
Rhythm interpretation: Normal sinus rhythm with one PAC (fifth complex)
Comment: A U wave is present

Strip 11.30
Rhythm: Regular (basic rhythm); irregular with PVCs
Rate: 72 to 75 beats/minute (basic rhythm)
P waves: Sinus (basic rhythm)
PR interval: 0.12 to 0.16 second
QRS complex: 0.12 second (basic rhythm and PVCs)
Rhythm interpretation: Normal sinus rhythm with bundle branch block and paired PVCs
Comment: A U wave is present

Strip 11.31
Rhythm: Regular (atrial and ventricular)
Rate: 240 beats/minute (atrial); 60 beats/minute (ventricular)
P waves: Four flutter waves before each QRS complex
PR interval: Not measurable
QRS complex: 0.08 to 0.10 second
Rhythm interpretation: Atrial flutter with 4:1 AV conduction

Strip 11.32
Rhythm: Regular (basic rhythm); irregular with pause
Rate: 54 beats/minute (basic rhythm)
P waves: Sinus (basic rhythm)
PR interval: 0.20 second (basic rhythm)
QRS complex: 0.06 to 0.08 second (basic rhythm); 0.06 second (junctional escape beats)
Rhythm interpretation: Sinus bradycardia with a pause followed by two junctional escape beats—the specific pause (sinus arrest or block) cannot be identified due to the presence of the escape beats.

Strip 11.33
Rhythm: Regular
Rate: 25 beats/minute
P waves: Absent
PR interval: Not measurable
QRS complex: 0.24 second or greater
Rhythm interpretation: Idioventricular rhythm

Strip 11.34
Rhythm: Regular (basic rhythm); irregular with pause
Rate: 65 beats/minute (basic rhythm)
P waves: Sinus (basic rhythm)
PR interval: 0.18 to 0.20 second
QRS complex: 0.06 to 0.08 second
Rhythm interpretation: Normal sinus rhythm with sinus arrest

Strip 11.35
Rhythm: Regular
Rate: 84 beats/minute
P waves: Absent
PR interval: Not measurable
QRS complex: 0.12 to 0.14 second
Rhythm interpretation: Accelerated idioventricular rhythm

Strip 11.36
Rhythm: Not measurable
Rate: Not measurable
P waves: Absent
PR interval: Not measurable
QRS complex: Absent
Rhythm interpretation: Ventricular standstill (asystole)

Strip 11.37
Rhythm: Regular
Rate: 40 beats/minute
P waves: Sinus
PR interval: 0.12 second
QRS complex: 0.08 second

Rhythm interpretation: Sinus bradycardia
Comment: A U wave is present

Strip 11.38
Rhythm: Regular
Rate: 100 beats/minute
P waves: Inverted before each QRS complex
PR interval: 0.08 to 0.10 second
QRS complex: 0.08 second
Rhythm interpretation: Accelerated junctional rhythm
Comment: Baseline artifact is present

Strip 11.39
Rhythm: Regular (basic rhythm); irregular with PAC
Rate: 72 beats/minute (basic rhythm)
P waves: Sinus (basic rhythm); premature, abnormal P wave with PAC
PR interval: 0.14 to 0.16 second (basic rhythm); 0.12 second (PAC)
QRS complex: 0.04 to 0.08 second (basic rhythm); 0.08 second (PAC)
Rhythm interpretation: Normal sinus rhythm with one PAC (third complex)

Strip 11.40
Rhythm: Regular (basic rhythm)
Rate: 84 beats/minute (basic rhythm)
P waves: Sinus (basic rhythm); premature, abnormal P wave without QRS complex after fifth QRS complex
PR interval; 0.18 to 0.20 second
QRS complex: 0.06 to 0.08 second (basic rhythm); 0.08 second (PJC)
Rhythm interpretation: Normal sinus rhythm with one nonconducted PAC (after fifth QRS complex) and one premature junctional contraction following the nonconducted PAC

Strip 11.41
Rhythm: Regular (atrial)
Rate: 88 beats/minute (atrial)
P waves: Sinus
PR interval: Not measurable
QRS complex: Absent
Rhythm interpretation: Ventricular standstill (asystole)

Strip 11.42
Rhythm: Regular (basic rhythm); irregular with PVCs
Rate: 63 beats/minute (basic rhythm)
P waves: Sinus (basic rhythm)
PR interval: 0.12 to 0.16 second
QRS complex: 0.08 second (basic rhythm); 0.12 to 0.16 second (PVC)

Rhythm interpretation: Normal sinus rhythm with paired multifocal PVCs (fourth and fifth complexes)

Strip 11.43
Rhythm: Regular (basic rhythm); irregular with PACs
Rate: 136 beats/minute (basic rhythm)
P waves: Sinus (basic rhythm); premature and pointed (PACs)
PR interval: 0.16 to 0.20 second (basic rhythm); 0.12 second (PACs)
QRS complex: 0.06 to 0.08 second (basic rhythm); 0.08 second (PACs)
Rhythm interpretation: Sinus tachycardia with two PACs (fourth and eighth complexes)

Strip 11.44
Rhythm: Regular (basic rhythm); irregular with pause
Rate: 84 beats/minute (basic rhythm); slows to 79 after pause due to temporary rate suppression
P waves: Sinus
PR interval: 0.20 second
QRS complex: 0.08 to 0.10 second
Rhythm interpretation: Normal sinus rhythm with sinus arrest
Comment: ST segment depression and T-wave inversion are present

Strip 11.45
Rhythm: Unable to measure (only one cardiac cycle)
Rate: 63 beats/minute (basic rhythm)
P wave: Sinus (basic rhythm); inverted with PJCs and ectopic junctional beat
PR interval: 0.14 to 0.16 second (basic rhythm); 0.08 second (junctional beats)
QRS complex: 0.08 to 0.10 second (basic rhythm); 0.08 second (junctional beats)
Rhythm interpretation: Normal sinus rhythm with two PJCs (second and sixth complexes) and one ectopic junctional beat (third complex)

Strip 11.46
Rhythm: Regular (basic rhythm)
Rate: 60 beats/minute (basic rhythm)
P waves: Sinus (basic rhythm)
PR interval: 0.12 to 0.16 second
QRS complex: 0.08 second (basic rhythm); 0.12 second (PVC)
Rhythm interpretation: Normal sinus rhythm with one interpolated PVC (between fifth and sixth normal QRS complexes)

Strip 11.47
Rhythm: Regular
Rate: 42 beats/minute
P wave: Hidden in QRS complexes
PR interval: Not measurable
QRS complex: 0.08 to 0.10 second
Rhythm interpretation: Junctional
rhythm

Strip 11.48
Rhythm: Regular (atrial); irregular
(ventricular)
Rate: 79 beats/minute (atrial); 50 beats/
minute (ventricular)
P waves: Sinus
PR interval: Lengthens from 0.20 to
0.32 second (PR varies)
QRS complex: 0.08 to 0.10 second
Rhythm interpretation: Second-degree AV
block, Mobitz I

Strip 11.49
Rhythm: Regular (basic rhythm); irregular
with PAC
Rate: 107 beats/minute (basic rhythm)
P waves: Inverted before each QRS
complex (basic rhythm); premature,
pointed P wave with PAC
PR interval: 0.08 to 0.10 second (basic
rhythm); 0.12 second (PAC)
QRS complex: 0.08 to 0.10 second (basic
rhythm); 0.08 second (PAC)
Rhythm interpretation: Junctional
tachycardia with one PAC (ninth
complex)

Strip 11.50
Rhythm: Regular (atrial and ventricular)
Rate: 84 beats/minute (atrial); 28 beats/
minute (ventricular)
P waves: Sinus (bear no relationship to
QRS complexes)
PR interval: PR varies
QRS complex: 0.12 second
Rhythm interpretation: Third-degree AV
block
Comment: ST segment depression is
present

Strip 11.51
Rhythm: Irregular
Rate: 70 beats/minute
P wave: Sinus
PR interval: 0.18 to 0.20 second
QRS complex: 0.08 to 0.10 second
Rhythm interpretation: Sinus arrhythmia

Strip 11.52
Rhythm: Regular (basic rhythm); irregular
with PVCs
Rate: 72 beats/minute (basic rhythm)
P waves: Sinus (basic rhythm)
PR interval: 0.14 to 0.16 second
QRS complex: 0.08 to 0.10 second (basic
rhythm); 0.12 second (PVCs)
Rhythm interpretation: Normal sinus rhythm
with univocal PVCs in a trigeminal pattern
Comment: ST segment depression and
T-wave inversion are present

Strip 11.53
Rhythm: Regular
Rate: 94 beats/minute (atrial); 31 beats/
minute (ventricular)
P waves: Three sinus P waves to each
QRS complex (one hidden in the T wave)
PR interval: 0.36 second (PR consistent)
QRS complex: 0.08 second
Rhythm interpretation: Second-degree AV
block, Mobitz II

Strip 11.54
Rhythm: Regular (basic rhythm); irregular
with PVCs
Rate: 72 beats/minute (basic rhythm)
P waves: Sinus (basic rhythm)
PR interval: 0.12 to 0.14 second
QRS complex: 0.08 second (basic rhythm);
0.12 second (PVCs)
Rhythm interpretation: Normal sinus
rhythm with multifocal PVCs

Strip 11.55
Rhythm: Regular (atrial and ventricular)
Rate: 65 beats/minute (atrial); 32 beats/
minute (ventricular)
P waves: Two sinus P waves before each
QRS complex
PR interval: 0.44 to 0.48 second (PR
consistent)
QRS complex: 0.14 to 0.16 second
Rhythm interpretation: Second-degree AV
block, Mobitz II

Strip 11.56
Rhythm: Regular
Rate: 65 beats/minute
P waves: Inverted before each QRS complex
PR interval: 0.10 second
QRS complex: 0.04 second
Rhythm interpretation: Accelerated
junctional rhythm
Comment: ST segment elevation is present

Strip 11.57
Rhythm: Regular (basic rhythm); irregular
with pause
Rate: 72 beats/minute (basic rhythm)
P waves: Sinus
PR interval: 0.22 to 0.24 second
(PR consistent)
QRS complex: 0.08 to 0.10 second
Rhythm interpretation: Normal sinus
rhythm with first-degree AV block and
sinus arrest
Comment: ST segment elevation is present

Strip 11.58
Rhythm: Irregular
Rate: Not measurable (atrial); 140 beats/
minute (ventricular)
P waves: Fibrillatory waves are present
PR interval: Not measurable
QRS complex: 0.04 to 0.06 second
Rhythm interpretation: Atrial fibrillation
(uncontrolled rate)

Strip 11.59
Rhythm: Regular
Rate: 188 beats/minute
P waves: Hidden in T waves
PR interval: Not measurable
QRS complex: 0.06 to 0.08 second
Rhythm interpretation: Paroxysmal atrial
tachycardia

Strip 11.60
Rhythm: Regular (basic rhythm)
Rate: 47 beats/minute (basic rhythm)
P waves: Sinus (basic rhythm)
PR interval: 0.34 to 0.36 second (PR
consistent)
QRS complex: 0.14 to 0.16 second
Rhythm interpretation: Sinus bradycardia
with bundle branch block, first-degree AV
block, and sinus arrest
Comment: ST segment depression and
T-wave inversion are present

Strip 11.61
Rhythm: Regular (atrial); irregular
(ventricular)
Rate: 84 beats/minute (atrial); 70 beats/
minute (ventricular)
P waves: Sinus
PR interval: Lengthens from 0.24 to
0.40 second (PR varies)
QRS complex: 0.06 to 0.08 second
Rhythm interpretation: Second-degree AV
block, Mobitz I

Strip 11.62
Rhythm: Regular (basic rhythm); irregular with nonconducted PACs
Rate: 100 beats/minute (basic rhythm)
P waves: Sinus (basic rhythm); two premature abnormal P waves without QRS complexes (after the fourth and eighth complexes)
PR interval: 0.12 to 0.14 second
QRS complex: 0.06 to 0.08 second
Rhythm interpretation: Normal sinus rhythm with two nonconducted PACs (after fourth and eighth complexes)
Comment: T-wave inversion is present

Strip 11.63
Rhythm: Regular (basic rhythm)
Rate: 65 beats/minute
P waves: Sinus (basic rhythm); premature, abnormal P wave without QRS complex after third QRS complex
PR interval: 0.16 second
QRS complex: 0.12 second
Rhythm interpretation: Normal sinus rhythm with bundle branch block and nonconducted PAC (after third QRS complex)

Strip 11.64
Rhythm: Regular (basic rhythm)
Rate: 50 beats/minute
P waves: Sinus (basic rhythm); inverted P wave with PJC
PR interval: 0.12 second (basic rhythm); 0.08 second (PJC)
QRS complex: 0.08 to 0.10 second (basic rhythm); 0.10 second (PJC)
Rhythm interpretation: Sinus bradycardia with one premature junctional contraction (third complex)

Strip 11.65
Rhythm: Regular (atrial and ventricular)
Rate: 84 beats/minute (atrial); 42 beats/minute (ventricular)
P waves: Two sinus P waves before each QRS complex
PR interval: 0.12 to 0.16 second (PR consistent)
QRS complex: 0.12 second
Rhythm interpretation: Second-degree AV block, Mobitz II with 2:1 AV conduction

Strip 11.66
Rhythm: Regular
Rate: 79 beats/minute (atrial); 39 beats/minute (ventricular)
P waves: Two sinus P waves to each QRS complex
PR interval: 0.24 second (PR consistent)
QRS complex: 0.12 to 0.16 second
Rhythm interpretation: Second-degree AV block, Mobitz II

Strip 11.67
Rhythm: Regular (basic rhythm)
Rate: 52 beats/minute
P waves: Hidden in QRS complex
PR interval: Not measurable
QRS complex: 0.04 to 0.08 second
Rhythm interpretation: Junctional rhythm
Comment: Baseline artifact is present

Strip 11.68
Rhythm: Irregular (basic rhythm)
Rate: 60 beats/minute (basic rhythm)
P waves: Sinus (basic rhythm); absent during pause
PR interval: 0.12 to 0.16 second (basic rhythm); absent during pause
QRS complex: 0.12 second (basic rhythm); absent during pause
Rhythm interpretation: Sinus arrhythmia with bundle branch block and a sinus pause
Comment: Because of the irregularity of the basic rhythm, sinus arrest cannot be differentiated from sinus block, and the rhythm is best interpreted using the term sinus pause, indicating either rhythm could be present; ST segment elevation is present.

Strip 11.69
Rhythm: Regular
Rate: 115 beats/minute
P waves: Inverted before each QRS complex
PR interval: 0.08 to 0.10 second
QRS complex: 0.04 to 0.06 second
Rhythm interpretation: Junctional tachycardia

Strip 11.70
Rhythm: Regular (basic rhythm); irregular with PJC
Rate: 58 beats/minute (basic rhythm)
P waves: Sinus (basic rhythm); inverted with PJC
PR interval: 0.12 to 0.16 second (basic rhythm); 0.10 second on (PJC)
QRS complex: 0.08 second (basic rhythm); 0.10 second (PJC)
Rhythm interpretation: Sinus bradycardia with one PJC (third complex)

Strip 11.71
Rhythm: Regular (basic rhythm); irregular with nonconducted PAC
Rate: 63 beats/minute (basic rhythm)
P waves: Sinus (basic rhythm); one premature, abnormal P wave without a QRS complex (after the fourth complex)
PR interval: 0.28 to 0.32 second (PR consistent)
QRS complex: 0.12 second
Rhythm interpretation: Normal sinus rhythm with first-degree AV block and bundle branch block with one nonconducted PAC after the fourth QRS complex
Comment: ST segment elevation and T-wave inversion are present

Strip 11.72
Rhythm: Regular (basic rhythm); irregular with PVC
Rate: 52 beats/minute (basic rhythm)
P waves: Sinus
PR interval: 0.12 to 0.16 second
QRS complex: 0.06 to 0.08 second (basic rhythm); 0.16 second (PVC)
Rhythm interpretation: Sinus bradycardia with one PVC (after third QRS complex)
Comment: ST segment elevation is present

Strip 11.73
Rhythm: Regular (basic rhythm)
Rate: 68 beats/minute (basic rhythm)
P waves: Sinus (basic rhythm)
PR interval: 0.12 second (basic rhythm)
QRS complex: 0.08 to 0.10 second (basic rhythm); 0.14 to 0.16 second (PVCs); 0.08 second (junctional escape beat)
Rhythm interpretation: Normal sinus rhythm with paired PVCs (fourth and fifth complexes) and one junctional escape beat (sixth complex)
Comment: ST segment depression and T-wave inversion are present

Strip 11.74
Rhythm: Regular
Rate: 50 beats/minute
P waves: Hidden in QRS complex
PR interval: Not measurable
QRS complex: 0.04 to 0.06 second
Rhythm interpretation: Junctional rhythm
Comment: ST segment depression and T-wave inversion are present

Strip 11.75
Rhythm: Irregular (atrial)
Rate: 40 beats/minute (atrial)
P waves: Sinus
PR interval: Not measurable
QRS complex: Absent
Rhythm interpretation: Ventricular standstill (asystole)

Strip 11.76
Rhythm: Irregular
Rate: 60 beats/minute
P wave: Sinus
PR interval: 0.12 to 0.14 second
QRS complex: 0.08 to 0.10 second
Rhythm interpretation: Sinus arrhythmia
Comment: ST segment elevation is present

Strip 11.77
Rhythm: Regular
Rate: 68 beats/minute
P waves: P waves vary in size, shape, and direction
PR interval: 0.14 to 0.16 second
QRS complex: 0.08 second
Rhythm interpretation: Wandering atrial pacemaker
Comment: T-wave inversion is present

Strip 11.78
Rhythm: Regular
Rate: 214 beats/minute
P waves: Hidden in T waves
PR interval: Not measurable
QRS complex: 0.06 to 0.08 second
Rhythm interpretation: Paroxysmal atrial tachycardia

Strip 11.79
Rhythm: Regular (basic rhythm); regular (VT)
Rate: 72 beats/minute (basic rhythm); 167 beats/minute (VT)
P waves: Sinus (basic rhythm)
PR interval: 0.14 to 0.16 second (basic rhythm)
QRS complex: 0.08 to 0.10 second (basic rhythm); 0.12 second (VT)
Rhythm interpretation: Normal sinus rhythm with a 10-beat run of ventricular tachycardia.

Strip 11.80
Rhythm: Regular (basic rhythm); irregular with VT and paired PVCs
Rate: 100 beats/minute (basic rhythm)
P waves: Sinus (basic rhythm)
PR interval: 0.16 second
QRS complex: 0.04 to 0.08 second (basic rhythm); 0.12 second or greater (ventricular beats)
Rhythm interpretation: Normal sinus rhythm with a four-beat run of ventricular tachycardia and paired PVCs

Strip 11.81
Rhythm: Irregular
Rate: 260 beats/minute (atrial); 70 beats/minute (ventricular)
P waves: Flutter waves are present
PR interval: Not measurable
QRS complex: 0.04 to 0.08 second
Rhythm interpretation: Atrial flutter with variable AV conduction

Strip 11.82
Rhythm: Irregular
Rate: 60 beats/minute
P waves: Sinus
PR interval: 0.14 to 0.16 second
QRS complex: 0.06 to 0.08 second
Rhythm interpretation: Sinus arrhythmia

Strip 11.83
Rhythm: Regular
Rate: 48 beats/minute
P waves: Sinus
PR interval: 0.12 to 0.16 second
QRS complex: 0.06 to 0.08 second
Rhythm interpretation: Sinus bradycardia
Comment: A small U wave is present

Strip 11.84
Rhythm: Regular
Rate: 136 beats/minute
P waves: Sinus
PR interval: 0.14 to 0.16 second
QRS complex: 0.06 to 0.08 second
Rhythm interpretation: Sinus tachycardia

Strip 11.85
Rhythm: Regular
Rate: 54 beats/minute
P waves: Sinus
PR interval: 0.24 to 0.28 second (PR consistent)
QRS complex: 0.04 to 0.06 second
Rhythm interpretation: Sinus bradycardia with first-degree AV block

Strip 11.86
Rhythm: Regular (atrial and ventricular)
Rate: 94 beats/minute (atrial); 37 beats/minute (ventricular)
P waves: Sinus (bear no relationship to QRS complexes)
PR interval: PR varies
QRS complex: 0.12 to 0.16 second
Rhythm interpretation: Third-degree AV block

Strip 11.87
Rhythm: Regular
Rate: 150 beats/minute
P waves: None identified
PR interval: Not measurable
QRS complex: 0.12 to 0.16 second
Rhythm interpretation: Ventricular tachycardia

Strip 11.88
Rhythm: Regular (basic rhythm); irregular with pause
Rate: 56 beats/minute (basic rhythm)
P waves: Sinus (basic rhythm); absent during pause
PR interval: 0.16 to 0.18 second (absent during pause)
QRS complex: 0.08 to 0.10 second (absent during pause)
Rhythm interpretation: Sinus bradycardia with sinus arrest
Comment: ST segment depression and T-wave inversion are present

Strip 11.89
Rhythm: Not measurable
Rate: Not measurable
P waves: Absent
PR interval: Not measurable
QRS complex: Absent
Rhythm interpretation: Ventricular standstill (asystole)

Strip 11.90
Rhythm: Regular (basic rhythm); off by two squares
Rate: 75 to 85 beats/minute
P waves: Sinus (basic rhythm)
PR interval: 0.18 to 0.20 second
QRS complex: 0.06 to 0.08 second (basic rhythm); 0.08 second (junctional escape beat); 0.18 second (PVC)
Rhythm interpretation: Normal sinus rhythm with nonconducted PAC (after third complex), junctional escape beat (following nonconducted PAC), and one PVC (sixth complex)

Strip 11.91
Rhythm: Regular (atrial and ventricular)
Rate: 84 beats/minute (atrial); 42 beats/minute (ventricular)
P waves: Sinus (bear no relationship to QRS complex)
PR interval: PR varies
QRS complex: 0.12 to 0.14 second
Rhythm interpretation: Third-degree AV block

Strip 11.92
Rhythm: Regular
Rate: 188 beats/minute
P waves: Hidden in T waves
PR interval: Not measurable
QRS complex: 0.08 to 0.10 second
Rhythm interpretation: Paroxysmal atrial tachycardia

Strip 11.93
Rhythm: Irregular and chaotic
Rate: Not measurable
P waves: Recognizable P waves are absent; wavy, irregular deflections are seen that vary in size, shape, and height
PR interval: Not measurable
QRS complex: Absent
Rhythm interpretation: Ventricular fibrillation (coarse)

Strip 11.94
Rhythm: Regular (basic rhythm); irregular with pause
Rate: 75 beats/minute (basic rhythm)
P waves: Sinus (basic rhythm); absent during pause
PR interval: 0.24 second (basic rhythm) (PR consistent); absent during pause
QRS complex: 0.06 to 0.08 second (basic rhythm); absent during pause
Rhythm interpretation: Normal sinus rhythm with first-degree AV block and sinus exit block

Strip 11.95
Rhythm: Regular
Rate: 100 beats/minute
P waves: Inverted before each QRS complex
PR interval: 0.08 second
QRS complex: 0.06 to 0.08 second
Rhythm interpretation: Accelerated junctional rhythm

Strip 11.96
Rhythm: Regular (atrial); irregular (ventricular)
Rate: 88 beats/minute (atrial); 70 beats/minute (ventricular)
P waves: Sinus
PR interval: Lengthens from 0.20 to 0.36 second (PR varies)
QRS complex: 0.08 to 0.10 second
Rhythm interpretation: Second-degree AV block, Mobitz I
Comment: ST segment depression is present

Strip 11.97
Rhythm: Irregular
Rate: Not measurable (atrial); 100 beats/minute (ventricular)
P waves: Fibrillatory waves are present
PR interval: Not measurable
QRS complex: 0.06 to 0.08 second (basic rhythm); 0.12 to 0.14 second (PVC)
Rhythm interpretation: Atrial fibrillation (controlled rate) with one PVC (seventh complex)

Strip 11.98
Rhythm: Irregular, chaotic
Rate: Not measurable
P waves: Recognizable P waves are absent; wavy, irregular deflections are seen that vary in size, shape, and height
PR interval: Not measurable
QRS complex: Absent
Rhythm interpretation: Ventricular fibrillation (coarse)

Strip 11.99
Rhythm: Regular (basic rhythm); irregular with PAC
Rate: 125 beats/minute (basic rhythm)
P waves: Sinus (basic rhythm); pointed, abnormal P wave with PAC
PR interval: 0.12 to 0.14 second (basic rhythm); 0.12 second (PAC)
QRS complex: 0.04 to 0.08 second (basic rhythm); 0.06 second (PAC)
Rhythm interpretation: Sinus tachycardia with one PAC (12th complex)

Strip 11.100
Rhythm: Regular
Rate: 272 beats/minute (atrial); 136 beats/minute (ventricular)
P waves: Two flutter waves to each QRS complex
PR interval: Not measurable
QRS complex: 0.04 second
Rhythm interpretation: Atrial flutter with 2:1 AV conduction

Strip 11.101
Rhythm: Irregular
Rate: 60 beats/minute
P waves: Sinus
PR interval: 0.24 to 0.28 second (PR consistent)
QRS complex: 0.06 to 0.08 second
Rhythm interpretation: Sinus arrhythmia with first-degree AV block

Strip 11.102
Rhythm: Regular (basic rhythm); irregular with PVC
Rate: 79 beats/minute basic rhythm
P waves: Sinus (basic rhythm)
PR interval: 0.16 to 0.18 second
QRS complex: 0.06 to 0.08 second (basic rhythm); 0.16 second (PVC)
Rhythm interpretation: Normal sinus rhythm with one PVC (sixth complex)

Strip 11.103
Rhythm: Regular
Rate: 214 beats/minute
P waves: Not identified
PR interval: Not measurable
QRS complex: 0.16 to 0.20 second
Rhythm interpretation: Ventricular tachycardia

Strip 11.104
Rhythm: Irregular
Rate: Not measurable (atrial); 70 beats/minute (ventricular)
P waves: Fibrillatory waves are present
PR interval: Not measurable
QRS complex: 0.12 second
Rhythm interpretation: Atrial fibrillation (controlled ventricular rate) with bundle branch block

Strip 11.105
Rhythm: Regular (basic rhythm)
Rate: 72 beats/minute (basic rhythm)
P waves: Sinus
PR interval: 0.16 to 0.20 second
QRS complex: 0.06 to 0.08 second (basic rhythm); 0.12 second (PVC)
Rhythm interpretation: Normal sinus rhythm with one interpolated PVC (between sixth and seventh normal QRS complexes)
Comment: ST segment depression and T-wave inversion are present

Strip 11.106
Rhythm: Regular (atrial); irregular (ventricular)
Rate: 100 beats/minute (atrial); 30 beats/minute (ventricular)
P waves: Sinus
PR interval: 0.16 to 0.20 second (PR consistent)
QRS complex: 0.08 second
Rhythm interpretation: Second-degree AV block, Mobitz II with 2:1 and 5:1 AV conduction

Strip 11.107
Rhythm: Regular (basic rhythm); irregular with PVCs
Rate: 88 beats/minute (basic rhythm)
P waves: Sinus
PR interval: 0.12 to 0.14 second (basic rhythm)
QRS complex: 0.04 to 0.06 second (basic rhythm); 0.12 second (PVCs)
Rhythm interpretation: Normal sinus rhythm with three unifocal PVCs

Glossary

Aberrant Abnormal

Aberrantly conducted supraventricular premature beats A premature electrical impulse originating in the atria or AV junction that arrives at the bundle of His so early that the bundle branches are not sufficiently repolarized. Ventricular depolarization is delayed, resulting in a wide QRS complex. Also known as PAC or PJC with *aberrancy*.

Absolute refractory period The period of time during ventricular depolarization and most of repolarization when cardiac cells cannot be stimulated to depolarize. This period begins with the onset of the QRS complex and ends at the peak of the T wave.

Accelerated idioventricular rhythm A rhythm originating in an ectopic site in the ventricles. Characterized by a regular rhythm, an absence of P waves, wide QRS complexes, and a rate between 50 and 100 beats per minute. The rate is faster than the inherent firing rate of the ventricles but is slower than ventricular tachycardia. Also known as *AIVR*.

Accelerated junctional rhythm A rhythm originating in the AV junction characterized by a regular rhythm; inverted P waves immediately before the QRS, immediately after the QRS, or hidden within the QRS complex; a short PR interval of 0.10 second or less; a normal duration QRS complex; and a rate between 60 and 100 beats per minute. The rate is faster than the inherent firing rate of the AV junction, but slower than junctional tachycardia.

Accessory conduction pathways Several abnormal electrical conduction pathways within the heart that allow electrical impulses to bypass the AV node before entering the ventricles.

Acetylcholine The chemical neurotransmitter for the parasympathetic nervous system.

Acute myocardial infarction Necrosis of the myocardium caused by prolonged and complete interruption of blood flow to an area of the myocardial muscle mass.

Agonal rhythm A rhythm seen in a dying heart, in which the QRS complexes deteriorate into irregular, wide, indistinguishable waveforms just prior to ventricular standstill.

AIVR abbr accelerated idioventricular rhythm

Amplitude The height or depth of a wave or complex on the ECG measured in millimeters (mm). Also known as *voltage*.

Angina The term used to describe the pain that results from a reduction in blood supply to the myocardium. The pain is typically described as chest heaviness, pressure, squeezing, or constriction. Associated symptoms include nausea and diaphoresis.

Angioplasty The insertion of a balloon-tipped catheter into an occluded or narrowed coronary artery to reopen the artery by inflating the balloon, compressing the atherosclerotic plaque, and dilating the lumen of the artery. Often followed by insertion of a coronary artery stent. Also known as *percutaneous transluminal coronary angioplasty or PTCA*.

Antegrade conduction Conduction of the electrical impulse in a forward direction.

Aortic valve One of two semilunar valves; located between the left ventricle and the aorta.

Apex of the heart The bottom of the heart formed by the tip of the left ventricle; located to the left of the sternum at approximately the fifth intercostal space, midclavicular line.

Arrhythmia A general term referring to any cardiac rhythm other than a normal sinus rhythm. Often used interchangeably with *dysrhythmia*, a more appropriate term, but one used less often.

Artifacts Distortion of the ECG tracing by activity that is noncardiac in origin. Common causes of artifacts include patient movement, seizure activity, loose electrode pads, disconnected lead wire, electrical interference, and muscle tremors. Also known as *interference* or *noise*.

Asystole Absence of ventricular electrical activity. Tracing will show either P waves or a straight line. Also known as *ventricular standstill*.

Atria The two thin-walled upper chambers of the heart. The right and left atria are separated from the ventricles by the mitral and tricuspid valves.

Atrial fibrillation A rhythm originating in an ectopic site (or numerous sites) in the atria characterized by an atrial rate of 400 beats per minute or more; atrial waveforms appearing as an irregular, wavy baseline; a normal QRS duration; a grossly irregular ventricular rhythm; and a ventricular rate that may be fast or slow depending on the number of impulses conducted through the AV node.

Atrial flutter A rhythm originating in an ectopic site in the atria characterized by an atrial rate between 250 and 400 beats per minute, atrial waveforms appearing in a sawtooth pattern, a normal QRS duration, a regular or irregular ventricular rhythm, and a ventricular rate that may be fast or slow depending on the number of impulses conducted through the AV node.

Atrial kick Blood pushed into the ventricles as a result of atrial contraction to complete filling of the ventricles just before the ventricles contract.

Atrioventricular block (AV block) A delay or failure of conduction of electrical impulses through the AV node.

Atrioventricular junction (AV junction) Consists of the AV node and the bundle of His.

Atrioventricular node (AV node) Located in the lower portion of the right atrium near the interatrial septum; only normal pathway for conduction of atrial impulses to the ventricles; primary function is to slow conduction of electrical impulses through the AV node to allow the atria to contract (atrial kick) and complete filling the ventricles.

Atrioventricular valves (AV valves) The two valves located between the atria and the ventricles. The tricuspid separates the right atrium from the right ventricle; the mitral separates the left atrium from the left ventricle.

Automaticity The ability of the pacemaker cells of the heart to spontaneously generate an electrical impulse.

Autonomic nervous system Regulates functions of the body that are involuntary (not under conscious control). Includes the sympathetic and parasympathetic nervous systems, each producing opposite effects when stimulated.

AV abbr atrioventricular

Bachmann bundle A branch of the internodal atrial conduction tracts that extends across the atria, conducting the electrical impulses from the SA node to the left atrium.

Baseline The straight line between ECG waveforms when no electrical activity is detected.

Base of the heart Top of the heart located at approximately the level of the second intercostal space.

Beta-blockers A group of drugs that block sympathetic activity. Used to treat tachyarrhythmias, MI, angina, and hypertension.

Bigeminy A rhythm in which every other beat is a premature ectopic beat. The premature beat may be atrial, junctional, or ventricular in origin (i.e., atrial bigeminy, junctional bigeminy, or ventricular bigeminy).

Biphasic deflection A waveform that is part positive and part negative.

Bradycardia A rhythm with a rate of less than 60 beats per minute.

Bundle-branch block A block of conduction of the electrical impulses through either the right or left bundle branch, resulting in a right or left bundle-branch block.

Bundle branches A part of the electrical conduction system consisting of the right and left bundle branches that conducts the electrical impulses to the right and left ventricles and the Purkinje network.

Bundle of His A part of the electrical conduction system that connects the AV node to the bundle branches.

Bursts Three or more consecutive premature ectopic beats (atrial, junctional, or ventricular). Also known as *salvo* or *run*.

Calcium channel blockers A group of drugs that block entry of calcium ions into cells, especially those of cardiac and vascular smooth muscle. Used to treat hypertension, angina, and as an antiarrhythmic.

Cardiac cells Cells of the heart consisting of the muscle (or "working") cells, responsible for contraction of the heart muscle, and the pacemaker cells of the electrical conduction system, which spontaneously generate electric impulses.

Cardiac cycle Consists of one heartbeat or one PQRST sequence. Represents atrial contraction and relaxation followed by ventricular contraction and relaxation.

Cardiac tamponade Compression of the heart due to the effusion of fluid or blood into the pericardial cavity.

Cardiomyopathy A disease of the heart muscle. Characterized by chamber dilation, wall thickening, decreased contractility, and conduction disturbances. End result is usually severe dysfunction of the heart muscle, resulting in heart failure.

Cardioversion An electric shock synchronized to fire on the R wave of the QRS complex. Used to convert rhythms such as atrial fibrillation or flutter, paroxysmal atrial tachycardia, or ventricular tachycardia with a pulse to NSR. Also known as *synchronized shock*.

Chordae tendineae Thin strands of fibrous connective tissue that extend from the cusps of the atrioventricular valves to the papillary muscles of the ventricles and prevent the AV valves from bulging back into the atria during ventricular contraction.

Chronic obstructive pulmonary disease A chronic disease of the lungs characterized by episodes of bronchitis, pneumonia, a chronic productive cough, and dyspnea. Also known as *COPD*.

Circulatory system A closed system consisting of two separate circuits: the pulmonary circuit and the systemic circuit. The pulmonary circuit is a small circuit and includes blood vessels within the lungs and those carrying blood between the heart and lungs. The systemic circuit is a large circuit and includes the coronary circulation, blood vessels within the body, and those carrying blood to and from the body.

Collateral circulation An accessory blood pathway developed through enlargement of secondary vessels after obstruction of a main channel.

Compensatory pause A pause following a premature beat. A compensatory pause is identified on the ECG by measuring from the R wave before the premature beat to the R wave following the premature beat—if that measurement equals the distance between two normal cardiac cycles (three normal beats), the pause is considered to be compensatory. Compensatory pauses are more common with PVCs. A compensatory pause cannot be identified if the underlying rhythm is irregular. Also known as *complete pause*.

Conductivity The ability of a cardiac cell to conduct an electrical impulse.

Congestive heart failure An overload of fluid in the lungs and/or body caused by inefficient pumping of the ventricles. Also known as *CHF*.

Contractility The ability of the muscle cells of the heart to cause myocardial muscle contraction in response to an electrical stimulus.

Coronary circulation The blood supply to the heart, consisting of the right coronary artery, the left coronary artery, and their branches.

Couplet Two consecutive premature beats. Also known as *pair*.

Cyanosis A purplish discoloration of the skin caused by the presence of unoxygenated blood.

Defibrillation An unsynchronized electrical shock used to terminate ventricular fibrillation and pulseless ventricular tachycardia; uses higher joules of electricity. Also known as *unsynchronized shock*.

Deflection Refers to the waveforms in the ECG tracing (P wave, QRS complex, T wave, and U wave). A deflection may be positive (upright), negative (inverted), biphasic (having both positive and negative components), or equiphasic (equally positive and negative).

Demand pacemaker A demand pacemaker fires only when the heart fails to depolarize on its own (fires only "on demand"). This mode of pacing is called synchronous pacing because it is synchronized to sense the patient's own rhythm.

Depolarization The spread of an electrical stimulus through the heart muscle producing the P wave from the atria and the QRS complex from the ventricles; an electrical event expected to result in muscle contraction.

Diaphoresis Profuse sweating.

Diastole The period of atrial or ventricular relaxation.

Dying heart See *agonal rhythm*.

Dyspnea Shortness of breath.

Dysrhythmia Any rhythm other than a sinus rhythm. Used interchangeably with *arrhythmia*.

Electrical conduction system of the heart A network of highly specialized muscle tissue that initiates and transmits electrical impulses throughout the heart resulting in muscle contraction. It includes the sinus node, the interatrial tract (Bachmann bundle), the internodal pathways, the AV node, the bundle of His, the right and left bundle branches, and the Purkinje fibers.

Ectopic A beat or rhythm originating from a source other than the SA node.

Electrocardiogram (ECG) A graphic recording of the electrical activity of the heart generated by the depolarization and repolarization of the atria and ventricles.

Electrolyte An element or compound that when dissolved in water dissociates into positive and negative ions and is able to conduct an electrical current. An ion with a positive charge is called a cation. An ion with a negative charge is called anion.

Endocardium The innermost layer of the heart wall that lines the inner surface of the heart muscle and the heart chambers.

Enhanced automaticity An abnormal condition of pacemaker cells in which their firing rate is increased beyond the inherent rate.

Epicardial pacing Delivery of a pacing stimulus to the heart through wires placed on the epicardial surface of the heart during cardiac surgery.

Escape beat An ectopic beat that occurs late (instead of early) following a pause in the underlying rhythm (usually sinus). Escape beats may arise from the atrium (atrial escape beat), the AV junction (junctional escape beat), or the ventricles (ventricular escape beat). Escape beats are protective mechanisms to protect the heart from slow rates.

Excitability The ability of a cardiac cell to respond to an electrical stimulus.

Fascicle A bundle of muscle or nerve fibers. The left bundle branch divides into an anterior fascicle and a posterior fascicle, which form the two major divisions of the left bundle branch before it divides into the Purkinje fibers.

First-degree AV block A rhythm in which the sinus impulses are delayed longer than normal in the AV node, but all impulses are conducted to the ventricles. It is characterized by a consistent, but prolonged PR interval (greater than 0.20 second).

Heart rate The number of heartbeats or QRS complexes per minute.

Heart valves Four structures within the heart that open and close to allow blood flow in one direction through the heart's chambers and prevent a backflow of blood. Changes in chamber pressure govern the opening and closing of the heart valves.

His-Purkinje system The part of the heart's electrical conduction system consisting of the bundle of His, the bundle branches, and the Purkinje fibers.

Hypertrophy An increase in the thickness of a heart chamber because of a chronic increase in pressure and/ or volume within the chamber. Hypertrophy may occur in both the atria and the ventricles.

Idioventricular rhythm A rhythm originating in an ectopic site in the ventricles. Characterized by a regular rhythm, an absence of P waves, wide QRS complexes, and a rate between 30 and 40 beats per minute (sometimes less). This is the inherent rhythm of the ventricles. Also known as *IVR*.

Implantable cardioverter-defibrillator An implanted device that has the ability to pace for bradycardia, overdrive pace for tachycardia (antitachycardia pacing), and deliver an electric shock if needed. Also called *ICD*.

Infarction Death (necrosis) of tissue caused by an interruption of blood supply to the affected tissue.

Inferior vena cava One of two large veins that empty venous blood into the right atrium.

Inherent Native to or occurring naturally in a specified area; also known as *intrinsic*.

Inherent firing rate The normal rate at which electrical impulses are generated in a pacemaker, whether it is the SA node or an ectopic pacemaker. Also known as *intrinsic firing rate*.

Interatrial septum The wall separating the right and left atria.

Internodal atrial conduction tracts Three pathways of specialized conducting tissue located in the walls of the right atrium, which conduct impulses from the SA node through the right atrium to the AV node.

Interpolated PVC A premature ventricular contraction (PVC) that falls between two QRS complexes without a pause.

Intraventricular septum The wall separating the right and left ventricles.

Intrinsic beat Beats produced by the heart's own natural electrical conduction system. Also known as *native beat*.

Ion Electrically charged particle.

Ischemia Reduced blood flow to tissue caused by narrowing or occlusion of the artery supplying blood to it.

Isoelectric line See *baseline*.

IVR abbr idioventricular rhythm

J point The point where the QRS complex and ST segment meet.

Junctional rhythm A rhythm arising in the AV junction characterized by a regular rhythm; inverted P waves immediately before the QRS, immediately after the QRS, or hidden within the QRS complex; a short PR interval of 0.10 second or less; a normal duration QRS complex; and a rate between 40 and 60 beats per minute. Junctional rhythm is the normal rhythm of the AV junction.

mA abbr milliampere

Mediastinum Located in the middle of the thoracic cavity. Contains the heart, trachea, esophagus, and great vessels (pulmonary arteries and veins, aorta, and the superior and inferior vena cava).

MI abbr myocardial infarction

Milliampere Unit of measure of electrical current needed to cause depolarization of the myocardium. A term used most often with pacemakers.

Mitral valve One of two atrioventricular valves. Located between the left atrium and left ventricle. Similar in structure to the tricuspid valve but has only two cusps.

Monomorphic A term used to describe ventricular tachycardia in which the QRS complexes look the same in the same lead.

Morphology The shape and size of a waveform.

Multifocal A rhythm originating in multiple pacemaker sites.

Multifocal PVCs PVCs that look different in the same lead.

Mural thrombi Clots in the chambers of the atria caused by ineffective atrial contractions (may occur in atrial fibrillation or flutter).

Myocardium The middle and thickest layer of the heart wall composed primarily of cardiac muscle cells. Responsible for the heart's ability to contract.

Negative deflection A waveform that is below baseline.

Noncompensatory pause A pause following a premature beat. A noncompensatory pause is identified on the ECG by measuring from the R wave before the premature beat to the R wave following the premature beat—if that measurement is less than the distance between two normal R-R intervals (three normal beats), the pause is considered to be noncompensatory. Noncompensatory pauses are more common with PACs and PJCs. A noncompensatory pause cannot be identified if the underlying rhythm is irregular. Also known as *incomplete pause*.

Nonconducted PAC A PAC that occurs so prematurely that the impulse is not conducted to the ventricles. The nonconducted PAC is characterized by a premature, abnormal P wave not accompanied by a QRS, but followed by a pause. The nonconducted PAC occurs in addition to an underlying rhythm.

Normal sinus rhythm The normal rhythm of the heart originating in the SA node characterized by a regular rhythm, normal P waves, normal PR interval, normal QRS duration, and a rate between 60 and 100 beats per minute.

Overdrive pacing Pacing the heart at a rate faster than the tachycardia to terminate a tachyarrhythmia.

PAC abbr premature atrial contraction

Pacemaker A device that delivers an electric current to the heart to stimulate depolarization.

Papillary muscles Projections of myocardium arising from the walls of the ventricles connected to fibrous cords called chordae tendineae, which are attached to the AV valve leaflets. During ventricular contraction, the papillary muscles contract and pull on the chordae tendineae, thus preventing inversion of the leaflets into the atria.

Parasympathetic nervous system A part of the autonomic nervous system. Stimulation of this system decreases the heart rate, slows conduction through the AV node, decreases the force of ventricular contraction, and causes a drop in blood pressure.

Paroxysmal A term used to describe the sudden onset or cessation of an arrhythmia.

Paroxysmal atrial tachycardia A rhythm originating in the atria characterized by abnormal P waves that are usually hidden in the preceding T waves, a normal QRS duration, and a regular rhythm between 140 and 250 beats per minute. Often occurs with abrupt onset and termination.

Paroxysmal junctional tachycardia A rhythm arising in the AV junction characterized by a regular rhythm; inverted P waves immediately before the QRS, immediately after the QRS, or hidden within the QRS complex; a short PR interval of 0.10 second or less; a normal duration QRS complex; and a rate greater than 100 beats per minute. Often occurs with abrupt onset and termination.

PAT abbr paroxysmal atrial tachycardia

Pericardium The outermost layer of the heart wall, a fibroserous sac that surrounds the heart and the roots of the great vessels. It consists of the fibrous pericardium and the serous pericardium.

PJC abbr premature junctional contraction

Point of maximal impulse The place where the apex of the heart can be palpated the strongest, usually at the fifth intercostal space of the thorax, left midclavicular line. Also known as *PMI*.

Polymorphic A term used to describe ventricular tachycardia in which the QRS complexes look different in the same lead.

Positive deflection A waveform that is above baseline.

Premature atrial contraction An early beat originating from an ectopic site in the atria. The premature beat is characterized by a premature, abnormal P wave and a normal or abnormal PR interval followed by a normal duration QRS and a pause. The premature beat occurs in addition to an underlying rhythm. Also known as *PAC*.

Premature junctional contraction An early beat originating from an ectopic site in the AV junction. The premature beat is characterized by a premature, inverted P wave occurring immediately before the QRS, immediately after the QRS, or hidden within the QRS complex; a short PR interval of 0.10 second or less; and a normal duration QRS complex followed by a pause. The premature beat occurs in addition to an underlying rhythm. Also known as *PJC*.

Premature ventricular contraction An early beat originating from an ectopic site in the ventricles. The premature beat is characterized by a premature, wide QRS complex with no associated P wave and an ST segment and T wave that slope opposite the main QRS deflection followed by a pause. Also known as *PVC*.

PR interval The section of the ECG between the onset of the P wave and the onset of the QRS complex. The normal PR interval is 0.12 to 0.20 second.

Prinzmetal angina A type of angina occurring when the coronary arteries experience spasms and constrict.

Proarrhythmic The effect of certain drugs (especially antiarrhythmics) to induce or worsen ventricular arrhythmias.

PR segment The short isoelectric line on the ECG between the end of the P wave and the onset of the QRS complex.

Pulmonic valve One of two semilunar valves. Located between the right ventricle and the pulmonary artery.

Pulseless electrical activity A clinical situation in which an organized cardiac rhythm (excluding pulseless ventricular tachycardia) is observed on the ECG, but no pulse is palpated. Treatment protocols are the same as for ventricular standstill. Also known as *PEA*.

Purkinje fibers Fibers that are present at the termination of the bundle branches, which conduct electrical impulses into the myocardial muscle of the ventricles.

P wave The first waveform of the cardiac cycle representing depolarization of the right and left atria.

Q wave The negative deflection of the QRS complex that precedes the R wave.

QRS complex A waveform on the ECG that represents depolarization of the ventricles. It is composed of three waves: the Q wave, the R wave, and the S wave. Normal duration is 0.10 second or less.

QT interval The portion of the ECG between the onset of the QRS complex and the end of the T wave, representing ventricular depolarization and repolarization.

Rate suppression A temporary decrease in the heart rate for several cycles following a pause in the basic rhythm.

Reciprocal change A change detected by the 12-lead ECG in a wall of the heart opposite the site of a myocardial infarction.

Refractory Inability to respond to a stimulus.

Relative refractory period The period of time during ventricular repolarization during which the ventricles can be stimulated to depolarize by an electrical impulse stronger than usual. This period begins at the peak of the T wave and ends with the end of the T wave. Also known as the *vulnerable period* of ventricular repolarization.

Reperfusion rhythms Rhythms that may occur following reperfusion therapy. Examples of reperfusion rhythms include sinus bradycardia, accelerated idioventricular rhythm, premature ventricular contractions, ventricular tachycardia, and ventricular fibrillation.

Reperfusion therapy Treatment to reopen an occluded coronary artery using a thrombolytic agent or coronary interventions, such as balloon angioplasty or coronary artery stenting.

Repolarization The recovery of the depolarized heart muscle to the resting state producing the ST segment, the T wave, and the U wave.

Retrograde Moving backward or in the opposite direction to that which is considered normal.

R-on-T PVC A PVC that falls on the downslope of the preceding T wave. Stimulation of the ventricle at this time may precipitate repetitive ventricular contractions, resulting in ventricular tachycardia or fibrillation.

R-R interval The period of time from one R wave to the next consecutive R wave.

R wave   The positive wave in the QRS complex.

SA   abbr sinoatrial

Second-degree AV block, Mobitz I   A rhythm in which most of the sinus impulses are conducted to the ventricles, but some are blocked. In Mobitz I, the sinus impulse is normally conducted to the AV node, but each successive impulse has increasing difficulty passing through the AV node, until finally an impulse is blocked and not conducted to the ventricles. Characterized by regularly occurring P waves (regular atrial rhythm); progressively lengthening of the PR interval until a P wave appears that is not followed by a QRS complex, but instead by a pause; a normal duration QRS; and an irregular ventricular rhythm. Also known as *Wenckebach*.

Second-degree AV block, Mobitz II   A rhythm in which some of the sinus impulses are conducted to the ventricles, but most are blocked. Characterized by regularly occurring P waves (regular atrial rhythm); consistent PR intervals with two, three, or more P waves before each QRS complex; a ventricular rhythm that may be regular or irregular depending on the number of impulses conducted to the ventricles; and a QRS complex that may be of normal duration or wide depending on the site of the conduction disturbance.

Sequential ventricular depolarization   One ventricle depolarizes before the other (instead of simultaneously), resulting in a wide QRS complex.

Sick sinus syndrome   Sinus node dysfunction characterized by severe sinus bradycardia alternating with tachycardia (especially atrial fibrillation). The most common symptoms include lethargy, weakness, light-headiness, dizziness, and syncope. At present, the only treatment is the implantation of a permanent pacemaker. Also called *tachy-brady syndrome*.

Sinus arrest   A rhythm caused by a failure of the SA node to initiate an impulse (a disorder of automaticity). The ECG tracing will show a sudden pause in the sinus rhythm in which one or more beats are missing. The underlying rhythm does not resume on time following the pause.

Sinus arrhythmia   A rhythm originating in the sinus node characterized by an irregular rhythm, normal P waves, normal PR interval, normal QRS complex, and a heart rate that is usually normal but may be slow. The rhythm is caused by changes in vagal tone that occur during the respiratory cycle with the heart rate gradually slowing down during expiration and gradually speeding up with inspiration.

Sinus bradycardia   A rhythm originating in the sinus node characterized by a regular rhythm, normal P waves, normal

PR interval, normal QRS duration, and a rate between 40 and 60 beats per minute.

Sinus exit block   A rhythm caused by a block in the conduction of the electrical impulse from the SA node to the atria (a disorder of conduction). The ECG tracing will show a sudden pause in the sinus rhythm in which one or more beats are missing. The underlying rhythm resumes on time following the pause.

Sinus node   The dominant pacemaker of the heart located in the wall of the right atrium close to the inlet of the superior vena cava.

Sinus tachycardia   A rhythm originating in the SA node characterized by a regular rhythm, normal P waves, normal PR interval, normal duration QRS complex, and a rate between 100 and 160 beats per minute.

ST segment   The flat line between the QRS complex and the T wave that represents early ventricular repolarization. The ST segment is normally at baseline.

Stokes-Adams attacks   Fainting episodes that occur when the heart rate suddenly slows or stops momentarily; common with second-degree AV block, Mobitz II, and third-degree heart block.

Superior vena cava   One of two large veins that empty venous blood into the right atrium.

Supraventricular   A general term used to describe rhythms that originate in sites above the bundle branches (i.e., sinus node, atria, and AV junction).

S wave   The negative deflection of the QRS complex that follows the R wave.

Sympathetic nervous system   A part of the autonomic nervous system. Stimulation of this system increases heart rate, speeds conduction through the AV node, increases the force of ventricular contraction, and causes an increase in blood pressure.

Syncope   Fainting, usually resulting from cardiac or neurologic events.

TCP   abbr transcutaneous pacing

TdP   abbr torsade de pointes

Third-degree AV block   A rhythm in which there is no conduction of electrical impulses through the AV node to the ventricles. There is independent beating of the atria and ventricles with the atria being paced by the SA node at a rate of 60 to 100 beats per minute and the ventricles paced either by the AV junction at a rate of 40 to 60 beats per minute or by a ventricular pacemaker at a rate of 30 to 40 beats per minute or less. Characterized by regularly occurring P waves (regular atrial rhythm), variable PR intervals with no consistent relationship between the P waves and QRS complexes, a regular ventricular rhythm, and a normal duration QRS complex if the ventricles are paced by the AV junction and a wide QRS complex if paced from a ventricular site. Also known as *complete heart block.*

Torsade de pointes A form of polymorphic ventricular tachycardia associated with a prolonged QT interval. Characterized by wide QRS complexes, which continuously change polarity (from positive to negative and negative to positive), varying QRS amplitude, and a very rapid ventricular rate (often greater than 250 beats per minute). Also known as *TdP.*

Transcutaneous pacing External cardiac pacing. Consists of two large electrode pads commonly placed in an anterior-posterior position on the patient's chest to conduct electrical impulses through the skin to the heart.

Transvenous pacing Delivery of a pacing stimulus through a vein. A lead wire is inserted into a large vein and positioned in the right ventricle. Electrical impulses are conducted from an external power source (pacing generator) through the lead wire to the right ventricle.

Tricuspid valve One of two AV valves. Located between the right atrium and the right ventricle. Similar in structure to the mitral valve but has three cusps.

Trigeminy A rhythm in which every third beat is a premature ectopic beat. The premature beats may be atrial, junctional, or ventricular in origin (i.e., atrial trigeminy, junctional trigeminy, ventricular trigeminy).

T wave A small wave that follows the ST segment. Represents ventricular repolarization.

Unifocal PVCs PVCs that look the same in the same lead.

U wave A small wave sometimes seen following the T wave. Represents late ventricular repolarization.

Vagal maneuvers Methods used to stimulate vagal (parasympathetic) tone in an attempt to slow the heart rate. Methods include coughing, bearing down (Valsalva maneuver), squatting, breath-holding, carotid sinus pressure, stimulation of the gag reflex, and immersion of the face in ice water.

Valsalva maneuver Forceful act of expiration with mouth and nose closed producing a "bearing down" action. One of several vagal maneuvers.

Vasovagal reaction An extreme body response that causes marked bradycardia (due to vagal stimulation) and marked hypotension (due to vasodilation). A vasovagal reaction may result in fainting (vasovagal syncope).

Ventricles The two thick-walled lower chambers of the heart. They receive blood from the atria and pump it into the pulmonary and systemic circulation. The ventricles are separated from the atria by the mitral and tricuspid valves.

Ventricular fibrillation A rhythm arising from a disorganized, chaotic electrical focus in the ventricles where the ventricles quiver instead of contracting effectively. Characterized by wavy, irregular deflections, which vary in shape and amplitude. No QRS complexes are present.

Ventricular standstill A rhythm in which there is no electrical activity in the ventricles. The ECG tracing will show either P waves or a straight line. Also known as *ventricular asystole.*

Ventricular tachycardia A rhythm originating in an ectopic site in the ventricles. Characterized by a regular rhythm, an absence of P waves, wide QRS complexes, and a rate between 140 and 250 beats per minute. Also known as *VT.*

Vulnerable period The period of time during ventricular repolarization in which the ventricles can be stimulated to depolarize by a strong electrical stimulus. This period corresponds to the downslope of the T wave (relative refractory period). Electrical stimuli occurring during the vulnerable period may lead to ventricular tachycardia or ventricular fibrillation.

Wandering atrial pacemaker A rhythm originating in multiple pacemakers sites that shift back and forth between the SA node and an ectopic site in the atria or AV junction. It is characterized by P waves, which vary in size, shape, and direction.

Index

Note: 'i' refers to an illustration; 't' refers to a table; 'b' refers to a box.

Note: 'i' refers to an illustration; 't' refers to a table; 'b' refers to a box.

Note: 'i' refers to an illustration; 't' refers to a table; 'b' refers to a box.

Note: 'i' refers to an illustration; 't' refers to a table; 'b' refers to a box.

table 6.1 Summary of Sinus Arrhythmias

Name	Rhythm	Rate (Beats/Minute)	P Waves (Lead II)	PR Interval	QRS	Appearance
Normal sinus rhythm (NSR)	Regular	60–100	Positive in lead II; normal in size, shape, and direction; one P wave precedes each QRS complex	Normal (0.12–0.20 sec)	Normal (0.10 sec or less)	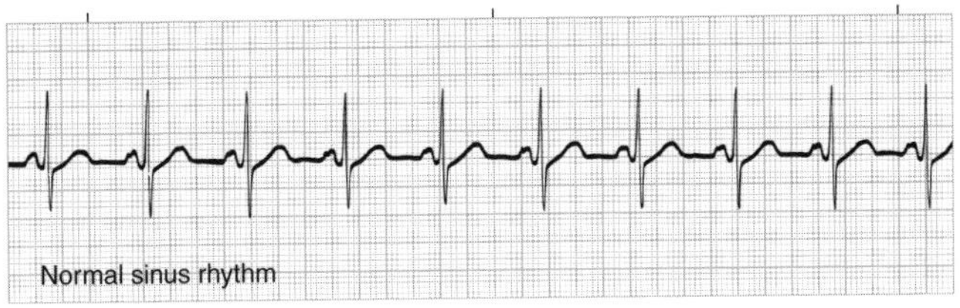 Normal sinus rhythm
Sinus bradycardia	Regular	40–60	Positive in lead II; normal in size, shape, and direction; one P wave precedes each QRS complex	Normal (0.12–0.20 sec)	Normal (0.10 sec or less)	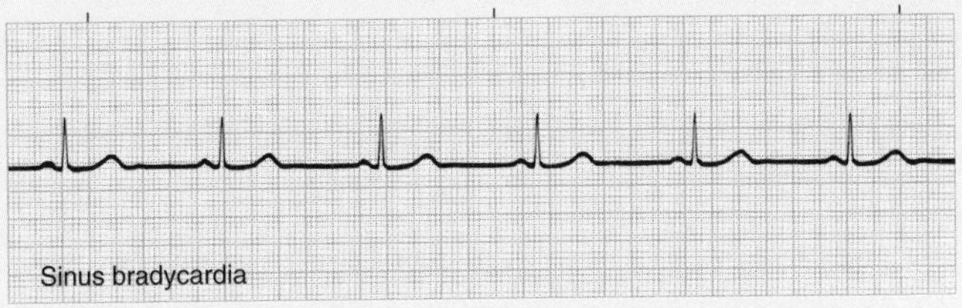 Sinus bradycardia
Sinus tachycardia	Regular	100–160	Positive in lead II; normal in size, shape, and direction; one P wave precedes each QRS complex	Normal (0.12–0.20 sec)	Normal (0.10 sec or less)	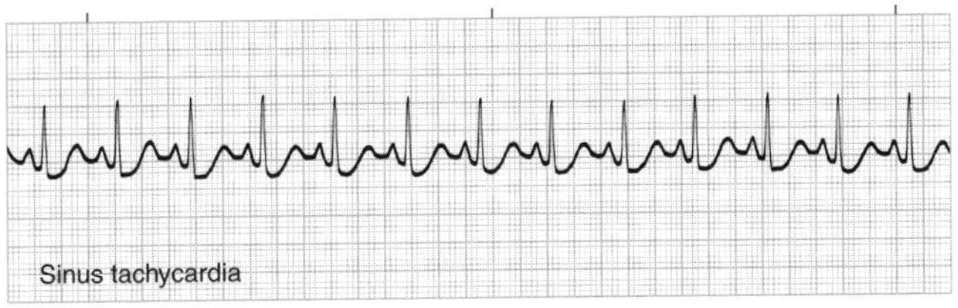 Sinus tachycardia
Sinus arrhythmia	Irregular	Normal (60–100) or slow (less than 60)	Positive in lead II; normal in size, shape, and direction; one P wave precedes each QRS complex	Normal (0.12–0.20 sec)	Normal (0.10 sec or less)	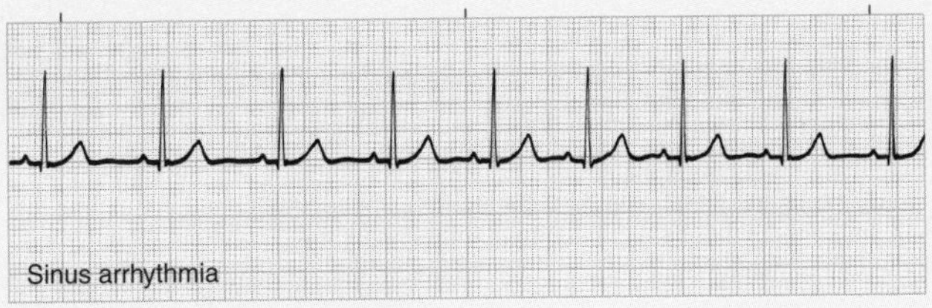 Sinus arrhythmia

table 6.1 Summary of Sinus Arrhythmias (Continued)

Name	Rhythm	Rate (Beats/Minute)	P Waves (Lead II)	PR Interval	QRS	Appearance
Sinus block and sinus arrest	Basic rhythm usually regular; there is a sudden pause in basic rhythm (causing irregularity) with one or more missing beats; after pause, heart rate may be slower (rate suppression) for several cycles but returns to basic rate	That of underlying sinus rhythm	Sinus P waves with basic rhythm; absent during pause	Normal (0.12–0.20 sec) with basic rhythm; absent during pause	Normal (0.10 sec or less) with basic rhythm; absent during pause	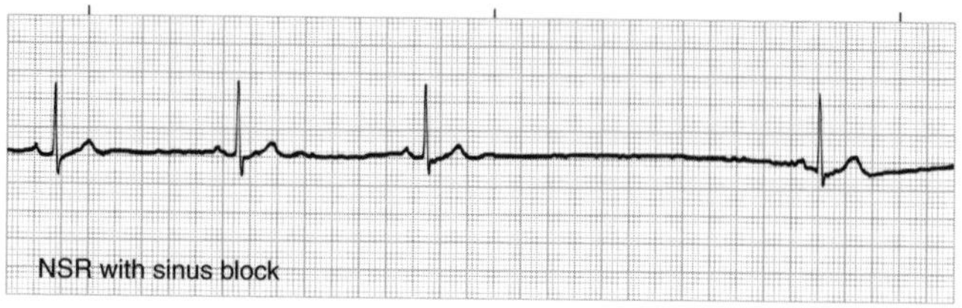 NSR with sinus block 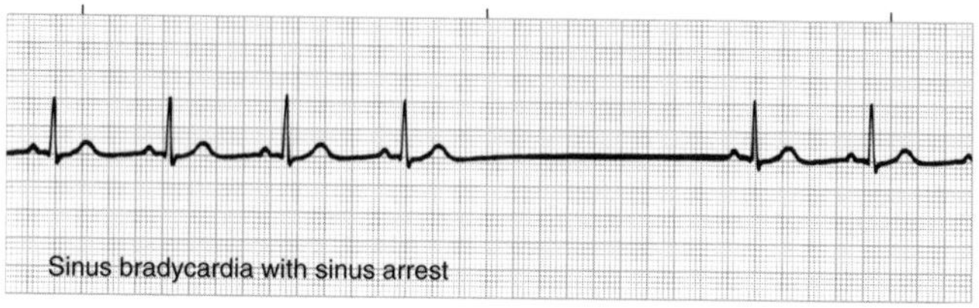 Sinus bradycardia with sinus arrest
Differentiating Features						
Sinus arrest:	Basic rhythm does not resume on time following pause.					
Sinus block:	Basic rhythm resumes on time following pause.					

Note: If the basic rhythm is irregular as in sinus arrhythmia, sinus block cannot be differentiated from sinus arrest. The event causing the pause would best be interpreted using the broad term sinus pause, indicating that either rhythm could be present.

table 7.1 Summary of Atrial Arrhythmias

Name	Rhythm	Rate (Beats/Minute)	P Waves (Lead II)	PR Interval	QRS	Appearance
Wandering atrial pacemaker (WAP)	Regular or irregular	Normal (60–100) or slow (less than 60)	Vary in size, shape, direction across strip; one P wave precedes each QRS	Usually normal; may be abnormal due to changing pacemaker location	Normal (0.10 sec or less)	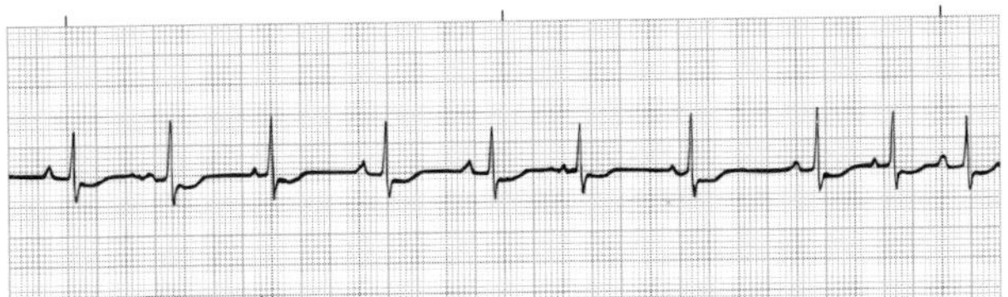 Wandering atrial pacemaker
Premature atrial contraction (PAC)	Basic rhythm usually regular; irregular with PAC	That of basic rhythm	Abnormal in size, shape, or direction; often found hidden in preceding T-wave distorting T-wave contour	Usually normal but may be abnormal; not measurable if hidden in preceding T wave	Normal (0.10 sec or less)	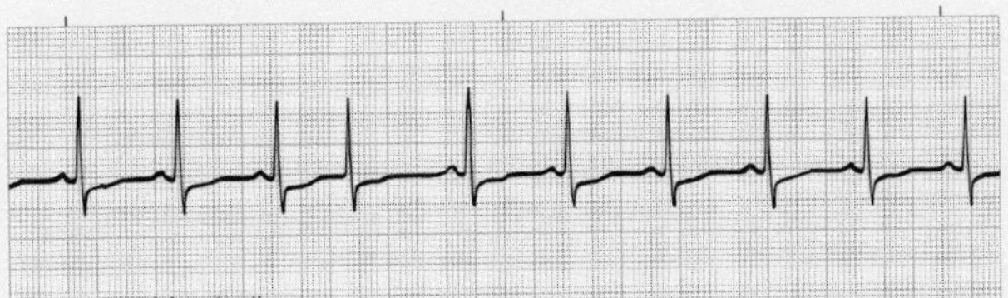 Premature atrial contraction 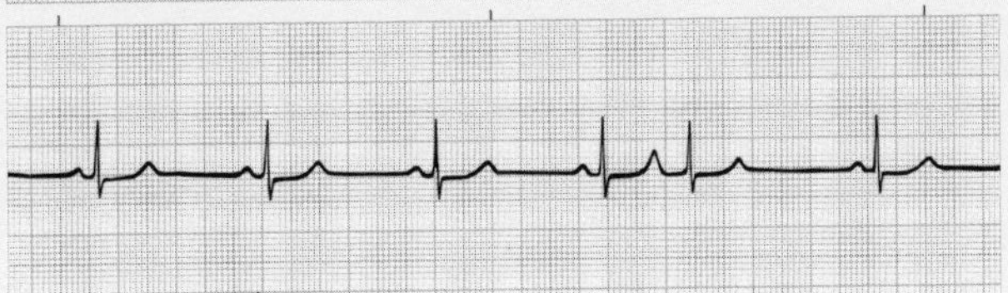 Premature atrial contraction
Nonconducted PAC	Basic rhythm usually regular; irregular with non-cond PAC	That of basic rhythm	Abnormal in size, shape, or direction; often found hidden in preceding T-wave distorting T-wave contour	Absent with non-cond PAC	Absent with non-cond PAC	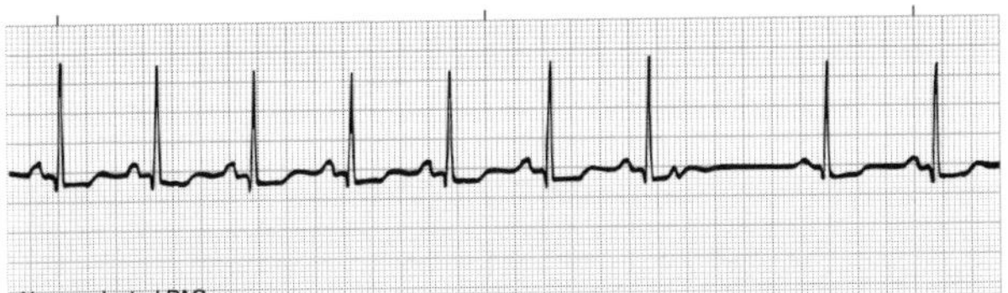 Nonconducted PAC 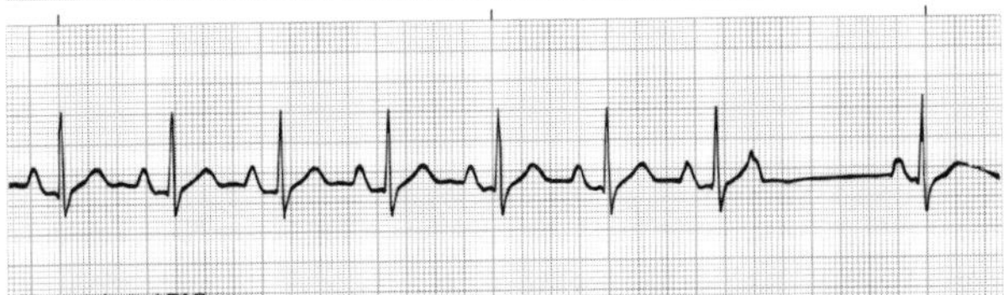 Nonconducted PAC
Paroxysmal atrial tachycardia (PAT)	Regular	140–250	Abnormal (often pointed); usually hidden in preceding T wave so that T and P waves appear as one deflection (TP wave)	Usually not measurable	Normal (0.10 sec or less)	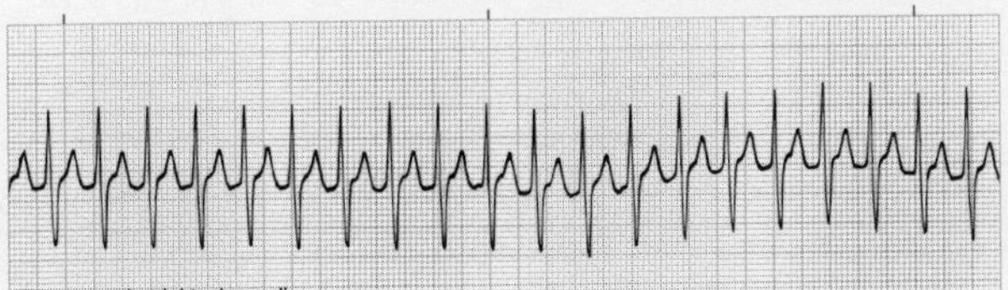 Paroxysmal atrial tachycardia

table 7.1 Summary of Atrial Arrhythmias (Continued)

Name	Rhythm	Rate (Beats/Minute)	P Waves (Lead II)	PR Interval	QRS	Appearance
Atrial flutter	Regular or irregular (depends on AV conduction ratios)	*Atrial:* 250–400 *Ventricular:* Varies with number of impulses conducted through AV node; will be less than the atrial rate	Sawtooth waves affecting entire baseline	Not measurable	Normal (0.10 sec or less)	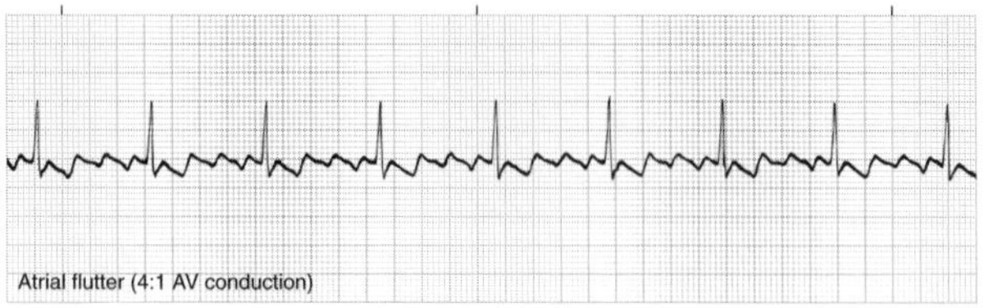 Atrial flutter (4:1 AV conduction) 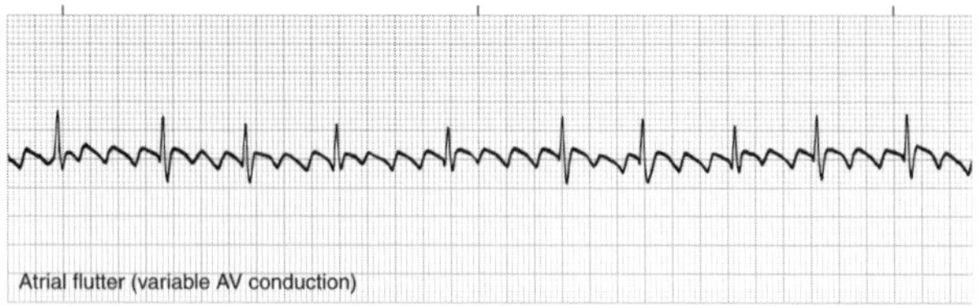 Atrial flutter (variable AV conduction)
Atrial fibrillation	Grossly irregular (unless vent rate is very rapid, in which case rhythm becomes more regular)	*Atrial:* Not measurable *Ventricular:* Varies with number of impulses conducted through AV node; will be less than the atrial rate	Wavy deflections affecting entire baseline	Not measurable	Normal (0.10 sec or less)	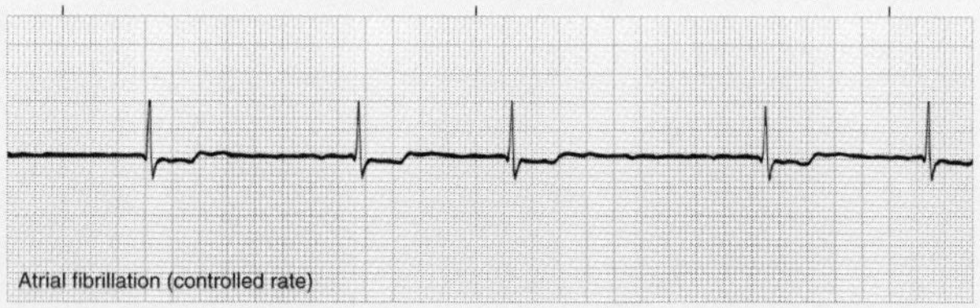 Atrial fibrillation (controlled rate) 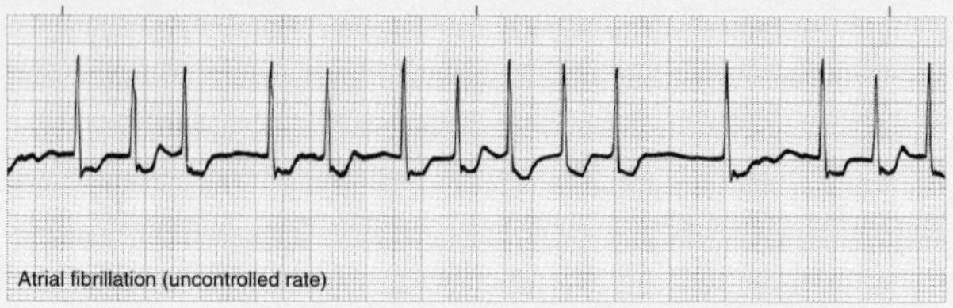 Atrial fibrillation (uncontrolled rate)

table 8.2 Summary of Junctional Arrhythmias and AV Blocks

Name	Rhythm	Rate (Beats/Minute)	P Waves (Lead II)	PR Interval	QRS	Appearance
Premature junctional contraction (PJC)	Basic rhythm usually regular; irregular with PJC	That of basic rhythm	Inverted in lead II; occurs immediately before QRS, immediately after QRS, or is hidden within QRS	Short (0.10 sec or less)	Normal (0.10 sec or less)	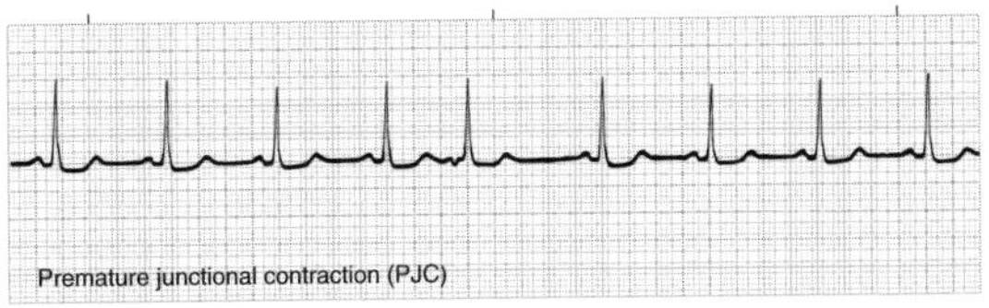 Premature junctional contraction (PJC)
Junctional rhythm	Regular	40–60	Inverted in lead II; occurs immediately before QRS, immediately after QRS, or is hidden within QRS	Short (0.10 sec or less)	Normal (0.10 sec or less)	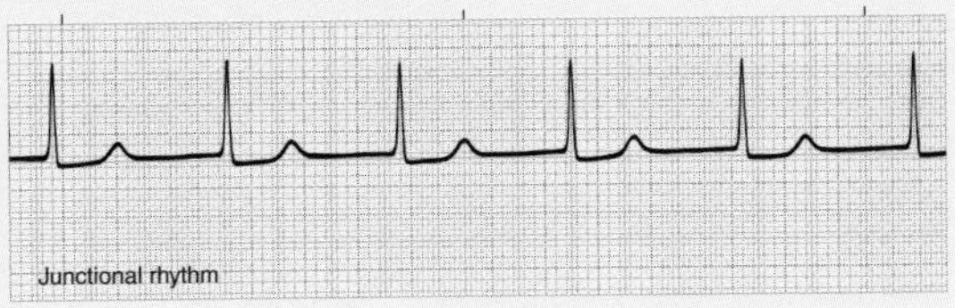 Junctional rhythm
Accelerated junctional rhythm	Regular	60–100	Inverted in lead II; occurs immediately before QRS, immediately after QRS, or is hidden within QRS	Short (0.10 sec or less)	Normal (0.10 sec or less)	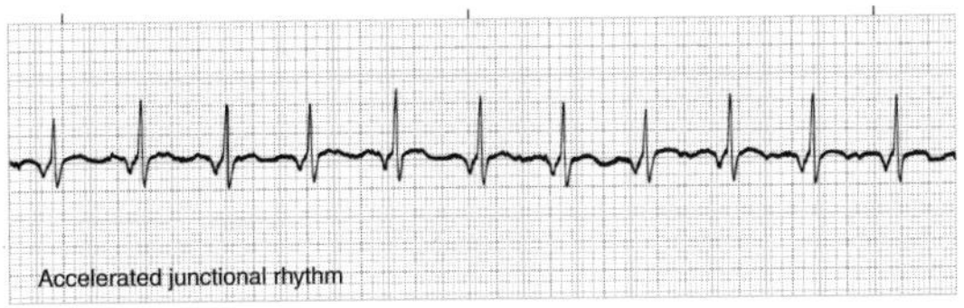 Accelerated junctional rhythm
Junctional tachycardia	Regular	>100	Inverted in lead II; occurs immediately before QRS, immediately after QRS, or is hidden within QRS	Short (0.10 sec or less)	Normal (0.10 sec or less)	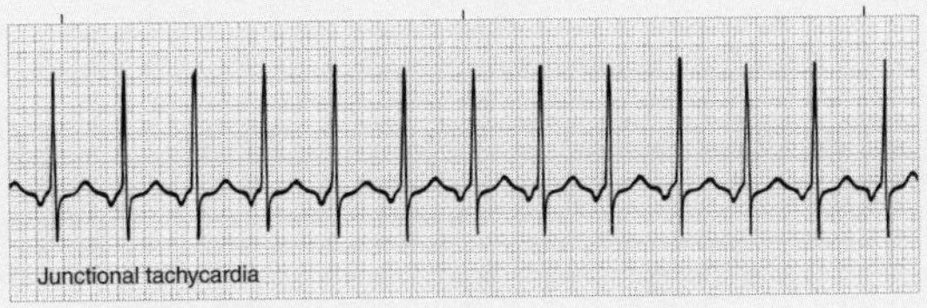 Junctional tachycardia

table 8.2 Summary of Junctional Arrhythmias and AV Blocks (Continued)

Name	Rhythm	Rate (Beats/Minute)	P Waves (Lead II)	PR Interval	QRS	Appearance
First-degree atrioventricular (AV) block	Regular	That of underlying sinus rhythm	Sinus origin; one P wave to each QRS	Prolonged (greater than 0.20 sec); remains consistent	Normal (0.10 sec or less)	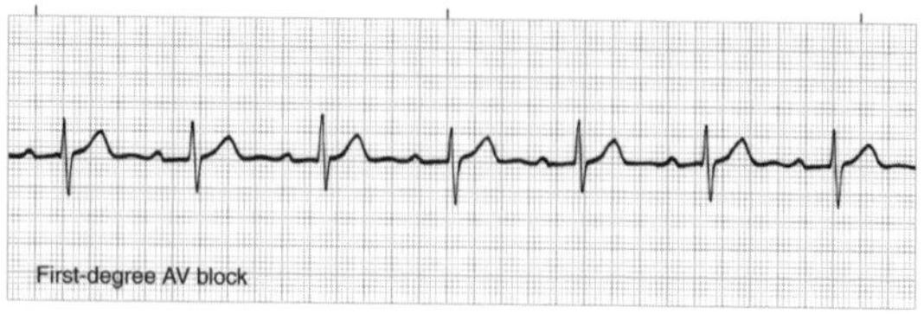 First-degree AV block
Second-degree AV block, Mobitz I	*Atrial:* Regular *Ventricular:* Irregular	*Atrial:* That of underlying sinus rhythm *Ventricular:* Varies with number of impulses conducted through AV node; will be less than atrial rate	Sinus origin	PR varies; PR progressively lengthens until a P wave is not conducted (P wave occurs without QRS); a pause follows the dropped QRS	Normal (0.10 sec or less)	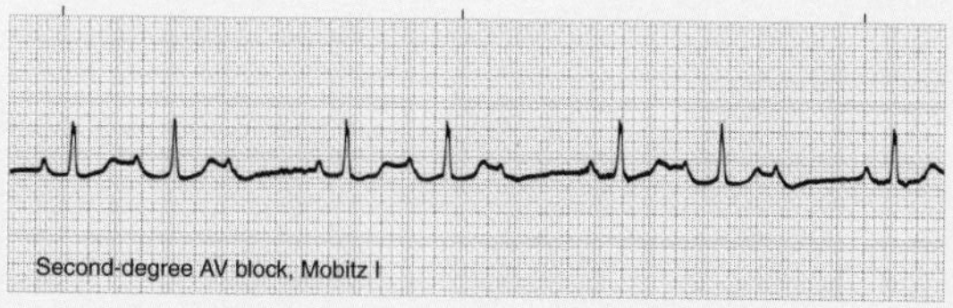 Second-degree AV block, Mobitz I
Second-degree AV block, Mobitz II	*Atrial:* Regular *Ventricular:* Usually regular; may be irregular if conduction ratios vary	*Atrial:* That of underlying sinus rhythm *Ventricular:* Varies with number of impulses conducted through AV node; will be less than atrial rate	Sinus origin; 2 or 3 P waves (sometimes more) before each QRS	Normal or prolonged; PR is consistent	Normal if block at AV node or bundle of His; wide if block in bundle branches	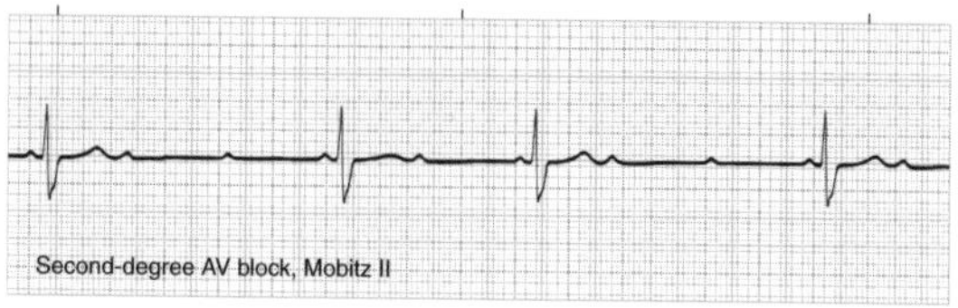 Second-degree AV block, Mobitz II
Third-degree AV block	*Atrial:* Regular *Ventricular:* Regular	*Atrial:* That of underlying sinus rhythm *Ventricular:* 40–60 if paced by AV node; 30–40 (sometimes less) if paced by ventricles	Sinus P waves with no constant relationship to QRS; some P waves hidden in QRS complexes, T waves, and in ST segments	Varies greatly	Normal if block at AV node or bundle of His; wide if block in bundle branches	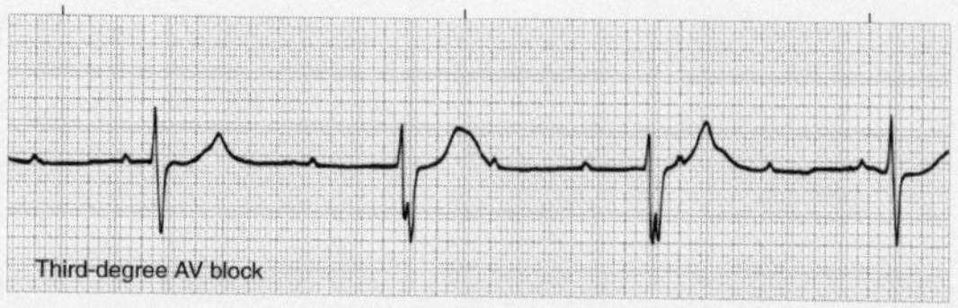 Third-degree AV block

table 9.1 Summary of Ventricular Rhythms and Bundle-Branch Block

Name	Rhythm	Rate (Beats/Minute)	P Waves (Lead II)	PR Interval	QRS Complex	Appearance
Bundle-branch block	Regular	That or underlying rhythm (usually sinus)	Sinus origin	Normal (0.12–0.20 sec)	Wide (0.12 sec or greater)	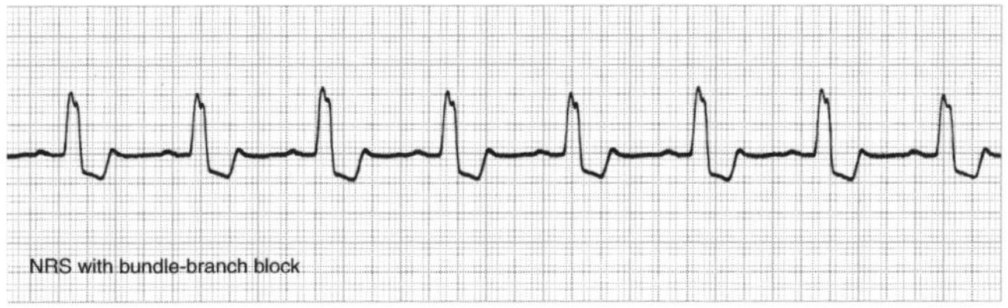 NRS with bundle-branch block
Premature ventricular contraction (PVC)	Basic rhythm usually regular; irregular with PVC	That of underlying rhythm	None associated with PVC	Not measurable	Premature, abnormal, and wide	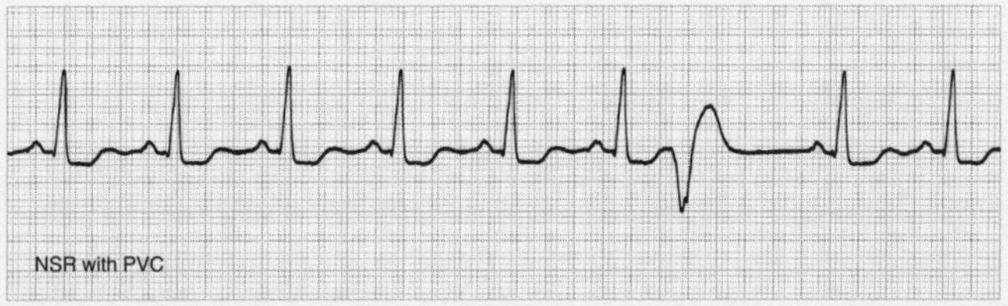 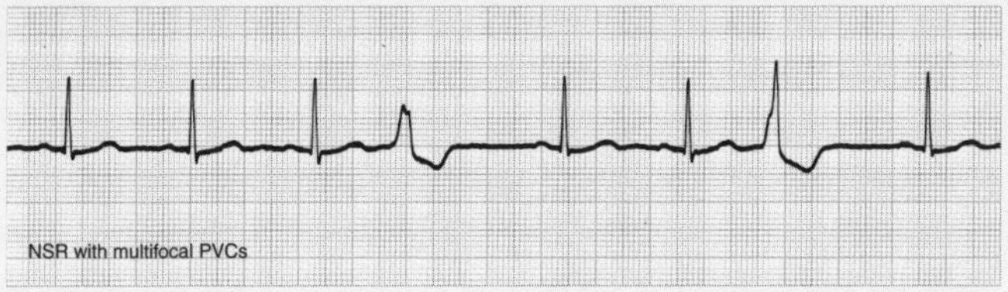 NSR with PVC NSR with multifocal PVCs
Idioventricular rhythm (IVR)	Regular	30–40 (sometimes less)	Absent	Not measurable	Wide (0.12 sec or greater)	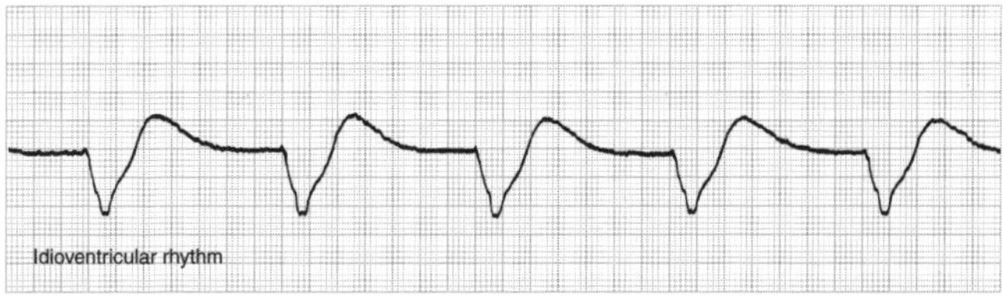 Idioventricular rhythm
Accelerated IVR	Regular	50–100	Absent	Not measurable	Wide (0.12 sec or greater)	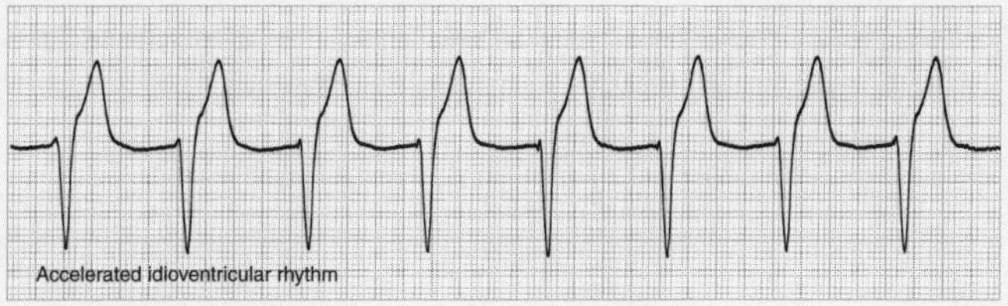 Accelerated idioventricular rhythm

table 9.1 Summary of Ventricular Rhythms and Bundle-Branch Block (Continued)

Name	Rhythm	Rate (Beats/Minute)	P Waves (Lead II)	PR Interval	QRS Complex	Appearance
Ventricular tachycardia (VT)	Regular	140–250	None associated with PVC	Not measurable	Wide (0.12 sec or greater)	Ventricular tachycardia
Ventricular fibrillation	None	None	Absent; wavy irregular deflections which may be "coarse" or "fine"	Not measurable	Absent	Ventricular fibrillation (coarse) Ventricular fibrillation (fine)
Ventricular standstill (asystole)	*Atrial:* If P waves present, will have atrial rhythm *Ventricular:* None	*Atrial:* If P waves present, will have atrial rate) *Ventricular:* None	Tracing will show P waves without QRS or a straight line	Not measurable	Absent	P-wave asystole. Straight line asystole